Also in the Variorum Collected Studies Series:

ANDREW CUNNINGHAM
The Identity of the History of Science and Medicine

JOHN HENRY
Religion, Magic, and the Origins of Science in Early Modern England

JOHN PARASCANDOLA
Studies in the History of Modern Pharmacology and Drug Therapy

JOHN GASCOIGNE
Science, Philosophy and Religion in the Age of the Enlightenment
British and Global Contexts

COLIN A. RUSSELL
From Atoms to Molecules
Studies in the History of Chemistry from the 19th Century

MAURICE CROSLAND
Scientific Institutions and Practice in France and Britain, c.1700–c.1870

EKMELEDDIN IHSANOGLU
Science, Technology and Learning in the Ottoman Empire
Western Influence, Local Institutions, and the Transfer of Knowledge

DAVID L. COWEN
Pharmacopoeias and Related Literature in Britain and America, 1618–1847

ROGER FRENCH
Ancients and Moderns in the Medical Sciences
From Hippocrates to Harvey

JOHN GASCOIGNE
Science, Politics and Universities in Europe, 1600–1800

ANDREW WEAR
Health and Healing in Early Modern England
Studies in Social and Intellectual History

JOHN KOMLOS
The Biological Standard of Living in Europe and America, 1700–1900
Studies in Anthropometric History

VARIORUM COLLECTED STUDIES SERIES

Ideas and Practices in the History of Medicine, 1650–1820

Adrian Wilson

Ideas and Practices in the History of Medicine, 1650–1820

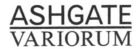

Published in the Variorum Collected Studies Series by

Ashgate Publishing Limited
Wey Court East
Union Road
Farnham, Surrey
GU9 7PT
England

Ashgate Publishing Company
Suite 3–1
110 Cherry Street
Burlington, VT 05401–3818
USA

www.ashgate.com

ISBN 9781409451563

British Library Cataloguing in Publication Data
A catalogue record for this book is available from the British Library.

The Library of Congress has cataloged the printed edition as follows: 2013947434

VARIORUM COLLECTED STUDIES SERIES CS1038

The paper used in this publication meets the minimum requirements of the American National Standard for Information Sciences – Permanence of Paper for Printed Library Materials, ANSI Z39.48–1984. ∞ ™

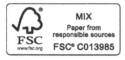

Printed in the United Kingdom by Henry Ling Limited, at the Dorset Press, Dorchester, DT1 1HD

CONTENTS

PART 3: MEDICAL CONCEPTS AND PRACTICES

INTRODUCTION

The title of this collection indicates the space that these essays inhabit: although they appeared across a span of over twenty years and deal with several different themes – childbirth/midwifery, hospitals, pathology – they share a concern with the mutual relations between ideas and practices, as becomes most apparent in the opening and closing chapters.

The three papers in Part 1 all seek to integrate the bodily and social aspects of early-modern childbirth – taking the 'bodily' not merely as a cultural construction, but rather as the actual, material body of the childbearing mother.[1] This they attempt by identifying micro-social processes, that is, transactions which were interpersonal in scale yet regular in form: the routines of the all-female childbirth ritual (Chapter II), and the different ways that practitioners both female and male were summoned to deliveries (Chapters III, I respectively). Such processes merit reconstruction, I hope to have shown, for at least three reasons. First, they turn out to be – whenever we take the trouble to investigate them – astonishingly rich, complex and diverse.[2] Second, their particularity is often – it is tempting to say always – consequential, yielding both insights and questions that would not otherwise have arisen.[3] And third, they were at least the sites, and sometimes also the engines, of large-scale historical change.

Although micro-social processes also feature in Part 2 (for instance in Chapter IV's diagram of voluntary-hospital functioning), these next three chapters are mainly concerned to link English medical institutions, especially voluntary hospitals, with the wider polity. Unlike nineteenth-century voluntary hospitals, which seem to have functioned as vehicles of middle-class identity,[4]

---

[1] On the difficulty of integrating the bodily and the social/cultural, see Dror Wahrman, 'Change and the corporeal in seventeenth- and eighteenth-century gender history: or, can cultural history be rigorous?' *Gender & History* 20 (2008), 584–602 and (for instance) Chris Shilling, *The Body and Social Theory* (first published 1993; second edition, London: Sage, 2003).

[2] For examples from other domains see Steven Shapin and Simon Schaffer, *Leviathan and the Air Pump: Hobbes, Boyle and the experimental life* (Princeton, N.J.: Princeton University Press, 1985), and Andrew Cunningham, *The Anatomist Anatomis'd: an experimental discipline in Enlightenment Europe* (Farnham: Ashgate, 2010).

[3] For instance, Cunningham in *The Anatomist Anatomis'd* brings to light the experimental character of eighteenth-century anatomy by attending to the actual activities of anatomists.

[4] Hilary Marland, *Medicine and Society in Wakefield and Huddersfield 1780–1870* (Cambridge: Cambridge University Press, 1987); R.J. Morris, *Class, Sect and Party: the making*

the medical charities of the eighteenth century – when of course the voluntary-subscription form was first created – were tied to faction and party.[5] Such connections between medicine and politics not only enrich our understanding of the medical institutions; they also serve as an argument against the division of history into thematic 'tunnels', a phenomenon long ago identified and cogently criticized by J.H. Hexter.[6] Thus these chapters propose that eighteenth-century English medical institutions offer opportunities to political historians on a much wider scale than has yet been appreciated.[7]

Part 3 concerns central questions of medical history's own identity, pertaining to the historical understanding of disease. These two chapters are connected in taking Michel Foucault – specifically his seminal *Birth of the Clinic* – as both inspiration and opponent: inspiration in respect of the ambition to elucidate historical change, opponent in respect of the way that Foucault went about it. Chapter VII argues that the history of ideas, though not sufficient in itself,[8] has to be depassed (that is, subsumed within a more inclusive apprehension),[9] not bypassed as Foucault proposed. Specifically, concepts of disease can and should be historicized, a claim that I seek to support using 'snapshots' from the history of pleurisy. And Chapter VIII proposes that what Foucault called the 'great break in the history of Western medicine' – that is, the mapping of disease onto the anatomical body – though indeed first fully realized in the early-nineteenth-century Paris *École de Santé*, by no means originated in that setting but rather had been developing, in a history that Foucault almost totally suppressed, for some two centuries before.

In the case of that final chapter I have appended a postscript which rectifies an unfortunate omission and points out that this failing ironically illustrates a key aspect of the chapter's argument.

ADRIAN WILSON

Leeds
August 2014

---

of the British middle class, Leeds 1820–1850 (Manchester: Manchester University Press, 1990).

[5] Bronwyn Croxson, 'The Public and Private Faces of Eighteenth-Century London Dispensary Charity', *Medical History* 41 (1997), 127–149, at 142–9.

[6] J.H. Hexter, *Reappraisals in History* (London: Longman, 1961), 194–5.

[7] Paul Langford, *Public Life and the Propertied Englishman, 1689–1798* (Oxford: Clarendon, 1991); Kathleen Wilson, *The Sense of the People: politics, culture and imperialism in England, 1715–1785* (Cambridge: Cambridge University Press, 1995).

[8] Cf. Andrew Cunningham, 'Identifying Disease in the Past: cutting the Gordian knot', *Asclepio* 54 (2002), 13–34.

[9] See R.D. Laing and D.G. Cooper, *Reason and Violence: a decade of Sartre's philosophy, 1950–1960* (London: Tavistock Publications, 1964).

ACKNOWLEDGEMENTS

I am grateful to Annie Jamieson for smoothing the way, to Chris Baxfield for helping with the index, to Jon Hodge for his constant encouragement, to everyone at Ashgate for their impressive professionalism, and to Cynthia for keeping me going. Special thanks go to Greg Radick for suggesting this edition in the first place and for mentoring me in the process of putting it together.

Grateful acknowledgement is also made to the following publishers for their kind permission to reproduce the papers included in this volume: Cambridge University Press (for Chapters I and IV); Taylor and Francis Books (II, VI); The History Press, Stroud (III); Oxford University Press (V); Science History Publications Ltd (VII); and Palgrave Macmillan, Basingstoke (VIII).

Every effort has been made to trace all the copyright holders, but if any have been inadvertently overlooked the publishers will be pleased to make the necessary arrangement at the first opportunity.

I

William Hunter and
the varieties of man-midwifery

Introduction

Historians tell us that the eighteenth century witnessed a 'revolution in obstetrics': From the 1730s there was a sudden increase in male attendance in childbirth, and the 'men-midwives' who thus came into being rapidly displaced the traditional midwife, instituted classes in midwifery, brought about an explosion of technical knowledge and further promoted their new activities by means of lying-in hospitals, wards and charities. The *causes* of this change (it is said) were the forceps and fashion. The design of the forceps was published in 1733; the instrument was taken up at once by male practitioners, for whom it served as 'the key to the lying-in room'. Fashion promoted the new man-midwifery, which began at the top of the social scale and spread inexorably downwards as each social rank aped its betters.[1]

William Hunter was himself a leading 'man-midwife' in mid-eighteenth-century London. Yet in trying to connect Hunter's practice with the wider 'revolution in obstetrics', we encounter an obstacle: Hunter's strenuous *opposition* to the midwifery forceps, made famous through remarks reproduced by Spencer in his *History of British Midwifery*. 'Where they save one, they murder twenty', Hunter said, adding that it was 'a thousand pities they were ever invented'. Can the forceps then have been the 'key to the lying-in room'? If not, how can the rise of man-midwifery be explained? And why did Hunter take this particular view – unlike such fellow men-midwives as William Smellie?[2]

---

1 The quoted phrases are from J. H. Aveling, *English Midwives: Their History and Prospects* (London, 1872), p. 86, and Walter Radcliffe, *Milestones in Midwifery* (Bristol, 1967), p. 30. See also Jean Donnison, *Midwives and Medical Men* (London, 1977), pp. 21–41; Audrey Eccles, *Obstetrics and Gynaecology in Tudor and Stuart England* (London, 1982), p. 124.
2 Herbert R. Spencer, *The History of British Midwifery from 1650 to 1800* (London, 1927), pp. 72–3.

The approach I shall take to these questions involves a focus on male obstetric practice rather than precept; a widening of view, to embrace the seventeenth century as well as the eighteenth; and, so far as is practicable, a shift of attention from 'obstetrics' or 'midwifery' to *childbirth*. To begin with, I shall outline certain features of childbirth itself that provide a necessary context for approaching the nature of male obstetric practice. The central section of the essay will be concerned with the different forms that man-midwifery could take; I shall then suggest provisional answers to the initial questions and conclude with some historiographical reflections.

The critical features of childbirth, in any society, are the social arrangements made for its routine management, the biological forms it can take and the technical means available for intervention. As to the social arrangements, childbirth in mid-eighteenth-century England was routinely managed not by male practitioners but by midwives, and it was usual for the birth to be attended by several other women – 'gossips', who were variously the friends, relatives and neighbours of the childbearing mother. Of the biology of childbirth the most important thing to be said is that most births, then as now, were normal and spontaneous, needing no assistance at all for a safe delivery. If difficulty arose, or was perceived to have arisen, there were three main techniques available: podalic version, craniotomy and forceps extraction.

The biological and technical dimensions deserve some amplification. From both modern and historical sources, we can derive the following picture of the incidence of different types of birth:

1. About 96 per cent of births were normal and spontaneous. Most of these (93 percent) came by the head, the remainder (about 3 per cent) by the breech.
2. The remaining 4 per cent of births involved serious obstruction and could not be delivered without intervention. Most of these cases of obstruction (around 3 per cent of all births) came by the head, just as did most of the spontaneous deliveries. The other 1 per cent of all births comprised roughly equal numbers of obstructed breech births (particularly footling breech, the rarest of the breech varieties but also the most dangerous) and cases of arm or shoulder presentation (all of which became obstructed, save only those few where the child was premature and thus very small).
3. Some births were subject to complications, either major or minor. The minor complications included fainting, vomiting and tearing of the perineum. The major complications, which were of much greater moment as they threatened the mother's life, were haem-

orrhage (flooding) and convulsions (what is now called eclampsia). The incidence of such minor complications is very difficult to assess, but a working guess of 1 per cent may not be too wide of the mark.

Complications were more likely in association with obstruction, and thus we cannot simply add the two together to assess the incidence of serious difficulty. Rickets, leading to a distorted female pelvis and thus to a greater likelihood of obstruction, seems to have been quite rare and thus not to have increased the likelihood of difficulty as much as might be expected. Thus, although there is some indeterminacy about this, we can say with confidence that serious difficulty (whether due to obstruction or to complications) was of the order of 4 per cent in frequency; that obstructed labour was the commonest source of difficulty; and that obstruction by the head was the most frequent form this took.

The different surgical techniques were designed for specific forms of obstruction, though they also had other applications. Both craniotomy and forceps extraction were used for obstructed births by the head; each in its different way permitted traction on the head (aiding the mechanical force of the uterus) and reduced the size of the head (permitting an easier passage through a fixed bony channel). Craniotomy could be used only on a dead child; it opened the skull. The midwifery forceps could be used if the child was alive or dead, for they grasped the head externally. The other chief technique, podalic version, was designed for malpresentations, notably for births presenting by the arm or shoulder; this method consisted literally in 'turning the birth to the feet' and it succeeded (in the hands of a skilled practitioner) because the feet of the child were both small (permitting an adult hand to pass) and easily grasped – in both respects unlike the head of the child, which was large, smooth and slippery. Thus, in theory, podalic version would have been used only for malpresentations, craniotomy only for delivering a dead child coming by the head, and the forceps for a child (living or dead) coming by the head. This was, on the whole, true, but in practice there were qualifications. For one thing, podalic version could be used for births by the head; for another there was the alternative technique of cephalic version (turning to the head) in malpresentations, though this was difficult to use and was seldom effectual; and third, it has to be added that craniotomy instruments were sometimes used on a living child, in the hope of saving the mother's life. (In very rare cases, with great luck and skill, a practitioner could even draw a living child with a craniotomy device.)

It is appropriate here to mention very briefly the well-known history of the midwifery forceps.[3] The instrument was invented, in the early seventeenth century, by one of the Chamberlens, a family of Huguenot refugees who had settled in England in the late sixteenth century. Practising in London throughout the seventeenth century, the Chamberlens kept the forceps a secret until about 1700 – after which date the design leaked out to a series of individual practitioners. By the 1720s the instrument had been demonstrated in Paris (though in a different form), and was being used by at least two London practitioners outside the Chamberlen family (and probably by many more than this). In the early 1730s the former secret burst into print, in the writings of Butter (1733), Chapman (1735) and Giffard (edited posthumously by Hody, 1734). Thereupon the forceps was widely available, and it was indeed taken up by large numbers of young surgeons. One such individual was William Smellie, who in the next decade settled in London and offered classes in midwifery at which the use of the forceps was taught. From this point on, man-midwifery and the forceps were widespread and also controversial.

The dramatic effects of the publication of the forceps design create the impression that man-midwifery was novel in the eighteenth century and that it was indeed the forceps that promoted man-midwifery. Yet the forceps story itself, beginning as it does a century earlier, qualifies this picture; and in fact there is abundant evidence of male obstetric practice in seventeenth-century England, *outside* the Chamberlen family. In the case of Percival Willughby of Derby, it is thanks to the lucky accident that he wrote a midwifery treatise which survived in manuscript that we know he had an extensive obstetric practice in the Midlands in the mid-seventeenth century. From other sources we learn of Willughby's counterparts, in the late seventeenth and early eighteenth centuries, in other county towns and also in large market towns. These seventeenth-century practitioners were not usually *called* men-midwives; rather, they were described by the routine practitioner-labels of the time, that is as physicians, surgeons, apothecaries.

Nonetheless, although male obstetric practice before the publication of the forceps was more common than has been thought, it was indeed unusual. The norm in childbirth was delivery by a midwife, and this remained true at least up to the middle of the eighteenth century, even in such centres of man-midwifery as London and Edinburgh. And it is this that sets for us the central question here: By what routes did male practitioners enter the lying-in chamber at all? What

3 See J. H. Aveling, *The Chamberlens and the Midwifery Forceps* (London, 1882); Kedarnath Das, *Obstetric Forceps* (Calcutta, 1929); Walter Radcliffe, *The Secret Instrument* (London, 1947).

were the *paths to childbirth* of men like Willughby in the seventeenth century, and Hunter in the eighteenth?

Eight paths to childbirth

The materials that most easily enable us to answer this question are the midwifery treatises written by these men, especially where such treatises include illustrative case histories. Such case histories are not necessarily representative of the practices from which they are drawn; yet for the present purpose this need not matter unduly, since we are concerned in the main with the 'range' of the phenomena, and rather less with their 'central tendency'. It is a reasonable assumption that male treatises will include at least some examples of all the major 'paths to childbirth' experienced by their authors. What follows is a descriptive account, based on that assumption. For this purpose I have used three treatises and one set of lecture notes. The treatises are those of Willughby, Giffard and Smellie; the lecture notes are from a student of Hunter's, and they are used in default of an actual treatise by Hunter himself.

A brief word is in order about these sources and their authors.[4] Percival Willughby (1596–1685) practised in Derby from about 1630 to at least 1672; he wrote his 'Observations in Midwifery' between 1660 and 1672, and it contains cases variously written down from recall (as far back as 1630 or earlier) and recorded as soon as they occurred (particularly from the 1660s). The treatise remained unpublished during Willughby's lifetime, but found its way into print in 1754, 1863 and 1972. It contains over a hundred deliveries performed by Willughby and introduced into the text to support his didactic arguments. The *Observations* was a polemic for non-intervention in normal births, and for podalic version in cases of obstruction. It claimed repeatedly that midwives, particularly young midwives in the countryside, were ignorant and injudicious practitioners.

William Giffard (fl. 1720s) was a London surgeon about whom little is known. He acquired an obstetric forceps during the 1720s, and

4 Percival Willughby, *Observations in Midwifery*, ed. Henry Blenkinsop (Warwick, 1863; reprinted with introduction by John L. Thornton, Wakefield, 1972). The 1754 edition was in Dutch; see Thornton's introduction. A slightly earlier, manuscript version of this treatise is in the British Library, Sloane MS 529, fols. 1–19, paginated 1–35. William Giffard, *Cases in Midwifery* . . . *Revis'd and publish'd by Edward Hody* (London, 1734). William Smellie, *A Treatise on the Theory and Practice of Midwifery*, 3 vols. (London, 1752, 1754, 1764; vols. 2–3 entitled *A Collection of Cases in Midwifery*). Reprinted (London, 1876–8), edited with annotations by Alfred H. McClintock. William Hunter: Royal College of Surgeons, London, MS 42.d.25, Lecture notes on midwifery taken from Hunter's lectures, n.d. (?1760s).

6

348

from that point (if not before) made a record of many of his obstetric cases, over 200 in all. After his death, these cases were edited and published by Edward Hody, FRS, as one of his first communications in print about the forceps.

William Smellie (1697–1763) was trained as an apothecary in Lanark, was acquainted with William Cullen, and practised obstetric surgery as part of a general rural practice in the 1720s and early 1730s. On learning of the forceps, he took steps to educate himself in their use, travelling first to London and then to Paris in a search for instruction. From Grégoire in Paris he gained the idea of using phantoms for teaching purposes, and he returned to London where he set up both as a practitioner and as a teacher. During the 1740s he had some 900 male pupils, who enrolled in courses of varying lengths for a sliding scale of fees; and he also taught some midwives, though it is not known how many. Subsequently, he wrote his *Treatise* for the further education of his former pupils. He retired from practice in 1759, and then produced two supplementary volumes of case histories – mostly his own, but a substantial number taken from other treatises (including Giffard's) and from his own ex-pupils' correspondence with him. There are over 500 cases in the treatise.

William Hunter needs no introduction in the present context, but two features of his career deserve mention. First, he began his medico-surgical education in the late 1730s, that is after the design of the forceps had been published. Second, he spent a year of training under Smellie, from late 1740 to late 1741. This was when Smellie's classes were just beginning, but it is safe to assume that his main ideas and practices were well settled by this time; Hunter, by contrast, was still learning. Hunter went on to become surgeon, physician, man-midwife and anatomist, and the lecture notes of his students show that he gave courses on all these topics with the possible exception of physic.

I shall also be referring briefly to two other male practitioners, both of the early eighteenth century.[5] Hugh Chamberlen was the last of the forceps family dynasty; something of his practice is known from aristocratic family papers investigated by Randolph Trumbach, and it is in this connection that I shall be mentioning him. James Houstoun attempted to become a man-midwife, but did not succeed; I shall

5 Randolph Trumbach, 'The Aristocratic Family in England, 1690–1780. Studies in Childhood and Kinship' (PhD thesis, Johns Hopkins University, 1972), p. 31. James Houstoun, *Memoirs of the Life and Travels of James Houstoun, M.D., Collected and Written by His Own Hand* (London, 1747), pp. 73–4.

consider his training in obstetrics, which he recounted in his autobiography.

When I began preparing this essay, it was my belief that men came to childbirth by just three distinct routes or 'paths'. As I worked through the material, however, it emerged that my theme was better chosen than I had actually imagined, for I found that the paths to childbirth numbered not three but eight. I wanted to contend that man-midwifery was complex, but the historical evidence surpassed my contention: The distinctions between different paths require to be drawn in three different dimensions. These dimensions concern the timing of the call for male attendance; whether or not the call had been anticipated; and finally, the presence or absence of a midwife in addition to the male practitioner.

The first dimension to consider – that of the timing – enables us to distinguish between three types of call, which I shall term advance calls, onset calls and emergency calls. In an *advance* call, the practitioner was summoned by the mother to come and reside in her house at some point during her pregnancy, to advise her on her diet and course of life, to remain until the birth itself, to be in attendance during the birth, and to continue for some time afterwards to supervise her post-partum recovery. An *onset* call summoned the practitioner to the delivery as soon as labour commenced; an *emergency* call sent for him only after some serious difficulty had arisen.

In the second dimension (anticipation), we have to distinguish between *booked* and *unbooked* calls. The male practitioner could be 'engaged'(as Willughby put it) or 'bespoke' (Smellie's term) for attendance, and this constituted a booked call; if there had been no such prior arrangement, the call was unbooked. All advance calls were by definition booked; onset and emergency calls, by contrast, could be either booked or unbooked. The booking amounted to an engagement to attend on the due summons; that summons could itself be of the onset or emergency type. This may seem strange in the case of an emergency call, yet it did indeed happen, at least in Willughby's practice. The effect of such an engagement was probably that he had to refuse all other calls, except emergencies close to hand.

Our third dimension concerns the presence or absence of a midwife. In both advance and onset calls, the male practitioner could be called either *in addition to* a midwife, or *in lieu of* a midwife; his own role differed radically in these two distinct situations. If a midwife was involved, the man's place was to be on hand in case difficulty arose; thus a further, subsidiary 'call' was required to bring him into

350

the delivery room itself. If, by contrast, there was no midwife, then the man's task was to effect the actual delivery. As for emergency calls, we may assume for the sake of initial simplicity that these always involved the prior attendance of a midwife, though we shall later see that this requires qualification.

Our sources by no means make it explicit in every case-description just which of these eight possible paths had been followed; the main difficulty lies in identifying onset calls and in specifying the particular variety within that broad category. Nonetheless, there is every indication that each of these eight distinct routes did in fact occur historically. The eight paths are summarised in Figure 12.1, and an illustration of each, drawn from the treatises of Willughby and Smellie, is given in the Appendix.

It is obvious that these calls will have been made to different extents amongst different social classes, and that they must have commanded different fees. *Advance* calls, in particular, could be made only by mothers of the gentry or merchant classes, since these women alone would have had the large houses required for entertaining the male practitioner as a living-in guest. Again, advance calls must have earned very large fees, since they tied the practitioner down; in theory, he was not permitted to accept any other engagement, although leave might be granted to answer an emergency call or to attend from its onset the delivery of a regular patient.[6] On the evidence of Willughby's cases, it would seem that *onset* calls came from a slightly wider circle of patients (the 'semi-gentry' or wives of clergymen and professionals as well as the gentry) and that *emergency* calls took him to mothers of all social classes; a preliminary examination of Giffard's and Smellie's cases suggests a similar picture for these two later practitioners. The size of the fees depended greatly upon the reputation and achievements of the individual practitioner, as well as on the wealth of the patient and on the type of call. It is impossible to be precise on this score, but it seems certain that there was a great difference in fees between advance calls, onset calls and emergency calls; and it is likely that advance calls commanded tens of pounds, onset calls one or a few pounds or guineas, and emergency calls perhaps a pound or less. On some occasions, particularly emergency calls, a practitioner might give his services free of charge.

Why were male practitioners called at all? On the evidence of Willughby's and Smellie's cases, it seems that both advance and onset calls were usually made because the mother (or someone else) ex-

6   See Willughby, *Observations,* p. 141, for an example of this.

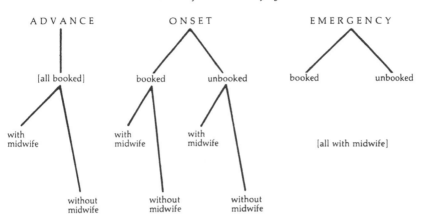

Fig. 12.1. Classification of paths to childbirth

pected that the birth would be difficult. This might be because of difficulty in previous births, through fear of the first birth or because there had been some problem in pregnancy such as a fever or discharge. Emergency calls, by definition, arose because of difficulty. Thus male practice, at least in its origins, was very largely connected with abnormal birth or with the expectation of such abnormality.

What I have presented so far is a framework of classification, designed to capture the 'varieties of man-midwifery' and at the same time to facilitate comparisons between different practitioners. But this framework leaves out the important question of *who made* the different types of call. Here I can only offer an impressionistic account, surveying the main features of the problem – together with the observation that this is a crucial question on which much more work is needed. First, it seems that whenever 'booking' was involved, it was done either by the mother herself or by her husband. Second, and similarly, it was again the mother or husband who made 'advance' and 'onset' calls *without a midwife*. Third, there is a further dimension in those 'advance' and 'onset' calls that were made *with* a midwife. For, as we have seen, in these cases the original task expected of the male practitioner was merely to stand by in case of difficulty; and so the question arises as to who decided that 'difficulty' had indeed occurred, and thus that the male practitioner standing by should be asked to lend his active services. In practice, it seems (though this is a preliminary conclusion) that it was usually *the midwife* who made this decision. Thus in these two of our eight 'varieties', the 'calling' of a male practitioner actually took place in two stages, and was undertaken by different parties: first, the original booking, which was made by the mother or her husband; and second, the further summons to the delivery room, which might or might not occur, but which if it were made was made by the midwife.

This leaves just one of our eight varieties, namely *unbooked emergencies*. In practice, these were the commonest kinds of calls in all our sources – and it is here that the act of calling was at its most complex. There were several possible 'calling agents': the mother, her husband, the midwife, the various women attending the birth, and finally people outside the delivery room who knew the mother and were associated with the given male practitioner. In Willughby's cases we find all of these different possible agents named as having initiated the call. There are some cases where *combinations* of calling agents are mentioned, such as the mother and midwife or 'all the women'; there are also a few instances of conflict, where one party wanted Willughby to be called but another was opposed to this. Further, there appears to have been a difference between Willughby's practice in Derby (where he spent most of his working life) and London (where he lived for some four years, practising 'among the meaner sort of women'). In Derby, few of the emergency calls came from midwives, and there are examples of midwives being opposed to his being called. In London, it was the midwives themselves who usually called him, and we also find that Willughby was much more kindly disposed towards London midwives than towards their Midlands counterparts. Interestingly, we find that Giffard's and Smellie's cases – occurring in London some seventy to ninety years later – also show many emergency calls by midwives. Thus there seems to have been a tradition in London of better relations between midwives and surgeons than obtained in the provinces.

There is a further issue, pertaining especially to emergency calls, and just as important as the question of who made the call: namely *when and why* the call was made. So far, I have been writing as if the definition of an 'emergency' was unproblematical; but in fact, as the sources make abundantly clear, this definition was itself a social act. An emergency could consist in flooding – but how much flooding? In obstructed labour – but obstructed for how long? In danger to the mother's life – but how was this danger assessed? It was the participants in the birth who answered these questions, following their own beliefs about the nature of childbirth and the role of the male practitioner. A man-midwife might be called to deliver a living child, or a dead one; after twelve hours, or after ten days; in hope, or in fear. An obstetric emergency was, in short, *defined by* the participants in the birth: It was not a biological 'given', even though it was (so to speak)

11

socially constructed out of biological raw materials. And the social 'definition' of an emergency was in fact highly complex, involving as it did a number of separate people in distinctive social roles.

A final set of complexities has to be mentioned in connection with emergency calls, particularly of the unbooked variety. So far, I have been assuming for the sake of simplicity that in such cases, the primary management of the birth had been in the hands of a midwife; but of course, emergencies could and did occur with a male practitioner in charge. Further, I have been assuming that in the event of an emergency, the first recourse was to a male practitioner; but in fact, a midwife could be called in this role. Indeed, certain midwives seem to have specialised in such emergency work, or at least enjoyed reputations for being able to deliver difficult births: Three such midwives are mentioned in Willughby's treatise. Sometimes a chain of practitioners was called: Willughby occasionally found three or more midwives present at a difficult birth, and Smellie records cases where he was the second or third male practitioner to have been summoned. Hunter described in his lectures a case that went from the midwife to a male practitioner to a second male practitioner and then back to the original midwife. This would appear to be unusual: So far as a pattern can be detected, this would seem to be for the delivery to pass from midwives to male practitioners, but not the other way around.

Further variants arose as by-products of man-midwifery itself, through lying-in hospitals on the one hand and through the teaching practice of William Smellie on the other. We can presumably regard delivery in a lying-in hospital as a special case of the onset call, but a definitive classification of such births must await research into the admission and management policies of the lying-in hospitals. Smellie devised for teaching purposes an ingenious arrangement: He induced poor women to permit him and his pupils to deliver them. The advantage for the mother was that the delivery was free (and indeed, Smellie arranged a maintenance fund for these women during their lying-in by subscriptions from his pupils). The advantage for Smellie and the pupils was a stock of natural labours for their instruction. These arrangements represented onset calls (presumably of the booked variety); often Smellie himself was left in the role of emergency consultant; and he kept a midwife employed to attend such labours if they proved normal but lingering.

Profiles of practice

Any individual practice can be conceived as having a specific *profile*, consisting of the relative and absolute frequencies of these different

354

Table 12.1. *Profiles of practice: types of calls known to have been accepted by various practitioners (Willughby in Derby, all others in London)*

	Willughby (1660s)	Chamberlen (c. 1720)	Giffard[a] (1726–8)	Smellie (1740s)	Hunter (1740s–60s)
Advance	+	+	·	·	+
Onset	+	+	+	+	+
Emergency	+	?	+	+	+

Key: + = known to have occurred
   · = known not to have occurred
   ? = occurrence uncertain
[a]Cases 1–37 only.
Sources: See footnotes 4 and 5.

types of calls. In considering this question, I shall simplify the matter considerably by attending only to the distinction between advance, onset and emergency calls (i.e., suppressing the issues of booking and midwife presence). Table 12.1 shows, for five practitioners, which of these types of calls they are known to have attended. Here Giffard and Smellie stand out as not, apparently, having enjoyed the lucrative advance calls; all the five practitioners in question, however, received onset and (probably) emergency calls. For three of these practitioners (Willughby, Giffard and Smellie) a quantitative estimate can be made, provided we may assume that the cases in their treatises are representative of those in their practices. Table 12.2 displays this information, giving for Giffard and Smellie only provisional estimates based on small samples of their cases, whereas for Willughby's recorded cases the picture is complete.

We cannot, of course, assume that the cases in any individual's treatise are representative of those in his practice. On the contrary, we would expect the cases to be recorded selectively; and such selection might well distort the picture in the very dimension that concerns us. For instance, male practitioners might be expected to record more cases involving serious difficulty, to the relative neglect of normal births, which would have the effect of exaggerating the proportion of emergency cases. This problem can be resolved only by detailed work on each particular treatise, reconstructing the composition of the text, the distribution over time of different types of case, the purposes of the author, and so far as possible the socio-geographical catchment area of his practice. I have carried this out only for Willughby's treatise, but the results are very encouraging. Table 12.3 displays three tests that

Table 12.2. *Relative frequencies of advance, onset*
and emergency calls in selected/sampled cases
of Willughby, Giffard and Smellie

	Willughby	Giffard	Smellie
Numbers of cases			
Advance	11	—	—
Onset	6	4	9[a]
Emergency	47	28	22
Unknown	—	3	3
Total	64	35	34
Percentages			
Advance + onset	27	11–20	26–35
Emergency	73	80–9	65–74

Note: Cases used: Willughby – all his childbirth cases from 1660–1672, i.e., those occurring during the writing of his treatise; Giffard – the first 35 childbirth cases (coming from cases 1–37) of his treatise; Smellie – a stratified random sample (1 case in 10) of all the cases in his treatise (vols. ii and iii), replacing non-childbirth/non-Smellie cases with Smellie childbirth cases where possible.

[a]Includes one case received by his pupils at onset of labour, but which they referred to Smellie because an emergency arose.

can be made of the representativeness of the cases included in the previous table; if there was some particular bias (such as a bias in favour of emergency cases), it would almost certainly be reflected in one or more of these tests. In fact these measures show no such distortion; what seems to have happened is that the variety of Willughby's arguments had the accidental effect of making him record different types of calls to roughly equal extents. We cannot, of course, naïvely extend this finding to Giffard and Smellie, yet it is possible prima facie that their case series, too, are approximately representative.

Thus encouraged, we may return to Table 12.2, from which two main features stand out. First, Willughby was distinctive amongst these three practitioners in receiving 'advance' calls at all. It may be that the other cases in Giffard's treatise show a few such calls, but even so the sample suggests that the incidence of these in Giffard's practice must have been much lower than in Willughby's. As for Smellie, I can confirm from a sifting of the cases that he records no

356

Table 12.3. *Reliability of the cases in Willughby's treatise as a source for his practice: numbers of cases in various categories*

Similarity of two phases of the case series:[a]	1660–6	1667–72
Advance	5	6
Onset	3	3
Emergency	24	23
Totals	32	32
Types of case recording:	Primary[b]	Secondary[b]
Advance + onset	14 (27%)	3 (23%)
Emergency	37 (73%)	10 (77%)
Comparison with catchment area:	Observed	Expected[c] (with $N = 64$)
Advance + onset	17	9–28
Emergency	47	36–55

[a]These can be regarded as distinct 'phases', because Willughby's topics of concern changed in 1667.

[b]Primary cases are those involving the delivery of a mother whom Willughby had not delivered before; secondary cases are follow-up deliveries, i.e., further deliveries of mothers he had already delivered. It is likely that Willughby recorded all secondary cases (hence these are probably representative); it is certain that he recorded only a small fraction, about ⅕, of his "primary" cases (hence these are very probably unrepresentative).

[c]Basis of 'expected': Emergency practice estimated by various routes at 25–30 per year. Advance and onset cases estimated at 5–20 per year, on the assumption that amongst the eligible social classes and within Willughby's catchment area, the incidence of such calls could have been as low as 5 per cent or as high as 20 per cent. The figures given represent the extremes from these assumptions.

explicitly 'advance' cases at all. There may be some under the 'unknowns', but it is unlikely that this would have been a significant component of Smellie's practice without the fact ever being explicitly acknowledged; and of course Smellie was so busy with his teaching, and with his onset and emergency calls, that he lacked the incentive to accept advance calls. As we have seen, the advance calls were lucrative – but so was Smellie's teaching, which stood handsomely in place of an advance-call practice.

The second point that emerges from Table 12.2 is the overwhelming predominance of emergency calls in all three sets of cases. Around three-quarters of the cases – more amongst Giffard's, less amongst Smellie's – were of this type. If we compare the three sets in this respect (that is, ignoring the distinction between 'advance' and 'onset' cases that is relevant only in Willughby's practice) then their *similarity* is the striking finding. This serves to extend and underline a point I have made already, namely that 'man-midwifery' tended to be concentrated upon difficult births. Normal births were brought into male practice only via advance and onset calls, and even these calls were usually made because difficulty was *expected*. But the main component of male practice – at least, that of Willughby, Giffard and Smellie – was emergency work, and here of course difficulty had *already occurred*.

Finally, a 'profile of practice' should also include some assessment of the overall *rate* of practice, that is of how many births the given man-midwife attended in a typical year. For Willughby, some of this has already emerged (in Table 12.3): He saw in all perhaps thirty-five to forty births per year, and this is consonant with his socio-geographical catchment area. Notice that we have here a strong constraint on provincial obstetric practice by men: Willughby had a big local reputation, was seated in a county town, and practised over a ten-mile radius, yet given the distribution of population and the general restriction of his practice to emergency work, he could not have expected to attend as many as fifty births per year. The likely rate of practice for men-midwives in market towns must therefore have been still lower. In sharp contrast were the prospects in London, which had fifteen times as many births in the metropolitan area as occurred within Willughby's ten-mile radius of practice. Thus it is not surprising to find that Giffard seems to have attended something of the order of 50 to 100 births a year.[7] The rate of Smellie's London practice awaits investigation, but it seems overwhelmingly likely that this was at least as high as Giffard's.

Practice and precept

The 'profile of practice' of any given man-midwife dictated the actual experience of childbirth he accumulated. A practice dominated by emergencies would lead to much experience of malpresentations, obstructed labours and major complications; a practice involving

7   There are long gaps in Giffard's case series (as in Willughby's). If we look only at those cases without such long gaps between them, then from the first 37 cases in Giffard's treatise we find an average of a case every eight days, just under 50 per year. But there was a heavy concentration of cases in August, 1728 (cases 27–36, i.e., ten cases in all), including six uses of the forceps; this month may well have been more representative, and it would suggest over 100 cases per year. The true rate probably lay somewhere between these estimates.

16

358

more advance and onset cases might give far more opportunities to see the mechanism of normal labour, yet this could also depend on whether these cases involved a midwife as well as the male practitioner. This influence of the type of practice on the experiences of the practitioner can be brought out dramatically by contrasting two specific individuals: Percival Willughby and James Houstoun. We have already seen the broad contours of Willughby's practice: a delivery every ten days or so, mostly emergencies, but about once a month an advance or onset case – usually delivered, however, not by Willughby but by the midwife.

Houstoun's brief experience in man-midwifery was gained at the Paris Hôtel-Dieu. There, in the position of house surgeon, which he gained after arduous lobbying, he delivered in four months about 300 births – for which he was personally responsible, even though he was working in tandem with some fellow-trainee female midwives. It is therefore likely that he gained more experience of *normal birth* than Willughby acquired in a decade of practice, perhaps even in a lifetime. Yet precisely the opposite is true of *difficult* cases. If we take the florid example of arm/shoulder presentation, Houstoun probably saw only one such delivery; he may have seen none, or two, or just possibly as many as three, but it is highly unlikely that he delivered more than this.[8] Willughby, by contrast, delivered about six such cases every year; he became so adept at them that he could effect the delivery by podalic version in just seven minutes, and in the course of his practice he devised his own method of turning, improving on Paré's technique, which was the one he had learned initially. Moreover, there were qualitative differences between Willughby's experience and Houstoun's. In difficult births, Willughby was the practitioner of last resort; Houstoun, by contrast, 'called in the master-surgeon of the Hospital's assistance'. In normal births, Willughby usually played a subordinate role to the midwife; Houstoun's position was complex, since on the one hand he performed the delivery himself, while on the other hand 'we assisted one another, and had a mistress midwife who directed the whole'.

The actual experiences of the practitioner, together with his previous education, are what we should expect to have conditioned the attitudes he developed. Willughby provides a clear case in point, for his *Observations* record how he arrived at his strenuous belief in non-

8 Assuming that cases of arm/shoulder presentation occurred at a rate of 1 in 200 deliveries, in 300 births the odds are 14 to 1 against more than three such cases, using binomial probabilities.

intervention. His training had been confined to the use of the crotchet for craniotomies, and consequently, in advance and onset cases he 'gave way to the midwife' to do whatever she pleased. But different midwives managed deliveries in different ways: Some placed the mother on a midwife's stool, others in bed, still others kneeling on a bolster on the floor; some stretched the labiae with their hands and pulled the child, while others left the delivery to proceed naturally; some wanted to hurry labour, others to defer it. All this meant that Willughby had a rich pool of experience from which to learn – if he so desired. And he did indeed wish to learn, for he was horrified both at the sufferings of women in childbed and at the grisly work of craniotomy he might be called on to perform. Thus propelled to observe, Willughby 'took this observation': 'That those women were easiest or soonest delivered, that kept themselves warm and quiet, in or on their beds or pallets, deferring their labours to the very last, and patiently suffering nature to bedew with humours those places, and so to mellow and open by degrees their bodies, without midwives' enforcements.' The preconditions for this piece of learning were first, the different practices of different midwives, and second, Willughby's position on the sidelines in advance and onset cases – the fact that he usually did not have responsibility for conducting the delivery.

Smellie, Hunter and the revolution in obstetrics

In this light, I suggest, we can better understand the questions with which we began, concerning William Hunter's role in the eighteenth-century 'revolution in obstetrics'. Again, this is best brought out by a contrast – in this case, the contrast between Hunter and his teacher, rival and fellow-*émigré* from Lanarkshire, William Smellie.

Smellie's introduction to obstetric practice came in Lanark itself in the 1720s; he was then unacquainted with the forceps but could perform podalic version, and he seems to have had an emergency practice much akin to Willughby's. This means that the routine obstetric work Smellie was performing, as part of a general practice, consisted mainly of craniotomies. Now, compared to craniotomy, the forceps was a far more humane instrument – which is why Smellie, on reading about the forceps, acquired it and went about learning how to use it. As we have seen, his subsequent London practice included a significant proportion of normal births, yet numerically these were far outweighed by emergency cases. As Smellie tended to entrust onset calls to his pupils, and to give himself a consultant role, this pattern

360

would have been enhanced. Given this pattern of experience, Smellie was likely to be a relative enthusiast for the forceps and for surgical intervention (whether manual or instrumental) in general.

William Hunter's development as a man-midwife, very different from Smellie's, can be summarised in terms of four stages. First, he came to medical practice (in 1737) after the design of the forceps had been published: He was not a man of the craniotomy era. Second, his initial training in midwifery came from Smellie himself, that is from the leading forceps practitioner of the day. Third, he left Smellie's household to live with James Douglas and thereby gained access (as Helen Brock has shown) not only to a vast wealth of anatomical techniques, ideas and preparations, but also to the polite, aristocratic practice of man-midwifery. Finally, from 1748 at the Middlesex Hospital, and then from 1749 at the newly founded Lying-in Hospital, Hunter had a position as a consultant man-midwife. We shall now see that the obstetric attitudes displayed in Hunter's lectures are intelligible as the product of these experiences.[9]

A striking feature of the lectures is the frequency with which Hunter referred to Smellie – and, no less so, the complexity of his attitude to Smellie. From the lecture notes, Smellie emerges not only as the foil against whom Hunter develops his own anti-interventionist stance, but also in the role of the great man. In the introductory, historical lecture Hunter referred to some thirteen authorities, Hippocrates being the first and Smellie (mentioned three times) the last; in the substantive part of the course, Smellie towered over all the rest, with twenty-seven citations as against eighteen for all other authors combined (La Motte with four citations being his nearest rival). Strikingly, Hunter made no mention at all of Ould, Exton or Burton, whereas he did refer to Chamberlen, Mauriceau and Daventer – proof enough that such references were highly selective. The thrust of the references to Smellie is much more evenly balanced than might have been expected: fourteen references are critical, ten are favourable and the remaining six are ambiguous or neutral. The criticisms are almost invariably in the direction of describing Smellie as too officious, too interventionist, and to this extent the received view is correct; but the presence of great praise alongside the blame, together

9   The lecture notes, cited in fn. 4, are paginated 1–176, followed by a few pages on the management of children. The themes I discuss are found on the following pages: references to Smellie, pp. 7, 8, 10, 25, 28, 32, 34, 35, 39 (twice), 47, 51, 59, 73f, 90, 92, 97, 101, 102, 104 (twice), 111, 115, 119, 122, 131, 134, 139, 147, 173. Forceps, pp. 102–16. Placenta, pp. 95 (from which I quote), 99f. Reputation and 'delicacy', pp. 39, 43, 44, 50, 51, 52, 53, 55, 58, 70, 79, 82f, 87f, 94, 95, 134, 150, 153, 168, 172–6 (my final quotation is from p. 176).

with the sheer weight of the references to Smellie, suggests something more: that in the sphere of midwifery, Smellie was something of a father-figure for Hunter.

What strengthens this picture is the fact that Hunter's own anti-interventionism was by no means as total or as doctrinaire as has sometimes been supposed. On the forceps, the lecture notes reveal that the classic quotation reproduced by Spencer has to be heavily qualified: Although inveighing several times against their injudicious and over-hasty use, Hunter devoted much time (some fifteen pages in the manuscript notes) to detailed instructions on how to apply the forceps. Similarly on the third stage of labour:

> If pains come on 20 minutes or half an hour after the delivery
> of the child, pull gently on the funis to extract the placenta; but
> in weak relaxed women with pendulous bellies, we should
> wait a long time before the uterus can recover its tone so as to
> be capable of contraction. If without attending to the state of
> the uterus . . . we should pull forcibly at the funis, the gaping
> sinuses may pour forth such a torrent of blood as to bring on a
> fatal syncope.

The key phrase here is 'without attending to the state of the uterus'. Far from putting forward a dogma or doctrine, Hunter was seeking to regulate practice by attentive observation: Sometimes, he held, manual removal of the placenta was appropriate, but at other times it was not. His famous anti-interventionism, then, consisted in a shift of emphasis and to some degree in self-presentation, rather than representing a total break with Smellie's teaching. Its rhetorical force was animated by Hunter's desire to demarcate himself from Smellie, to establish his own separate identity as a practitioner.

But if Smellie left a mark on Hunter, so too, in a different way, did James Douglas. The aristocratic practice in midwifery that Hunter initially owed to Douglas was largely made up of onset calls. This would have shifted the balance of Hunter's obstetric experiences sharply in the direction of normal birth and away from obstructed labours. Moreover, Hunter's consultancy work, too, would also have exposed him to normal births – and incidentally, through enhancing his reputation and status, probably helped him to develop his private onset practice as well. It is plausible to suppose that as Hunter gained more and more experience of normal birth, he became more and more conscious of those powers of nature that were to be a conspicuous theme of the argument of his lectures.

These experiences make it intelligible that Hunter's proclaimed approach to midwifery consisted in distancing himself from Smellie in the specific direction of arguing for less hasty intervention. But something more was to strengthen this attitude. Hunter's lectures reveal an overwhelming concern with what he called the 'dress and address' of the practitioner. In lecture after lecture he returned to such themes as the reputation of the *accoucheur*, the devices needed to create and to maintain the reputation, and the delicacy this enterprise required. Hunter was, in fact, teaching his pupils man-midwifery, not merely as a technical skill, but also as a social role. It was to this topic that the last words of the lecture course were devoted: 'Advice to young accoucheurs' takes up several pages of the notes, and it ends with this slogan: 'It is not the mere safe delivery of the woman will recommend an accoucheur, but a sagacious well-conducted behaviour of tenderness, assiduity and delicacy.' Here we have the man-midwife who wants to get into the delivery room, and to deliver normal births amongst wealthy patients – a far cry indeed from the emergency practice of a previous generation. And it seems likely that this strengthened Hunter's reliance upon nature, his anti-interventionism: To touch a lady was a different matter from touching the wife of a tradesman. At one point in the lectures this becomes explicit; fittingly, this is one of Hunter's criticisms of Smellie. It concerns the diagnosis of pregnancy:

> Smellie advises introducing a finger in ano which will more likely ascertain the pressure, but the indelicacy of this operation has exploded its practice in private. Such practice is improper when you are called to satisfy a lady. Here you should for your own reputation's sake endeavour to use some ambiguous answer, and by prescribing some inoffensive medicine . . . to amuse her a month longer.

Hunter's developing experience, his attitudes to technical obstetric issues, and his approach to the social role of the man-midwife were thus all of a piece. To some extent he inherited this particular niche from James Douglas and (indirectly) from such predecessors as Hamilton and Manningham; but by his own lectures and by the force of his own highly successful example, he must have enlarged it enormously. That he eventually delivered the queen herself was a fitting symbol of his triumph.

The picture that has emerged here is consistent with the accepted view that the 'revolution in obstetrics' was promoted both by the forceps and by fashion, but it would seem that these two influences worked within different spheres of practice. The role of the forceps was primarily in emergency work; fashionable practice involved onset and advance calls. What Smellie was for the obstetric surgeon, the emergency practitioner, Hunter was for the physician-man-midwife. With the distinction drawn between these different types of practice, and with Hunter's own development understood in these terms, there is no longer a paradox about Hunter's attitude to the forceps.

Conclusion: man-midwifery and its historiography

It will be apparent that my approach to William Hunter, and to man-midwifery in general, differs in several respects from Professor Shorter's interpretation, elsewhere in this volume (Chap. 13). In the first place, we have different historiographical objectives: Shorter writes in evaluative terms, whereas I have limited myself to description. Second, we have different pictures of the long-term developments: Swayed as I am by Willughby's *Observations*, I do not find the anti-interventionism of the late eighteenth century a wholly novel development. I am inclined to believe that not all midwives were meddlesome, and I have claimed that midwives could influence male practitioners as well as learning from them.[10] Third, with regard to the eighteenth century, we have studied different things: Shorter has extracted from treatises specific doctrines about the management of the separate stages of labour, whereas I have focused upon the overall stance or approach of individual practitioners. Fourth, in contextualising our findings, we have again gone different ways: Shorter has related text to text, whereas I have sought the intelligibility of texts in obstetric practice. Finally, as to that practice, we have different underlying images of its nature: For Professor Shorter it is largely a technical, biological matter, whereas I have depicted it as a series of social acts. Our approaches, it seems, are not so much complementary as incommensurable – no doubt a tribute to the richness of the subject.

The burden of my argument has been that the word 'man-midwifery' conceals more than it reveals. It meant eight different things – different paths to childbirth, as I have called them – and these were themselves complex. Any individual practice comprised a specific mixture of these different elements, and there was great room for differences between different individuals. Not only were there changes over time (notably the publication of the forceps) and specificities of place (such as the different opportunities for practice in London and elsewhere), but also there were different attitudes on the

10 Jean L'Esperance suggests that it is the 'central message' of Professor Shorter's *A History of Women's Bodies* (New York, 1982) that 'women owe their current happy situation in society to the superior knowledge and kindness of the opposite sex'. See *Ontario History*, LXXV (1983), 98–103 (I quote from p. 100), and ibid. 298–9 for the author's reply.

364

part of the men-midwives themselves. Precepts and experiences were interwoven in complex ways: Given the wealth of treatises and case-records, together with the diversity of attitudes exhibited by male practitioners, there is ample scope here for further research.

If we are confused by the term man-midwifery, that is an artefact of our distance in time from the period. Contemporaries knew what they meant and would have experienced no sense of contradiction in using the same word in different ways. We do the same – witness how many different things are covered by such words as 'historian' or 'doctor' – but when studying the past, we stand outside the relevant speech-community and thus are misled by the appearances of words.

It is equally significant that a man could be, to all intents and purposes, a man-midwife – a man much engaged in delivering women – without ever being described as such. The most striking example of this is Percival Willughby, a specialist in deliveries in the 1660s. Willughby is more accessible to historical view than many other seventeenth-century practitioners (whether obstetric or not), yet the several ways he was described include no hint of his obstetric work. At different times and in different contexts he was called 'surgeon', 'physician', 'extra-licentiate', 'gentleman', and (on his tombstone, apparently erroneously) 'M.D'. Thus, just as we cannot read off the nature of man-midwifery from the word 'man-midwife', so too we cannot infer the absence of male obstetric practice from the absence of the word later used to describe it. This goes a long way to support the viewpoint, variously advanced by Roberts, Pelling and Webster, and Cunningham, that the content of practice is not to be naively inferred from any practitioner-label.[11] What such labels meant, at any point in the early-modern period, remains to be discovered – as does the full meaning of 'man-midwifery'.

Acknowledgements

I wish to acknowledge the help of Helen Brock, who has been very generous in supplying me with references and drew my attention in

11   R. S. Roberts, 'The Personnel and Practice of Medicine in Tudor and Stuart England', *Medical History*, VI (1962), 363–82, and VIII (1964), 217–34 (see particularly pp. 375–6 of the first of these two parts of the article); Margaret Pelling and Charles Webster, 'Medical Practitioners', in Webster, ed., *Health, Medicine and Mortality in the Sixteenth Century* (Cambridge, 1979), pp. 165–235 (see esp. p. 235); Andrew Cunningham, 'The Medical Professions and the Pattern of Medical Care: The Case of Edinburgh, c.1670–c.1700', in Wolfgang Eckart and Johanna Geyer-Kordesch, eds., *Heilberufe und Kranke im 17. und 18. Jahrhundert die Quellen- und Forschungssituation* (Münster, 1982), pp. 9–28. Cunningham writes (p. 17) that 'we just do not know which particular functions were undertaken by someone calling himself a "surgeon" or "apothecary": and we will not know them until such time as we try to discover them – from a position of confessed ignorance'.

particular to the Hunter lecture notes in the Royal College of Surgeons library; Andrew Cunningham, for his criticisms and advice; and the librarian and staff of the Royal College of Surgeons library, for facilitating my research. Where a reference is not supplied, supporting details will be found in A. F. Wilson, 'Childbirth in Seventeenth- and Eighteenth-Century England', (D. Phil. thesis, University of Sussex, 1982). This is to be published as *A Safe Deliverance* (Cambridge, in press).

Appendix: illustrative examples of different paths to childbirth

These cases are taken from the treatises of Willughby and Smellie (see footnote 4). References to Smellie's cases are to the case numbers supplied by McClintock to his edition.

One of the Willughby cases used here is described in both of the extant versions of his treatise, and I have reproduced both accounts since they give different though compatible details. These particular descriptions (example 3) are given in full. All the other examples are abridged to bring into greater prominence the theme with which I am concerned. I have modernised spelling and punctuation throughout.

Notice that in examples 2, 4 and 6 the absence of a midwife is not stated but can be inferred by contrast with examples 1, 3 and 5 respectively. In examples 5 and 6, the fact that the call was unbooked is inferred by contrast with examples 3 and 4. Again, in example 1 it is not stated explicitly who delivered the child (the midwife or Willughby), but it can be inferred that it was the midwife, both because there is no description of the birth itself and by contrast with his account of the third stage of labour. Finally, notice in examples 1, 7 and 8 the participation of two or more agents in bringing Willughby to the birth and getting him to act.

1.Advance call, with midwife (Willughby, Observations, 64–7)

I was sent for by a Lady and kinswoman, who thought that she was within a fortnight of her account, but she continued above that time seven weeks . . .

Friday 29 November 1661 about four in the afternoon, she forced herself to have a stool in her closet. By this great striving . . . her waters did break . . . [but] she had no labour at all . . . I persuaded her, on Saturday night, to go to bed, and was called again to her [on Sunday] December 1 early in the morning . . . In the afternoon . . . she had a hard stool, but it must [have been] concealed from me.

Her labour being long and tedious, I entreated her to take the Earl of Chesterfield's powder to move the birth . . . The child was born . . . between four and five, that Sunday [afternoon].

The child was stillborn. The midwife made much ado to revive the child, but in vain. I caused her to separate it from the after-burden . . . The midwife was fearful to fetch the after-burden, so I was put upon the work by her husband, the which I quickly performed.

366

2. *Advance call, without midwife (Willughby,* Observations, *40–2)*

A young, good conditioned lady (the Lady Byron) . . . desired my company, and entreated me to be with her, and to assist her in the time of her travail, and in the mean space to direct her what was convenient to be done or observed by her . . . She had a thin and weak body, and was troubled with great fears, never having any child before.

August the thirteenth [1661] the moon changed; that night she had some grumbling disquiets, and the ensuing night they increased. Thursday, August the fifteenth, I came early in the morning to her, and finding some foregoing signs of labour, at her desire she was removed into another chamber, and laid into a truckle bed about seven in the morning.

. . . In the afternoon, about one o'clock, the womb began to open . . . About a quarter past four she was delivered of a daughter. It was troublesome to fetch the after-burden as she lay on her back. She was put to her knees, and then it was obtained easily, and so she was then removed to another bed.

. . . The child was baptized Aug. 22 1661 . . . Aug. 23, I left this lady, giving her thanks for her loving favours to me.

3. *Onset call, booked, with midwife (Willughby,* Observations, *37–8; and British Library, Sloane MS 529, p. 3)*

Printed version. . . . being in Staffordshire with a worthy good man, I saw his wife great with child. [Lady Broughton, margin] She told me what terrible afflictions she had suffered in the birth of her first child, and wept much at the remembrance of them. She entreated me that I would come to her in the time of her labour, and for that purpose she would send good horses for me. I gave her instructions to lie quietly in or on her bed until I could come to her, and not suddenly put herself under her midwife's hands. She sent me horses. I went eight miles to her. In the mean time she kept her body warm, and lay quiet. So soon as I was come she sent for me into her chamber. Going with her midwife apart from the company, I asked how this gentlewoman was, and what she thought of the birth. She replied that she could not tell, and that in all her days she never was with so peevish a woman, and that she would not suffer her to touch her body. I sat by this gentlewoman a little space, and, perceiving that labour came upon her, I went forth of the room, putting her under the midwife's hands. The waters issued without enforcement, presently the child followed them, and she was easily and quickly delivered.

When I went away, she gave God thanks, and said that her pains were nothing in comparison to what she had formerly suffered.

Manuscript version. Anno 1648: There was a worthy good Lady, yet living, that had much suffered under the midwife's hands at the birth of her first child. As I walked with her, she made great moans, with tears in her eyes, thinking what afflictions she had suffered before she could be delivered, and feared what would become of her, being great with child. I comforted her and advised her not to let her midwife too suddenly meddle with her. Being not past 8 miles from her house, she sent 2 horses to bring me, and rejoiced at my coming. I asked the midwife how the labour proceeded; she said that she knew not, and that in all her days, she never came nigh so peevish a creature as this Lady was; and that she would not let her touch her. I was glad to hear it; I whispered the Lady in her ear, and went down into the parlour. I had not long been there, but the waters flowed, and the child followed, as she lay on her truckle-bed, and all sorrow was quickly past; for which when I came into the chamber to take my leave, with a smiling countenance she gave me thanks and rewarded my coming with gold.

4. Onset call, booked, without midwife (Smellie, case 100)

In the year 1748, I was bespoke to attend a woman in her first child; and received a call about the middle of the ninth month, when she complained of pains in her head and back . . . I found the os internum soft, but not open; from which circumstance I declared she was not in labour; then I ordered her to be blooded to a quantity of eight ounces; and a clyster being injected, she was relieved of her complaints. In a fortnight after this visit, I was again called, and found the labour begun . . .

For three or four days she had been subject to slight pains, which returned at long intervals; then they became more frequent, recurring every two hours; and by the time I was called, they had grown stronger, and came faster . . . I prescribed an emollient clyster . . . and then the labour proceeded in a slow and kindly manner . . . I did not confine her to any particular position, but allowed her to walk about, and undergo her pains whether sitting or lying in bed.

[Smellie then recounts the course of the labour in detail.]

I have given a particular detail of this case, in order to make young practitioners acquainted with the common method of acting in natural labours, these being the circumstances that usually occur to a healthy woman in bearing her first child.

5. Onset call, unbooked, with midwife (Smellie, case 186)

In the year 1742, I was called to a patient about the age of forty, in labour of her first child; though I was not permitted to examine, but was obliged to wait in another apartment, in case of accidents. By the midwife's information from time to time, I understood the child advanced very slowly . . . and that the pains, though seldom, were pretty strong.

In this manner labour proceeded for the space of twelve hours, at the expiration of which the midwife told me that . . . she was afraid [the child] was now dead . . . However, the child was delivered soon after she gave me this account, and appeared to have been but a very little time dead . . .

I afterwards learned that the shyness of the patient proceeded from the artful insinuations of the midwife, who terrified her with dreadful accounts of the use of instruments.

6. Onset call, unbooked, without midwife (Smellie, case 123)

I was called to a patient in labour of her first child. The membranes broke in the evening, and she had frequent pains all night; but would not allow me to examine till about eight o'clock next morning . . .

368

She enjoyed no rest all night, the pains grew excessively strong and frequent, and the child's head had not advanced in the least. Being apprehensive from her violent complaints of the abdomen that the uterus would burst by such strong efforts, I prescribed a paregoric draught to allay the violence of the pain and procure sleep . . .

About twelve that night, when the effect of the opiate was worn off, her violent pains recurring, I was allowed to examine again; and finding the head still in the same situation, the draught was repeated. This kept her tolerably easy till eight in the morning, when the pains returning, it was again administered; for the same reason it was repeated at six in the evening and four in the morning. About eight, I was permitted to examine the third time.

At length I was, in the evening, suddenly called from another apartment, and finding the head almost delivered, I had just time to prevent the laceration of the external parts . . . After delivery, her urine was obstructed for three days; and for eight weeks afterwards she lost the power of retention, which, however, returned with her strength. As for the child, it was probably lost by her timorous disposition, in consequence of which she refused all assistance at the latter end of labour.

7. Emergency call, booked (Willughby, Observations, 112–4)

January the 12 Anno 1669 I was entreated, and at that time engaged, by a worthy, good, loving gentleman, to be ready to attend his good wife [Mrs Alestry, margin], and to assist her and her midwife (if need required) in the time of her travail, with the best and utmost of my endeavours.

January the 30th, travail came upon her, about eleven o'clock at night, and so continued with throws and pains all that night and the next day, without any descent of the child. The pains continued all the time in her back only.

At night January the 31 I was sent for, and, upon discourse with her and the midwife, I conceived that the labour would be difficult, and full of danger . . . I entreated her to take a gentle clyster . . . and I stayed all that night in the house with her.

The next morning, Feb 1, I caused a Doctor of Physic to be sent for, and the Divines were entreated their prayers . . . [The Dr and I] concluded to appoint with external applications, to dilate the passages, and also internal medicines, to promote labour. But, through the ill position of her body, these ways nothing at all availing, I was earnestly entreated by the Doctor, from her husband, with several others of her relations, to use the operation of the hand, to try, if possible, the birth might be forced. Whereupon I did attempt it.

. . . I endeavoured to turn the birth, and would willingly have laid her by the infant's feet, but could not possibly effect it . . . [Subsequently,] by her husband, and friends, and the Doctor, with several women, I was much persuaded and entreated by them all to draw the child with instruments, and she was willing to submit, in hopes to be delivered.

But, through the narrow passage of her body, I could not get up my hand over any part of the head to fix the instrument, nor in any other part of it to make a breach . . . So I was necessitated to desist, without any hopes of delivery, not knowing which way to relieve her, and she died . . . And my not delivering her was occasioned by the straitness of the passages, and the unusual ill conformation of the bones . . . She had been afflicted, in her infancy, with the rickets. She had very great, swelled ankle-bones, she went waddling, and her left leg was shorter than the other, and the middle of her back was much inverted, from the hips to the shoulders. She was of a very low . . . stature.

8. *Emergency call, unbooked (Willughby,* Observations, *82–3)*

August 4 1668 Mrs Mary Harley of Walton in the Wolds, being in labour and having suffered much affliction; her husband, with her desire, caused me to be sent for. The child came right, with the head pitched towards the bones. She had, several times, strong forcing throws, but they nothing availed. To move more strongly the expulsive faculty, I gave her several doses of the midwife's powder, acuted with a large quantity of Borax.

Therefore I thought it good to put back the child's head, and to deliver her by the child's feet, the which I did about twelve o'clock that night . . . All of us thought the child had been dead. But . . . the child revived . . .

As for the good woman. She was very well for the space of an hour after her delivery, and for her preservation she gave God thanks and for my care of her she also thanked me.

After this time she fainted . . . But, through God's permission, with cordial spirits she was again restored . . . She was subject to a scouring, which I disliked. I gave her several medicines to prevent it . . . At her friends' desire I stayed with her ten days. I would willingly have stayed longer, for I feared her weakness. But, perceiving that they were willing to let me go, I took leave and departed, after I had left them some directions.

It was reported that she was afflicted with convulsions toward the end of the month, and so died.

II

The ceremony of childbirth
and its interpretation

In this chapter I want to argue that a woman's becoming and
being a mother in seventeenth-century England was suffused
with political meaning; and specifically, that the ritual
management of childbirth reflected the wider context of
gender relations in what has been called 'the world we have
lost'.[1] In order to develop this claim, which represents a shift in
my own thinking about the subject of childbirth, I will describe
what is known of the popular birth-ritual, and then survey some
modern interpretations of that ritual. It will emerge that these
interpretations exhibit a certain gender-specificity: women
historians have been more willing than their male colleagues to
grasp the political meaning of the 'rite of passage' surrounding
childbirth. We will also see that the procedures which made up
the customary ritual – procedures later condemned on medical
grounds – are intelligible as rational responses to the material
demands of seventeenth-century motherhood. In this respect
the management of childbirth fits well with the studies on
breastfeeding conducted by Dorothy McLaren, whose memory
we honour in this volume.

Let us first remind ourselves of the central role which
childbirth played in the lives of seventeenth-century women. In
a sense a woman's whole life revolved around the act of giving
birth. Not that women were continuously engaged in
'breeding': on the contrary, a typical married women could
expect to give birth only four or five times after getting married
in her mid- twenties.[2] Nevertheless, her life as a servant from her
teenage years would have been devoted to accumulating the
'portion' she brought to marriage;[3] and marriage itself was
centred upon the bearing of children. It was materially

disastrous for a woman to become an unmarried mother: if her lover could not be found or 'named', she would experience not only the difficulty of supporting herself and her baby, but also a variety of pressures from the authorities of parish and manor, which might make it difficult for her own parents or relatives to assist her in her plight.[4] The loss of her 'honour' thus amounted to the loss of her means of subsistence. All the more impressive, therefore, that very few unmarried mothers seem to have resorted to infanticide to escape such difficulties.[5] Instead, such mothers either made shift as best they could to bring up their children, or 'dropped' their babies in some well-chosen place where there was a good chance that the children would be found and maintained by others: on the doorstep of a wealthy family (*Tom Jones*), on the church porch (where the parish officers would find the child), or, in London, in the vicinity of Christ's Hospital (as if to remind its seventeenth-century governors that their sixteenth-century predecessors had accepted foundling children).[6] The sometimes large numbers of foundlings, particularly in towns and especially in London, testify not to maternal 'indifference' but rather to the desperate plight of the unmarried mother.[7] Hence the willingness with which women accepted the bonds of marriage. In exchange for legal inequalities, for a vow of obedience, for conferring on the husband an absolute property in her goods, labour, and sexuality, marriage offered the mother-to-be a vital security.[8] For most women, the role of wife was the best prospect which life offered.

Thus, the key context of seventeenth-century childbirth was the material role of women within the social institution of marriage. This fundamental fact is obscured for us as historians by the particular construction of childbirth in our own society. For us, childbirth is a *medical* event, located in the medical space of the hospital, managed by medical personnel, apprehended by medical categories. Correspondingly, its history has been seen as a medical matter. What results is a double historiography: on the one hand, a dense and technical history, rich in obstetric detail and devoid of context; and on the other hand, in works of general or social history (including the history of the family), a symmetrically opposite laconic glance, dismissing childbirth in a page, a paragraph, or a mere sentence.[9] Yet different though they are, these two historiographies nevertheless share a language: the language of evaluation. We speak of childbirth as midwifery/obstetrics, and we do so in terms of welfare, efficiency, progress, improvement; in terms of cruelty, ignorance, superstition, backwardness, inadequate care. Such evaluative formulations rest upon the medical concept of childbirth and help to confirm us in our own attachment to that model.

We can begin to detach ourselves from this medical conception if we note, following Jean Donnison and Audrey Eccles, that the medicalization of childbirth was itself a historical process, a process which effectively began in the eighteenth century.[10] For seventeenth-century mothers, childbirth had many different meanings: it might become a medical event, but was not inherently so; and indeed, male medical access to childbirth was highly restricted and very much on women's terms.[11] Thus, before childbirth belonged to medicine, it belonged to women. As we shall now see, women had constructed a coherent system for the management of childbirth, a system based on their own collective culture and satisfying their own material needs.

The ceremony of childbirth

Childbirth in seventeenth-century England was a social occasion, specifically an occasion for women. In the later months of her pregnancy, the mother-to-be would issue invitations to her female friends, relatives, and neighbours. Her midwife would probably know when the birth was due; as a rule, the midwife lived in the same village as the mother, and she might well have been giving advice on the management of the pregnancy.[12] When the mother's labour pains began, there fell upon her husband (perhaps assisted by a servant or neighbour) the duty of what in East Anglia was known as 'nidgeting': that is, going about from house to house to summon the midwife and the other women to the birth.[13] Within an hour or so, the group of women would be assembled in the mother's bedroom. Meanwhile, the husband would have to make his own arrangements for passing the ensuing hours – perhaps in the parlour downstairs, talking and drinking with a group of male friends, the situation later immortalized as the setting of Sterne's *Tristram Shandy*.[14] We have no equivalent literary account of the scene upstairs, around the mother in labour, but every indication suggests that this was the precise female complement of the all-male parlour scene depicted, and richly exploited, by Sterne. With the company of women assembled, the ceremony of childbirth could begin.

What was happening in these rapid preparations was that the mother was moving into a different social space: away from the world of men (centrally, her husband) and into the world of women. It was here, within the collective culture of women, that birth belonged. If, as sometimes occurred, the labour proceeded so swiftly that the child was born before all the invited women were present, this could occasion anxiety: Ralph Josselin wrote in his diary[15] that at his wife's eighth delivery (14 January 1658), after the arrival of the midwife and nurse, 'her labour came on so strongly and speedily that . . . only 2 or 3 women more in to her, *but* god supplied all' (emphasis added). It would seem, from this and other rare fragments of evidence, that over five women were usually present. The collective character of the ritual was manifest from the onset.

The invited women often included the mother's own mother: for instance, in late October 1678 Jane Josselin rode to London to be with her daughter Mrs Elizabeth Smith at Elizabeth's first delivery.[16] As to the other women, the evidence I have so far compiled (all of it indirect) suggests that these comprised the mother's closest personal friends. Thus, some mothers apparently later felt guilty at not having invited a particular woman – which implies that the invitation was a compliment, that to omit it was a slight, and that the mother made her own choices in the matter.[17] Especially revealing is the word used to describe the invited women, its origins and its wider usage. They were known as 'gossips' and it is from this that we get our word 'gossip' – originally, a male description of what women did when they got together.[18] The word 'gossip' was a corruption of 'god-sib', or 'god-sibling' – that is, someone invited to witness the birth for the subsequent purpose of the child's baptism. It retained a usage with respect to baptism (and here could refer to men as well as to women), but by the seventeenth century had acquired a wider meaning which referred specifically to women. Thus, when Nicholas Culpeper wrote about 'the melancholy of virgins and widows', he recommended as the chief protective against this illness or ill-humour that the women should 'rejoice with her gossips' – that is, that she should take delight in the company of her female friends.[19] Such usage suggests that the collective ritual of childbirth was an integral part of a wider women's culture.

As essential as the gossips was the *midwife*, or, as she was known in some areas, the 'gracewife'.[20] Admittedly, some births did take place without the midwife. On occasion, she might not arrive in time, as when Jane Josselin gave birth in 1649 to her fifth child.[21] Again, some villages were too small to have their own midwives. The churchwardens of Dry Drayton, Cambridgeshire, replied to the visitation articles of 1662 that 'we have none . . . that practice midwifery but charitably; our neighbours as we conceive help one another'.[22] However, it is more likely that births in Dry Drayton were attended by a midwife from a neighbouring village – or perhaps that the churchwardens were simply protecting their own midwife from the considerable expense of taking out a bishop's licence in midwifery. William Harvey, arguing that midwives were too interventionist, wrote in the mid-seventeenth century that 'the business is far better managed among the poor and among those who have become pregnant in secret and are delivered in private without . . . any midwife'.[23] This seems to imply that all 'poor' women managed without midwives. Yet Harvey's friend Percival Willughby, who shared Harvey's attitude to midwives (and may in fact have been the source of this conviction on Harvey's part), had to go to some lengths to find particular stories of delivery without a midwife.[24] Indeed, other evidence shows that even unmarried mothers might well make use of a midwife: thus, in February 1668 Jane Barton, wife of Thomas, of Uttoxeter, was being 'sought for' by the consistory court apparitor, for having acted as midwife to a bastard-bearer.[25] Deliveries without a midwife, then, were rare; the presence of the midwife was the customary norm.

Etymologically, the midwife was the 'with-woman': the woman whose task it was to *be with* the mother during the delivery.[26] In practice, her tasks were more specific than this. The midwife took charge as soon as she arrived, and expected to remain in charge thereafter. It was even possible for a young and inexperienced midwife, probably of no higher than yeoman status, to defy a mother who was a lady – that is, the wife of a gentleman, a member of the ruling class.[27] *Power*, then, was a defining feature of the midwife's office. Correspondingly, the midwife was *paid* for her services, the sum depending greatly on the wealth and social standing of the mother. For the delivery of a pauper woman, the midwife might be paid 2 shillings by the parish officers; for a typical delivery in a town, perhaps 6 shillings; for delivering a gentlewoman or the wife of an aristocrat, a fee measured in guineas; for delivering the Queen, £100.[28] Daniel Fleming of Oxford always paid the midwife 10 shillings, and did so 'at my first going in to see my wife after her delivery'.[29] The midwife's remuneration did not end here, for she would later receive tips from the godparents (and possibly from others as well) at the baptism of the child. If the godfather were as wealthy as Samuel Pepys, the midwife would thereby receive another 10 shillings.[30] Beyond power and payment, the midwife probably had a further defining characteristic: it seems likely that she alone was entrusted with the *right to touch* the mother's labiae, vagina, and cervix. Certainly some midwives did handle the labiae: midwives were enjoined (by male practitioners) to investigate the state of the birth by touching the cervix; and while the gossips could and did handle the child and cut the umbilical cord, I know of no instance of a gossip's touching the mother's 'privities'.[31]

The social space of the birth, then, was a collective female space, constituted on the one hand by the presence of gossips and midwife, and on the other hand by the absence of men. It was however equally important to demarcate the *physical* space of the birth: to confer upon the room a different character, signifying its special function. This was achieved by physically and symbolically enclosing the chamber. Air was excluded by blocking up the keyholes; daylight was shut out by means of heavy curtains; the darkness within was illuminated by means of candles, which were therefore part of the standard requirements for a delivery.[32] Thus reconstituted, the room became the *lying-in chamber*, the physical counterpart of the female social space to which the mother now belonged. The flickering candlelight must have given the darkened room an atmosphere not unlike that of a rather busy and crowded little chapel. Somewhere in this room, if it had a fireplace, or perhaps elsewhere in the house, some of the gossips were preparing the mother's *caudle* – the special drink which was associated with childbirth, consisting of ale or wine, warmed with sugar and spices.[33] The mother drank the caudle to keep up her strength and spirits: no doubt the midwife instructed her on how much of it to drink and when, and the gossips kept themselves busy by maintaining the supply. (Caudle was also used as a nourishing drink for sick patients, sometimes enhanced with the yolk of an egg.[34] That it was very pleasant to taste is indicated by the manner of its use in a certain male ritual, recorded by Anthony Wood at Oxford: each freshman had to make a little speech, 'which if well done, the person that spoke it was to have a cup of caudle; if dull . . . salted drink'.[35])

As the gossips and midwife arrived, as the room and the caudle were being prepared, the birth itself was gradually advancing. However, even the entry of the child into the world was a matter of culture, not simply of Nature. The midwife had her own technique, perhaps acquired by instruction from another midwife whom she had served as a deputy, perhaps learnt by reading in a 'midwife's book': this technique she would generally have used before, and she would be convinced that it worked. Accordingly, midwives seem to have had great confidence in their own chosen methods, and those methods varied enormously.[36] There were some midwives who simply left the birth to Nature, keeping the mother warm in her bed and waiting for the delivery to proceed. Others, by contrast, stretched the labiae to dilate the passage, pulled on the child as soon as some part presented itself, and made such efforts that (in Willughby's words) 'the sweat did run down their faces, in performing of their work'.[37] The midwife might carry about with her a midwife's stool, on which the mother sat for the delivery. However, this custom, common in seventeenth-century London (and known in other localities, such as Derby), seems to have fallen out of favour with midwives by the eighteenth century.[38] There were many alternatives: the mother could lie in bed, either on her back or on her side; she could sit in another woman's lap; or she could kneel on a bolster on the floor, either with her head down (what Willughby called 'a slope, bending posture descending') or with her head supported on the lap of one of the gossips ('a slope, bending posture ascending').[39]

In a small minority of births, such differences of technique were probably consequential. The midwife had other choices to make as well: whether to extract the placenta by hand or to leave its expulsion to Nature; whether to search for a possible second child and, if a twin were found, whether to leave this or attempt to deliver it. There were also a few births (probably about one in thirty) where the delivery became obstructed or (still more rarely) where some accident such as bleeding occurred.[40] In the vast majority of deliveries, however, whatever the midwife's technique, the birth proceeded smoothly and swiftly, producing a living child in a matter of hours. If the child seemed faint or weakly, the midwife and gossips had various methods of reviving it; such expertise was apparently an important part of the midwife's work.[41] Once the child had been delivered, the 'navel-string' tied and cut (perhaps, as we have seen, by one of the gossips), and the child washed, the birth was completed by *swaddling* the child. Though the methods of swaddling (the tightness and length of the bandage, for instance) may well have varied, the fact of swaddling was one of the constant features of the management of birth. Swaddling was apparently either performed by the midwife, or at least supervised by her; once the child was swaddled, it was at last shown to the mother.[42]

With the act of swaddling, the birth was completed, but the ceremony of childbirth was only beginning: for the full childbirth ritual comprised not just the delivery itself, but the ensuing *lying-in*, a process which took some 3 weeks to a month. It was for this, as much as for the birth itself, that the room had been prepared; hence its description as the lying-in chamber. The mother had been 'brought to bed', she had completed her 'crying out'; but she was still 'in the straw', and she would remain in that state for what was called 'the month' or 'her month'.[43] In many respects the mother was now treated as if she were an invalid: above all, she was given a prolonged period of rest, in which her body could recover from the trauma of delivery. However, just as her bodily state was gradually altering, so too she shifted, in the course of 'the month', in social and physical space.

Physically, lying-in appears to have comprised three stages. At first, the mother was confined to her bed, for a period which varied from 3 days to as long as a fortnight. During this time, the room remained darkened; thus, in 1608 we find a lying-in chamber described, over 5 days after the delivery, as a 'dark lodging'.[44] Throughout this time the bed linen was kept unchanged, but the mother's 'privities' were kept clean by poultices or by bathing with herbal decoctions.[45] Then came her 'upsitting', when the bed linen was first changed; after this the mother remained in her room for a further week or 10 days, not confined to bed but still enjoying physical rest. In the third and final stage of lying-in, the mother could move freely about the house, but did not venture out of doors: this stage, too, seems to have lasted for about a week or 10 days. The *timing* of the different stages depended on the mother's perception of her physical strength. Jane Josselin was 'about the house' within 22 days of the birth of her ninth child, but after her previous delivery it had been 38 days before Ralph could record in his diary that she was 'up and down in the house, god's name be praised'.[46] Nevertheless, the *sequence* of stages seems to have been constant, so far as our fragmentary evidence suggests.

Corresponding to these shifts in physical space were a series of movements in social space. At first, only women could visit the mother, probably only in ones or twos, and perhaps only those women who had been present during the delivery itself. The 'upsitting' appears to have been an important social occasion, to judge by the examples under this word in the *Oxford English Dictionary*.[47] There is some evidence to suggest that a women's feast took place a little later, during the second stage of lying-in.[48] On the thirteenth day after one delivery, Ralph Josselin noted in his diary that his wife had been visited by some local women. Similarly, but at greater length, Samuel Sewall in New England wrote on 16 January 1702 (2 weeks after a delivery): 'My wife treats her midwife and women: had a good dinner, boiled pork, beef, fowls; very good roast beef, turkey-pie, tarts. Madam Usher carved; Mrs Hannah Greenleaf; Ellis, Cowell, Wheeler . . . ' The list of names ran on to a total of seventeen women. In addition to such group occasions, there were individual visits, during which the female guest would be invited to drink the mother's caudle. Thus, the celebratory, collective female character of the birth was continued into the process of lying-in. Correspondingly, male access to the mother was restricted: initially, only men who were the mother's own relatives could visit her, though by the final stage of lying-in this restriction was apparently relaxed.[49] It may have been easier for a man to pay a visit if he was accompanied by his wife; thus, Samuel and Elizabeth Pepys visited Betty Michell on 3 May 1667, only 10 days after her delivery.[50]

A further dimension of the lying-in transition concerned the mother's physical work. In the first stages of lying-in, it was impossible for her to perform any household tasks. Accordingly, it was standard practice for a *nurse* to be recruited.[51] A relative or friend would sometimes come to assist about the house and to look after the mother; on other occasions the nurse would be hired. Jane Josselin made use of a hired nurse after at least three of her deliveries; and on a further occasion her friend Mrs Harlakanden stayed with her, lending charitable help. As an alternative, one of the children could serve, as Penelope Mordaunt suggested her young daughter Pen could do: 'I grow very uneasy [she wrote to her husband in 1699] . . . which has made me this day send . . . for blankets and things for the child, lest I should be caught; and if I be, Pen must be nurse for I have none yet.' The hired nurse was known in the nineteenth century as the 'monthly nurse', a phrase which suggests that her services persisted for the full lying-in period. Though the term was first used from about the 1840s, the practice of employing such nurses long predated the word: the adjective 'monthly' was probably added at this time to distinguish this kind of nursing from other types, and especially hospital nursing.[52] However, the nurse might be hired for only 2 to 3 weeks; and in fact mothers were probably working at household tasks in the third stage of lying-in. This was the practical meaning of Jane Josselin's being 'about in the house' or 'up and down in the house' – as her husband Ralph made explicit on a further occasion, when he wrote (on the 29th day) 'my wife busy through mercy in the family'.[53] Yet the mother could not work out of doors; and thus, even with the help of a nurse, the husband had to carry out some of the traditional tasks of the wife. In 1570, William Kirke of Stow-cum-Quy, Cambridgeshire, admitting the charge that he had been absent from church, explained that his wife was 'lying in childbed, and also his children wanted succor, for which he was then compelled to travail in fetching meal from the mill and such other like.' This was regarded as a reasonable excuse: the case against him in the ecclesiastical court was dismissed.[54]

In addition to these progressive changes of bodily state, of physical location, of social contacts, and of involvement in household tasks, the mother's lying-in may have involved a further distinction from normal married life, a distinction in the sphere of *sexual activity*. Here our evidence is, understandably, at its most fragmentary; yet the picture which emerges is a consistent one. According to Jane Sharp's midwifery treatise, husband and wife should not have sexual intercourse until after the completion of lying-in.[55] Correspondingly, the diarist Nicholas Blundell wrote in 1704 that 'my wife's month being now out we lay together'. The only other reference to this matter which I have encountered comes from Ralph Josselin, who wrote on 8 March 1648: 'at night my wife in kindness came and lay in my bed'.

At this stage Jane Josselin was 25 days into her lying-in after the birth of her fourth child. It was another 11 days before Ralph could write in his diary: 'This day . . . my wife went to church with me; the lord be praised for this mercy in raising her up again.' Her other deliveries indicate that Jane's lying-in 'month' always lasted for over 30 days, just as it did on this occasion.[56] Here, then, it would seem that she was sleeping with her husband – whether carnally or chastely hardly matters, I suggest – earlier than the norm. The key point to observe is that Ralph Josselin recorded this as a 'kindness'. Because his wife was still lying-in, still sleeping in a separate bed, his normal conjugal rights were suspended. It is the presence of this norm, rather than the unanswerable question as to how often it was obeyed or transgressed, which is the critical point. If in this respect Josselin and Blundell were representative, then we can take the sexual prohibition outlined by Jane Sharp as genuinely reflecting popular expectations.

The end of the lying-in 'month' was marked by the ecclesiastical rite of *churching*. The churching of women had been practised in the Christian churches, both Catholic and Orthodox, for centuries. In the medieval Catholic Church, its official title was 'purification'; in 1552 the Reformed Church of England changed this to 'the thanksgiving of women after childbirth', and added 'commonly called the churching of women'. [57] In theory, the mother could not go outdoors until she was churched – which poses a curious conundrum: how did she get from her house to the church? The traditional form was that she went in the company of women – her midwife, and a number of others, presumably the same gossips who had attended the birth itself.[58] She also wore a veil: this can be interpreted as a remnant of the Catholic rubric of 'purification', and it was indeed so seen by certain Puritans; but it is also possible to regard the veil simply as a device of symbolic enclosure, suitable for the journey from house to church. Seen in this light, the journey continued the themes of the lying-in itself: physical enclosure on the one hand, and social enclosure in the company of women on the other. (Did her husband accompany her too? The evidence I have compiled on this point is conflicting; perhaps different customs obtained in different localities and at different times.[59])

The ceremony of childbirth

Once inside the church, the woman would kneel 'in some convenient place, as hath been accustomed, or as the Ordinary shall direct'.[60] (Such was the rubric of 1662 – a flexible compromise between the pre-Reformation rule that she should kneel at the church door, and the 1552 specification that this should take place near the holy table. Some parishes had a specific 'uprising seat'/ 'child-bed pew'/ 'childwife pew'/ 'churching pew' for mothers who were about to be churched.[61]) The priest then exhorted her to 'give hearty thanks unto God' for her 'safe deliverance . . . in the great danger of childbirth', and recited to her an appropriate psalm: in the early seventeenth century, Psalm 121 (criticized by the Puritans); from 1662, either Psalm 116 or Psalm 127. There followed a *kyrie eleison*, the Lord's Prayer, three specific versicles and responses, and a concluding short prayer of thanks and supplication. Finally, the woman had to make her 'accustomed offerings' to the priest and to the parish clerk. (What was ' accustomed' varied from parish to parish; at Cheswardine, Shropshire, according to a terrier of 1722, the vicar received 4d and the clerk either 2d or two white loaves.[62]) The churching service probably took about 10 minutes. It could be held at any time, by arrangement with the incumbent, but it seems that women usually came to be churched during divine service. If this was on a Sunday, when communion was held, then as the Book of Common Prayer delicately put it, 'it is convenient that she receive the holy Communion' immediately after the completion of the churching service.

Far more is known about churching than about any other aspect of lying-in, both because the churching ritual brought the mother into contact with a male and record-keeping institution (the Church of England), and because churching was a major focus of the controversy between the ritualist established Church and its Puritan opponents. For these reasons, and because of the stigma of 'purification' which had been attached to the medieval ritual, it is easy to see churching as purely an imposition from without, as a male and clerical burden laid upon mothers. However, the significance of the churching service can only be grasped in the context of the popular ceremony of childbirth as a whole. We shall therefore return to the subject of churching a little later in this chapter, after considering the meaning of the wider ritual.

Before the mother's churching, there had occurred another ecclesiastical rite, the sacrament of *baptism*, which amounted to

the social birth of the child, its entry into the human community
– and which had traditionally taken place within a few days of
the physical birth.[63] In theory, neither the mother nor the
father had any place at baptism; instead, the three godparents
or 'sponsors' took their place. Thus, the fact that baptism was
(supposedly, at least) performed in the church, whereas the
mother was confined to the house, should not have been of any
consequence. However, mothers may have wanted to be present
at the baptism of their newborn children.[64] Some women
delayed the child's baptism until the day of their own
churching. Other families practised private baptism – baptism
at home – and made of this a cheerful family ritual, in which the
mother herself took part. In such a case, baptism was probably
delayed until at least the second stage of lying-in.[65] Pepys offers
us an example: in 1667, at the christening of Betty Michell's
child (12 days after its birth, and 2 days after Samuel and
Elizabeth had paid Betty the visit which was mentioned earlier),
they found the house 'full of his [Mr Michell's] fathers and
mothers and all the kindred, hardly any else, and mighty merry
in this innocent company; and Betty mighty pretty in bed.'
There were in fact certain links between baptism, churching,
and lying-in. Before the Reformation, the newly baptized child
was wrapped in a special 'chrisom cloth': the mother returned
this cloth to the priest as part of her offerings when she was
churched.[66] Again, as we have already seen, the midwife would
receive tips from the sponsors at the baptism – and so too would
the nurse. Indeed, W. E. Tate claimed that some baptismal fonts
had special 'midwives' seats' adjoining them.[67] Thus, the
customs surrounding baptism deserve to be considered in
relation to lying-in and churching. (This is one of many reasons
for wishing that we possessed a modern scholarly study of the
history of baptism in early-modern England.)

I have been implying that the ceremony of childbirth was
followed by women of all social classes. Yet most of the evidence
I have been citing pertains to mothers of high social status – the
wives of the aristocracy, the gentry, and what can be called the
semi-gentry.[68] Did mothers lower down the social scale behave
in the same way? Living as they did in one- or two-roomed
cottages they cannot have used a separate room; they may well
have been unable to afford the curtains, perhaps the candles,
and possibly the paid nurse. Yet there were many possibilities
for adaptation and improvisation. The 'month' could be

shortened in duration; in place of a separate room the bed itself could serve as the lying-in space; the mother could lie in at the house of a more wealthy relative (perhaps her own mother) or friend.[69] Each of these practices is documented; and in fact there is every reason to think that the ceremony of childbirth was effectively universal amongst married mothers. One oblique indication of this is the fact that wealthy mothers made an expensive display of their lying-in chamber: the mere fact of lying-in did not demonstrate their social status, and that status accordingly had to be shown by other means.[70] Again, we shall subsequently see that churching was observed by almost all mothers, and that the interval between birth and churching was generally about 4 weeks. The 'monthly nurses' of the nineteenth century worked amongst the poor as well as the rich.[71] Glimpses of the lives of the poor in the seventeenth and eighteenth centuries are rare indeed, but we know that Mary Toft – undoubtedly extremely poor – had a nurse during her lying-in before her famous superfetation of rabbits in 1726. (Mary was, incidentally, churched a fortnight after her initial delivery, a miscarriage.[72]) The parish overseers of the poor could subsidize the drinking associated with childbirth, supplying 'a pint of liquor for Anne Barne's lying-in'.[73] For the penurious 1790s, we have more systematic evidence in the form of agricultural labourers' budgets collected by middle-class observers sympathetic to the plight of the poor. The Anglican minister David Davies reckoned the expenses of lying-in at 20 shillings, assumed that this happened once in 2 years, and so concluded that 10 shillings per year was required. Out of a total family budget of £7 per year this was a very large sum.[74] The lying-in expenses included the midwife's fee, 'attendance of a nurse for a few days', 'a bottle of gin or brandy always had upon this occasion', and 'half a bushel of malt brewed, and hops'. The fact that these expenses were standard amongst the poorest families in a time of extreme hardship strongly suggests that the lying-in ritual was universally observed.[75]

What did *men* make of this exclusively female ritual? As usual, we have only fragmentary indications. Diarists referred rather casually and patchily to birth and lying-in. Thus, Ralph Josselin, perhaps the most meticulous recorder of such mundane matters, mentioned some of the stages of lying-in after some of his wife's ten deliveries, but never wrote down the whole story for any single confinement, only ever identified one of the gossips by name, never named the midwife or recorded her fee (unlike his contemporary Daniel Fleming) – and never made any comment on the customs of lying-in.[76] Medical writers of the seventeenth century were similarly laconic; they seem in general to have accepted and endorsed the practices of women. A case in point is Percival Willughby.[77] He believed that the chamber should be dark and warm: '[As] for the labouring woman's chamber, let it be made dark, having a glimmering light, or candle-light, placed partly behind the woman, or on one side, and a moderate warming fire in it.' The numbers of women, he went on, should not be excessive: 'and let it not be filled with much company, or many women; five or six women assisting will be sufficient.' Thus, Willughby simply assumed that the birth would be a collective female affair; male advice could aspire only to regulating the numbers. Similarly, though he criticized midwives at great length and regarded the midwife's practical tasks as slight, he believed that midwives were the appropriate practitioners to manage childbirth, and disapproved of 'men-midwives' – that is, of men replacing the female midwife. As for the timing of 'upsitting', Willughby agreed with James Wolveridge that this should be *later* than the customary 3 or 4 days after birth.[78] Other matters such as caudle, swaddling, the further stages of lying-in, or the duration of the whole process, Willughby did not discuss at all. Here (and in other medical treatises of the period) we seem to find an attitude of passive acceptance.[79]

However, there are also some signs of male hostility. The Puritans of the early seventeenth century criticized churching along with other ecclesiastical ceremonies: as we shall see a little later, some male Puritan attacks on churching extended to the whole process of lying-in. After the Restoration, we find William Sermon constructing the fantasy that lying-in was not observed by American wives, and suggesting that English women should similarly return to their wifely duties immediately after birth.[80] *The Woman's Advocate* of 1683 attributes to a husband some aversion to women's sociability during lying-in, and then defends the women in the following terms:

> for gossips to meet . . . at a lying-in, and not to talk, you may as well dam up the arches of London Bridge, as stop their mouths at such a time. 'Tis a time of freedom, when women . . . have a privilege to talk petty treason.[81]

The ceremony of childbirth

In the eighteenth century, as a result of the new 'man-midwifery', male medical practitioners began to criticize many aspects of the ceremony of childbirth: swaddling, the enclosed room, eventually even the presence of gossips.[82] We know that these criticisms were supported by some husbands; nevertheless much of the childbirth ritual remained intact well into the nineteenth century. William Cobbett, in his *Advice to Young Men* of 1830, implied that young husbands resented the duty of having to fetch gossips and midwife at the onset of labour. Characteristically, Cobbett went on to say that they should learn to accept that duty.[83] Here we have a few hints that men's acceptance of the ritual practices of women could be tinged with a certain resentment. It is perhaps significant that these criticisms tended to be voiced indirectly. Cobbett, writing in 1830, followed the same convention as the anonymous male author of *The Woman's Advocate* a century and a half before him: attributing to husbands a critical attitude, and then arguing against that attitude. It is as if the ceremony of childbirth were so well established in custom as to be almost beyond the reach of explicit criticism in print.

Both of these male responses – passive acceptance and muffled resentment – serve to underline the universality and hegemony of the ritual. Herein lies a significant irony for the historian: for these responses, while attesting to the normative power of the ceremony of childbirth, also had the effect that only scattered and fragmentary documentary traces were left. There is no single document, so far as I am aware, which describes the process in full: a reconstruction such as I have attempted here has to be based on assembling disparate details from a wide range of sources. And it is striking that even texts relatively rich in such details – such as Josselin's diary and Willughby's midwifery treatise – omit many aspects of the ritual. Thus, our sources systematically conceal from us the central importance of the ceremony of childbirth in the lives of seventeenth-century women.

The meaning of the ritual

The early-modern ceremony of childbirth followed a coherent and consistent structure: it comprised an ordered pattern of actions governed by a discernible set of rules. But where did

these rules arise? How had the ritual come into being, and why
was it maintained? What were its origins, and what was its
meaning? In turning to these questions, we enter a territory in
which the historian has almost no documentary evidence; in
which his or her interpretations therefore stand naked. When it
was a matter of reconstructing the ritual (the task of the
previous section), our evidence was fragmentary; here at the
level of investigating its meaning, we pass from fragments to
documentary silence. Though the documents are silent,
however, the historian will speak; and in fact, three distinct
interpretations of the ceremony of childbirth can be found in
the literature.

One interpretation (to which I formerly adhered) assimilates
this specific ritual to the general pattern of 'rites of passage',
classically delineated by Arnold van Gennep.[84] According to this
reading, certain critical life-events – such as birth, puberty,
death – are always, in every society, surrounded by ritual
procedures. The existence of the ritual is unsurprising: it
stemmed simply from 'ancient folk tradition'.[85] It was necessary
for such an 'event of nature' to be 'immersed in culture', since
this 'made the birth a social and human act'.[86] Thus, the
meaning of the various specific activities was that these
comprised the necessary stages of rites of passage in general. All
such rites, according to van Gennep, entailed three stages:
separation, transition, reincorporation. The early-modern
ceremony of childbirth conformed to this pattern, with the
demarcation of the lying-in room achieving separation, the
'month' of isolation accomplishing transition, and the final
churching ceremony making for reincorporation. Thus, this
specific historical ritual bears out van Gennep's
anthropological argument, even though van Gennep himself
had not applied that argument in this particular direction.

A second interpretation (that of Keith Thomas) offers a
more specific reading. Here the focus is upon popular attitudes:
the customs of lying-in and churching, it is argued, flowed from
these attitudes, so that the attitudes themselves can in turn be
read off from the popular customs. Specifically, the meaning of
lying-in and churching was that these reflected concepts of
women's inferiority and impurity:[87]

> medieval churchmen had . . . devoted a good deal of
> energy to refuting such popular superstitions as the belief

that it was improper for the mother to emerge from her house ... before she had been purified ... The church ... was reluctant to countenance any prescribed interval after birth before [churching] could take place ... But *for people at large churching was indubitably a ritual of purification closely linked to its Jewish predecessor* (emphasis added).

Thus, lying-in satisfied a popular demand for the ritual puri-fication of women after childbirth. The 'origin' of the ritual of churching was 'the primitive view of woman as shameful and unclean'. This in turn was an aspect of a seventeenth-century 'universal belief in [women's] inferior capacity', a belief which determined the subordinate place of women in the social order. Consequently, Puritans' criticisms of the churching ritual 'had done something to raise women's status'.[88]

The weakness of these two interpretations is that they have little or no explanatory force. We may grant, for the sake of argument, that a 'rite of passage' was involved; but why did the rite take the particular form it did? Alternatively, we may accept that a popular belief in women's 'impurity' was at work; but this will not explain the complex structure of customs outlined in the previous section. Above all, neither of these interpretations can come to grips with the two central facts about the ceremony of childbirth – namely, the fact that this ritual was exclusively *female* and the fact that it was *collective*. These basic features of the ritual have no significance within the 'rites of passage' framework; and they can be taken to contradict the 'impurity' reading, since the women who thronged around the mother during and after the delivery did not behave as if *they* felt her to be impure. Thus, while Thomas and I have both managed to bring to light some valuable information about the management of childbirth, the particular readings which we have given to this material do not stand up to critical assessment.

The third interpretation, which has a very different thrust, was offered by Natalie Zemon Davis in the course of her essay 'Women on top'.[89] Davis's material came chiefly from continental Europe in the early-modern period, but much of her argument applies also to England, including her brief and telling observations on the ritual of childbirth. The essay as a whole was concerned with a popular tradition, displayed in stories, paintings, and carnivals, in which women were depicted in roles of dominance over men. Exploring the complex meanings and uses of this imagery, Davis asked what the 'woman-on-top' image might have meant to 'the majority of unexceptional women living within their families'. She pointed out that the subjection of wives to husbands, prescribed within marriage, was not always obeyed, and speculated that 'the ambiguous woman-on-top of the world of play made the unruly option a more conceivable one within the family'. And in the course of this argument, Davis wrote: 'In actual marriage, subjection . . . might be reversed temporarily during the lying-in period, when the new mother could boss her husband around with impunity.' In a note to this passage, Davis acknowledged the contribution to this argument of three other scholars, all women, and added: 'Italian birth-salvers (that is, trays used to bring women drinks during labour and the lying-in) dating from the fifteenth and sixteenth centuries were decorated with classical and Biblical scenes showing women dominating men.'

Davis was suggesting, then, that the process of lying-in accomplished a reversal of the normal power-relations between wife and husband; that the mother's lying-in month was indeed 'her month'; that the ceremony of childbirth placed the woman 'on top' amidst *all* families. Here we have a very different interpretation from the two readings of the ritual discussed above. Those readings portrayed women as essentially obedient to the ritual; Davis's reading depicts the ritual itself as reflecting the interests of women. As I shall now argue, it is this interpretation which offers the key to the meaning of the ceremony of childbirth.

Since the ceremony of childbirth withdrew the mother from the world of men, and placed her within the world of women, its significance will emerge only if we attend to the general context of relations between the sexes in seventeenth-century England. Those relations were patriarchal: that is, men had power over women. A central aspect of male power, one which operated in daily life and which was also used as a significant ideological resource,[90] was the authority of the husband over the wife. As we saw earlier, marriage was a contract of inequality: the wife vowed to 'obey and serve' her husband.[91] More specifically, the common law conferred on the husband an absolute property in the wife's worldly goods; in her physical labour and its fruits; and last but not least, in her sexuality.[92] Thus, if conjugal relationships went to law – as they sometimes did – the husband's ownership was endorsed and his power over his wife reinforced. This structural inequality of conjugal life did not preclude loving relationships between husband and wife, any more than the authority of parents over children today precludes love between the generations within the family. On the contrary, love and power were closely related, a fact made explicit in images of God: God *was* both Power and Love – that is, power and love attained a relationship of identity at the apex of the natural order. The male ideal of conjugal relations involved female submission to male power, enabling that power to be wielded with gentleness and consideration. Thus, in the event of a personal contest between husband and wife, the husband would behave as Samuel Pepys did on such an occasion: he first 'desired' Elizabeth, 'and then commanded her', to do his bidding.[93] Husbands had a rich range of resources to deploy: their very abstention from the iron fist of patriarchy was itself an instrument of power, a kindness which should command acceptance of their wishes.[94]

The effect of the lying-in month was to withdraw from the husband two of the customary fruits of marriage: his wife's physical labour and her sexual services. From the woman's point of view this made possible a period of rest and recovery. Her physical labour, both inside and outside the house, was replaced by that of the monthly nurse: the payment made to the nurse was effectively a subsidy to the wife on the part of the husband. Thus, the ceremony of childbirth inverted the normal pattern of conjugal relations: the wife's bodily energies and sexuality now, for the space of 'the month', belonged to her; what marriage had taken away from her, the ceremony of childbirth temporarily restored. This makes intelligible the fact that the ritual was a collective female event. The presence of other women may have served to police the lying-in – to ensure that the husband respected the norms. More generally, the immersion of the mother in a female collectivity elegantly inverted the central feature of patriarchy, namely its basis in individual male property.

All this goes to support Davis's interpretation of the ceremony of childbirth. The strength of that interpretation is that it enables us to situate the management of childbirth within the context of women's actual lives: lives of hard physical labour, performed under a rubric of love and an ethos of service, on behalf of an individual male master, the husband.

The ceremony of childbirth

The ritual of childbirth was constructed and maintained by women *because it was in the interests of women*; and it represented a successful form of women's *resistance* to patriarchal authority.

The churching of women

If the main lines of the ceremony of childbirth were constructed by women in this way, what are we to make of the ecclesiastical ritual which marked the completion of lying-in – the occasional service of churching?: for the churching service has every appearance of having emanated from the world of men. It was an ecclesiastical ceremony; it had been described in the Middle Ages as a ritual of 'purification'; after the English Reformation, it still involved various features which in the eyes of the Puritans bore the same stigma of defilement-by-birth; it required the mother to pay money to the priest and to the parish clerk.[95] At first glance, then, churching seems an alien and male imposition on what was otherwise a female ritual. However, a more careful investigation suggests the very opposite, as we shall now see.

Perhaps the first thing to note about churching is that this was a highly *popular* service. Even in strongly Puritan London parishes, it was followed by over 90 per cent of mothers in the early seventeenth century, probably about 4 weeks after the birth.[96] Such precise evidence is difficult to find for the eighteenth century, but we know that it was specifically the need for churchings and baptisms which was given as the reason for establishing a sub-parochial chapel at Brentwood hamlet in 1715.[97] Again, in the nineteenth century, when the irreligion of the working class was the central lament of the Anglican Church, churching apparently remained just as popular as ever.[98] As late as the 1950s, it was still being practised by forty-one out of forty-five married women in Bethnal Green, interviewed by Michael Young and Peter Willmott.[99] To bring the picture almost up to the present, however anecdotally, let me report two stories.[100] One came from a large British hospital in the late 1970s; here an Anglican minister visited the maternity ward, offering to church the mothers *in situ*, and all the women but one took up his offer. (Not all these women were Anglicans.) The second anecdote comes from a married woman friend of mine who hails from an Anglican family. She is not a church-goer, and when she had her two children (in the 1970s) she was not churched. However, after the second delivery she had a particular experience which, with hindsight, she regards as relevant to the question of churching. For perhaps 5 weeks after the birth, she felt emotionally confused – not 'postnatally depressed', simply overwhelmed by the range and intensity of the feelings she was experiencing. Once she had recovered her equilibrium, she had a strong desire *to go and give thanks to somebody for her recovery.* Interestingly, she did not at the time connect this with churching, even though she had been brought up an Anglican and had even attended at least one churching. Instead, she simply experienced this as a spontaneous and rather inchoate wish, one which she did not know how to satisfy and therefore never did satisfy.

I have already introduced, surreptitiously, a second point: that if churching was (and perhaps still is) popular, its popularity was specifically amongst *women.* This can be illustrated by what Young and Willmott reported from Bethnal Green.[101] One woman's explanation (amongst several) will suffice as an example: '*It's the Mums.* It's not that I actually believe in it, but I'd get an uneasy feeling if I didn't do it. You don't like to break tradition.' (emphasis added) The attitude of husbands, by contrast, was hostile. Mr Jeffreys sneered (after his wife had said, 'It's your religion, isn't it? I mean you've got to do it') – 'Your Mum's done it – you do it. They're all the same.' We are beginning to glimpse that attitudes to churching are gendered; and so it was in the late sixteenth century. As is well known, churching was vigorously opposed by the Puritans; and in the case of Henry Barrow, his denunciation of churching extended to an ironic critique of the whole lying-in process:[102]

After they have been safely delivered of childbirth, and have lain in, and been shut up, their month of days accomplished; then are they to repair to church and to kneel down in some place nigh to the communion table (not to speak how she cometh wimpled and muffled, accompanied with her wives, and dare not look upon the sun nor sky . . .) unto whom (thus placed in the church) comes Sir Priest . . . [etc.] . . . And then, she having offered her accustomed offerings unto him for his labour, God speed her well, she is a woman on foot again, as holy as ever she was; she may now put off her veiling kerchief, and

50

The ceremony of childbirth

look her husband and neighbours in the face again . . .
What can be a more apish imitation, or rather a more
reviving of the Jewish purification than this?

Such were the words of a Puritan *man*. Puritan women, on the
other hand seem to have satirized the ecclesiastical ritual as to
its form, while adhering to the lying-in period and using the act
of coming to church as a means of publicly announcing its
completion. Thus, in 1578 Katherine Whithed, according to the
churchwardens of Danbury,[103]

> came into the church, with a kerchief over her head, to
> give thanks for her childbearing, at the sermon time,
> [and] whilst [the minister] was at the sermon, she with a
> loud voice demanded of him if he were ready to do his
> duty she was ready to do hers; whereby she troubled him
> in his sermon and caused the people to make a laughter.

Similarly, in 1597 Jane Minors of Barking not only kept her
child unbaptized for a month after birth, but also[104]

> very unwomanlike, came to be churched at the end of the
> said month, together with her child to be baptised, and
> feasted at a tavern 4 or 5 hours in the forenoon; and [in
> the] afternoon came to the church . . . to be seen . . .
> [and] went out of the church, unchurched, unto the
> tavern again. And when she was spoken unto by the clerk
> to return to church again and to give God thanks after her
> delivery, she answered it was a ceremony.

Or again Mrs Pinson of Wolverhampton, at some point in the
1630s, went with her husband[105]

> and her midwife, and other women . . . to be churched,
> but being demanded by the priest why she did not wear a
> veil, she answered she would not; and being told by the
> priest that he was commanded by the ordinary not to
> church any but such as came thither reverently and lowly
> in their veils, she in the church, after prayers ended,
> scornfully pulled off her hat and put a table napkin on her
> head, and put on her hat again, and so departed from the
> church.

90

The ceremony of childbirth

In two of these three cases (the first and third), the husband was described as being involved in the wife's defiance; in the case of Jane Minors, the husband was not mentioned. What is common to all these cases is that the women in question *wanted to be churched*; and where there are further details, we find that the lying-in month had been observed and that the midwife and other women attended the mother on the way to the church.

The key to Puritan responses, I suggest, is provided by the defiant words of Richard Morley of Grantham, who in February 1589 was reported as saying that[106] 'the churching of women is a beggarly ceremony, and that all those which do use it do in some respect forsake Christ, and *if he could have persuaded his wife she should never have given thanks*' (emphasis added).

All the available evidence in fact suggests that while both men and women amongst the Puritans criticized the *form* of churching, it was men and men only who criticized the *fact* of it. We have here, couched in different language and centring on different issues, the same gender-division of responses that appeared, over three centuries later, in Bethnal Green. As far as the Puritans go, we might say that one *man's* 'purification' was another *woman's* popular ritual. Here lies a crucial point: that popular attitudes to an ecclesiastical ritual were and are by no means a simple matter.[107] We certainly cannot read off women's attitudes to churching from male denunciations of the practice, nor from the words of the ceremony itself. It was perfectly possible for a woman to regard the ecclesiastical rite as a piece of meaningless nonsense, while also wanting very badly to go through that rite. After all, the officiating clergyman was only one of the people present: the church ritual involved the presence of the congregation, and it may well have been this which mattered.[108] In short, observance of churching could mean many different things. The ritual for the mother herself was what she and her gossips made of it.

However, this point can be pressed a little further. It is not just that women accepted the churching ritual and made of it what they wished; more than this, there were many aspects of that ritual which in fact had probably been created by women in the first place. So far as can be ascertained, the various surrounding customs were precisely *customs*; they derived their force not from canon law but from popular usage. It was thus that the woman was accompanied by her 'wives', including the midwife; thus that the period of a month was followed; it may

The ceremony of childbirth

have been for this reason that an 'uprising seat' was placed in some churches; even the veil itself was possibly of popular rather than ecclesiastical origin.[109] (The question of the veil came to law in 'Shipden's case' of 1622: it was decreed that the wearing of the veil was compulsory, but only on the grounds 'that it was the ancient usage of the church of England'.[110]) Seen through male Puritan eyes, these various trappings were all Popish or Jewish. However, the eye which sees in order to denounce is no key to the origins. In particular, the regular presence in the churching procession of the company of women links the ecclesiastical ritual firmly with the lay ceremony of childbirth – hence the popularity of churching. Women liked it because it was a women's ritual.

Let us take one final step further down this interpretative road, and ask a question: how and why did churching enter the rites of the Christian Church in the first place? Works of Church history answer this chiefly by reference to the fact that Jesus's mother was purified (a nice paradox, this) after his birth. Textual warrant does not however constitute efficient cause; and churching was in fact introduced into medieval Christian practice, without any apparent apostolic or patristic basis. Why was it introduced at all, and indeed when was it introduced? These questions require an expert answer, which I cannot attempt. However, the suggestion can be made, for the medievalists to refine or refute, that the purification of women was an ecclesiastical response to some *prior popular ritual*. If, as seems plausible, the ritual of lying-in was practised not just in England but all over Europe, and dates from the Middle Ages or earlier, then there is every reason to suppose that the lying-in interval was concluded by some collective rite, some act of 'reincorporation' (in the terminology of van Gennep). It would not be surprising to find the Church responding to this by offering its own ritual, Christian instead of pagan, and absorbing some elements of the pagan ritual in the process. Moreover, we should expect such a process to have been fraught with struggle and contest; such contest might well produce documentation; and thus it may become possible to test this hypothesis. Certainly, the origins of churching would be well worth investigating, in view of its long-lived later popularity amongst the women of England.

Churching enjoyed this popularity, I suggest, because it legitimated the wider ceremony of childbirth. The concept of the lying-in month achieved an elegant fusion between Biblical precedent (the Jewish ritual of purification) and the material needs of women (for rest and recovery after childbirth). That fusion broke down, of course, in the Reformation, and the consequent struggles over churching enable us to see what women's priorities were: they wanted churching, but not the veil; lying- in, but not purification. Once we focus in this way on the gender specificity of Puritan responses to churching, it becomes clear that the history of churching provides strong support for Natalie Zemon Davis's interpretation of lying-in: that the ceremony of childbirth placed 'the woman on top'.

Conclusion

It is likely that not only the general structure of the childbirth ritual, but also its specific details, will turn out to be intelligible in terms of the material lives of women. If we view the procedures of the ritual through modern medical concepts, those procedures are likely to appear irrational and even dangerous; thus, bed-rest for a week is now supposed to be attended with risks to the mother's health. Once situated in the context of women's lives, however, those same procedures will emerge in a very different light. One case in point is the swaddling of the child. Swaddling is precisely a child-care practice which women would favour, for it does no harm to children but confers an immense benefit upon mothers – since its central effect is to send the child to sleep. Moreover, swaddling is much more acceptable to children if they have been accustomed to it from the moment of birth.[111] This is exactly the way in which women actually implemented swaddling in early-modern England. Here we see that an immense rationality underlay swaddling, a rationality which inhered in the needs of *both* the mother *and* the child. Along these lines, I suggest, we may later be able to explain the other features of the ceremony of childbirth – just as François Loux has disclosed the rationality of many French peasant customs of child-care.[112] Those customs, Loux has found, were denounced as 'irrational' by nineteenth-century observers who came from a different social milieu and deployed different criteria of welfare. In fact, it is not a question of the rational versus the irrational; rather, it is a question of *whose* rationality will prevail.

Such is the burden of Loux's findings; and I suggest that the same will apply to all the details of the ceremony of childbirth when these have been adequately reconstructed and contextualized. The darkened room, the caudle, the presiding midwife, the timing of 'upsitting' and of the subsequent stages of lying-in – all these invite explanation in terms of the material needs of women.

It would be valuable to compare the early-modern English ceremony of childbirth with the childbirth rituals of other societies, and to subject these, too, to a political reading. There are some indications of national differences with early-modern Europe; and there is a large and open question as to how the early-modern English ritual was transformed, by the mid-twentieth century, into the hospitalized ritual of today. So far as I am aware, very little research has been undertaken in this area by historians.[113] The discipline which has focused on ritual in great detail is of course anthropology; and from this quarter there derives some qualified and indirect support for the reading of ritual I have developed in this chapter. In a recent study, Karen and Jeffery Paige have interpreted 'reproductive rituals' as 'a continuation of politics by another means'.[114] On their analysis, every such ritual results from an underlying conflict, and is a way of expressing that conflict while also containing it within manageable bounds. In interpreting ritual as the result of political conflict, this approach is similar to the interpretation offered here. However, the meaning assigned to politics differs radically between the present reading of early-modern English childbirth, on the one hand, and the Paiges' comparative analysis of ethnographic material on the other. On their reading, reproductive politics reduces to competition *between men* over the limited available 'resources' of women and children. Here all agency is seen as residing in men; women are passive, the objects and not the subjects of reproductive rituals. In the words of Paige and Paige,[115] 'men are the most important political actors in preindustrial societies'. Correspondingly, the underlying conflicts are individual ones: they partake of the social only in so far as this individuation is universal. Preindustrial 'man' thus acquires a somewhat Benthamite character. By contrast, taking my lead from Natalie Zemon Davis, I have interpreted the politics of ritual as a matter of contest *between the sexes*, stressing the active agency of women. As a result, the underlying conflict appears as a social one, with the conjugal power of the individual husband representing simply the particular instantiation of a set of structural relations. No doubt there is much room here for further exploration. On the one hand, the interpretation of tribal 'reproductive rituals' needs to take account of the agency of women. On the other hand, much could doubtless be learnt about historical ritual by placing this in a comparative setting, drawing upon the very rich ethnographic literature which Paige and Paige have surveyed and analysed.

The historiographic context of the present argument is of course the increasing impact on early-modern history of women scholars, who are bringing into focus a variety of themes which male historians have tended to neglect, to marginalize, or to misunderstand. Many studies in this tradition have influenced this essay. Valerie Fildes and the late Dorothy McLaren, for instance, have demonstrated both the coherence and the demographic impact of the activities of women as mothers in the past.[116] Again, Jean Donnison and Audrey Eccles have enabled us to see the historical importance of midwives, opening up a different perspective from that of traditional medical history.[117] Natalie Zemon Davis and her colleagues initiated the interpretation of lying-in as resistance. Several women scholars have produced important critiques of the 'history-of-the-family' tradition.[118] More generally, Linda Gordon and Sally Alexander have called for a historiography of gender-*relations*, and for a focus upon women as active agents, as subjects rather than passive objects of historical processes.[119] This opens up a very large agenda for historians of the early-modern period. It is true that for this period, direct documentation of the lives of women is relatively sparse and diffuse. Nevertheless, as Sara Mendelson and Patricia Crawford have demonstrated, there is available a considerable corpus of both manuscript and printed material from the pens of seventeenth-century women: and this testimony is only beginning to be exploited.[120] Moreover, the indirect imprint of women can be found across a vast range of historical documents,[121] particularly if we attend to the *genesis* of our sources,[122] remembering in doing so that relations of gender were constitutive of the social order.

These considerations must prompt us to ask whether women's resistance to patriarchal power, so effectively

56

The ceremony of childbirth

organized in the ceremony of childbirth, was manifested in other ways and in other areas. In fact there is every reason to believe that this resistance was widespread in early-modern England; that women mounted a *counter-power* against male control, long before the advent of an organized feminist movement and literature. Patriarchy evolved in a series of *contests*: there were innumerable individual struggles like those of Elizabeth Pepys, and collective struggles like those of the London women petitioners of the 1640s and 1650s.[123] The 'woman on top' tradition, demonstrated by Davis, not only nourished but also reflected these struggles. This phenomenon of women's resistance to patriarchal power is immensely important in at least two ways: first, as a striking instance of women's agency; second, because this resistance and the responses it provoked effect for us a real-life analytical dissection of patriarchal power, permitting us to investigate the structuring of gender relations.[124] Intense interest therefore attaches to the project of systematically reconstructing the struggles of women against familial and civic forms of male power. Historians are only beginning to recapture these episodes: as yet it is too early to attempt either a typology of their occasions, or a chronological analysis of the unfolding of patriarchy within the early-modern period. Nevertheless two basic points are already clear. First, the struggles of women were far more effective when collective support could be mobilized. The individual wife could seldom triumph over her husband, since the husband held the final sanction of the law; but collective action could wrest back for women certain rights and victories. Second, such collective action could often transcend divisions of social class and of marital status. The propertied widow could make common cause with married women; married women could support the unmarried bastard-bearer; respectable wives and poor women could join together in political action.[125]

What made such solidarity possible was the fact that women of many different stations in life shared certain central experiences, such as the pains of childbearing, the inequality of marriage, or at least the expectation or memory of these. But what gave force to these shared experiences was something else: a collective culture of women. A network of so-called 'gossip' bound together the women of each locality in a web of relationships which partly mirrored the male hierarchy (squire,

96

tenant farmer, husbandman, landless labourer), yet partly cut across that hierarchy.[126] Wider networks, made possible by the continual migration which characterized English populations, conferred a national character upon many aspects of this culture. Gender roles were socially constructed, and the collective culture of women played an important part in this process.[127] Until the mid-eighteenth century, this culture was probably more important, for most women, than the culture of social class; and it was to this shared women's culture that the ceremony of childbirth belonged.

Indeed, it is tempting to suggest that the childbirth ritual not only reflected women's general culture, but also played an important part in the construction and maintenance of that culture. Childbirth was sufficiently frequent, and lying-in sufficiently protracted, that a typical English village would have had at least one mother 'in the straw' at most times of the year. Thus, childbirth provided frequent and more or less continuous opportunities for women to get together; and these opportunities were probably unique in the separateness from men which they made possible. Perhaps, then, the expanding meanings of 'gossip' – childbirth witness, female friend, getting together of women, hostility to men – reflect an underlying social reality, a range of women's activities in which childbirth was as central in real life as it seems to have been in the history of this word. If so, we may wonder whether the role of midwives was restricted to childbirth and associated healing activities. Perhaps the midwife's authority in childbirth was but one aspect of some wider role she played in maintaining the collective culture of women.[128] At all events, these possibilities offer us a rich and interesting field for further investigation.

Acknowledgements

The research for this chapter has been supported by the generosity of the Wellcome Trust. The staff of Cambridge University Library and of the Lichfield Joint Record Office have extended invaluable facilities. Linda Pollock has very kindly made available a wealth of material from family papers – far more than I have had space to cite here. For detailed advice I wish to thank Anna Abulafia, Timothy Ashplant, Jeremy Boulton, David Cressy, Andrew Cunningham, Anna Davin,

Valerie Fildes, John Henderson, Ann Hess, Gill Hudson, Henry Krips, Valerie Krips, Philippa Levine, Susan Magarey, Jane Morgan, John Morrill, Roy Porter, Wilf Prest, Miri Rubin, Simon Schaffer, Shulamith Shahar, Hendrik van der Weef, and Mike Woodhouse, Finally, I am particularly grateful to Rosalind Bayham and to Hugh McLeod for their indispensable help in the development of the argument.

Notes

1. P. Laslett, *The World We Have Lost* (London, 1965); *The World We Have Lost Further Explored* (London, 1983). Throughout this chapter, dates are given according to New Style year, and spelling and punctuation are modernized.

2. C. Wilson, 'The proximate determinants of marital fertility in England 1600–1799', in L. Bonfield, R. M. Smith, and K. Wrightson (eds), *The World We Have Gained: Histories of Population and Social Structure* (Oxford, 1986), 203–30.

3. R. A. Houlbrooke, *The English Family 1450–1700* (London, 1984), 72–3, 83–4; A. Macfarlane, *Marriage and Love in England: Modes of Reproduction 1300–1840* (Oxford, 1986), 267–8, 276–7.

4. M. Chaytor, 'Household and kinship: Ryton in the 16th and 17th centuries', *Hist. Workshop J.*, 10 (1980), 25–60, p. 48; K. Wrightson, 'The nadir of English illegitimacy in the seventeenth century', in P. Laslett, K. Oosterveen, and R. M. Smith (eds), *Bastardy and Its Comparative History*, (London, 1980), 176–91, p. 179.

5. R. W. Malcolmson, 'Infanticide in the eighteenth century', in J. S. Cockburn (ed.), *Crime in England, 1550–1800* (London, 1977), 187–209.

6. H. Fielding, *The History of Tom Jones, a Foundling* (London, 1749); W. E. Tate, *The Parish Chest: A Study of the Records of Parochial Administration in England* (Cambridge, 1969), 61–2; R. K. McClure, *Coram's Children: The London Foundling Hospital in the Eighteenth Century* (New Haven, 1981), 8–9.

7. See A. Wilson 'Illegitimacy and its implications in mid-eighteenth century London: the evidence of the Foundling Hospital', *Cont. & Change*, 4 (1989), 103–64.

8. J. H. Baker, *An Introduction to English Legal History* (2nd edn, London, 1979), 391–407. For an overview of women's position, see P. Crawford, 'From the woman's view: pre-industrial England, 1500–1750', in Crawford (ed.), *Exploring Women's Past* (2nd edn, Sydney, 1984), 49–85.

9. Examples of the former genre include H. R. Spencer, *The History of British Midwifery from 1650 to 1800* (London, 1927); H. Thoms, *Our Obstetric Heritage: The Story of Safe Childbirth* (Handen, Conn., 1960); W. Radcliffe, *Milestones in Midwifery* (Bristol, 1967). Childbirth received 6 pages in R. Trumbach, *The Rise of the*

Egalitarian Family: Aristocratic Kinship and Domestic Relations in Eighteenth-century England (New York, 1978), 180–5; but a page or less in M. D. George, *London Life in the Eighteenth Century* (first pub. 1925; Harmondsworth, 1966), 60–61; G. M. Trevelyan, *English Social History* (London, 1944), 65, 345; L. Stone, *The Family, Sex and Marriage in England 1500–1800* (London, 1977); R. Porter, *English Society in the Eighteenth Century* (Harmondsworth, 1982), 41, 294; Houlbrooke, *The English Family*, 129–30.

10. J. Donnison, *Midwives and Medical Men: A History of Inter-professional Rivalries and Women's Rights* (London, 1977); A. Eccles, *Obstetrics and Gynaecology in Tudor and Stuart England* (London, 1982).

11. The specific 'paths' by which male practitioners were called to childbirth in seventeenth- and eighteenth-century England are outlined in A. Wilson, 'William Hunter and the varieties of man-midwifery', in W. F. Bynum and R. Porter (eds), *William Hunter and the 18th-century Medical World* (Cambridge 1985), 343–70, esp. 349–57, 365–9.

12. P. Willughby, *Observations in Midwifery*, ed. H. Blenkinsop (Warwick, 1863; repr. ed. J. L. Thornton, Wakefield, 1972), 184, 197; Trumbach, *The Rise of the Egalitarian Family*, 181.

13. *OED* (12 vols, Oxford 1933), under 'nidget', verb (2). Ralph Josselin directly mentioned his own activity in summoning the women for only two (the third and eighth) of his wife's ten deliveries; however, in a further case (the fourth birth) a chance indirect reference makes it clear that this was his customary role. This is an excellent example of the very patchy nature of our evidence. See A. Macfarlane (ed.), *The Diary of Ralph Josselin* (London, 1976), 50, 415, 118.

14. L. Sterne, *The Life and Opinions of Tristram Shandy, Gentleman* (9 vols, York and London, 1760–7). In fact, it is by no means clear how the father-to-be passed the time. The most explicit indications I have encountered both come from America: Samuel Sewall, in 1677, was sitting with his father 'in the great hall' when he heard the cry of the newborn child; William Byrd, in 1709, having sent for the midwife at about 9 o'clock, did not wait up but went to bed an hour later. See L. Pollock (ed.), *A Lasting Relationship: Parents and Children Over Three Centuries* (London, 1987), 33, 35.

15. Macfarlane, *Diary of Ralph Josselin*, 415.

16. Ibid., 615. See also Willughby, *Observations*, 186, 205, 215–16 (mother); 218 (husband's mother); 235 (sister); 238 (kinswoman).

17. See M. Macdonald, *Mystical Bedlam: Madness, Anxiety and Healing in Seventeenth-century England* (Cambridge, 1981), 109; cf. K. Thomas, *Religion and the Decline of Magic: Studies in Popular Beliefs in Sixteenth- and Seventeenth-century England* (first pub. 1971; Harmondsworth, 1978), 665.

18. *OED*, 'gossip', noun (1a, 1c, 2a, 2b), verb (1,2); and 'gossiping', noun (1,2).

19. N. Culpeper, *A Directory for Midwives* (first edn 1651; London, 1675), 119.

The ceremony of childbirth

20. *OED*, 'grace', noun (21b).

21. Macfarlane, *Diary of Ralph Josselin*, 165.

22. CUL, Ely diocesan records, B/9/1 (25 September 1662).

23. W. Harvey, *Exercitationes de generatione animalium* (London, 1651), trans. G. Whitteridge (*Disputations Touching the Generation of Animals*, Oxford, 1981), 404.

24. Willughby, *Observations*, 11, 31–6, 233–4.

25. LJRO, Lichfield diocesan records, B/V/4, bundle for Staffs., 1667–8.

26. *OED*, 'midwife'.

27. Willughby, *Observations*, 142–5, 226.

28. J. Lane, 'The administration of an eighteenth century Warwickshire parish: Butlers Marston', *Dugdale Soc. Occ. Pap.*, 21 (1973), 20; Donnison, *Midwives and Medical Men*, 9–10, 208 (note 66); Trumbach, *The Rise of the Egalitarian Family*, 181; J. H. Aveling, *English Midwives: Their History and Prospects* (1872; London, 1967), 31.

29. J. R. Magrath (ed.), *The Flemings in Oxford* (3 vols, Oxford, 1904–24), vol. 1, 451 and *passim*.

30. R. C. Matthews and W. Latham (eds), *The Dairy of Samuel Pepys* (11 vols, London, 1970–83) quoted (with further examples) in Donnison, *Midwives and Medical Men*, 10.

31. Willughby, *Observations*, 4, 25, 158–60; Eccles, *Obstetrics and Gynaecology*, 87–8; H. Bracken, *The Midwife's Companion* (Lancaster, 1737), 105, 207.

32. C. White, *A Treatise on the Management of Pregnant and Lying-in Women* (London, 1772), 4–5, 248–9; Willughby, *Observations*, 65; J. Cooke, *Mellificium Chirurgiae, or the Marrow of Chirurgery* (London, 1648), 257; M. Thale (ed.), *The Autobiography of Francis Place* (Cambridge, 1972), 184.

33. *OED*, 'caudle' (noun, verb).

34. Ibid.

35. A. Clark (ed.), *The Life and Times of Anthony Wood, Antiquary, of Oxford, 1632–1695, Described by Himself* (5 vols, Oxford, 1891–1900), vol. 1, 138–41.

36. J. H. Aveling, *The Chamberlens and the Midwifery Forceps: Memorials of the Family and an Essay on the Invention of the Instrument* (London, 1882), 37; Donnison, *Midwives and Medical Men*, 8–9; Willughby, *Observations*, 72, 126.

37. Willughby, *Observations*, 6–7, 19, 73–4. The quote which follows is from ibid., 32.

38. Ibid., 8, 71, 73–4; Cooke, *Mellificium Chirurgiae*, 1685 edn, 255; W. Smellie, *A Treatise on the Theory and Practice of Midwifery* (3 vols, London, 1752–64), vol. 1, 199.

39. Willughby, *Observations*, 328–9.

40. Eccles, *Obstetrics and Gynaecology*, 92–3, 107, 125–30; Willughby, *Observations*, 43–51, esp. 45; Wilson, 'William Hunter', 344–5.

41. Willughby, *Observations*, 40, 66, 82 (note also the revival of the mother: ibid., 49, 234, 256); Donnison, *Midwives and Medical Men*, 50–1; Macfarlane, *Diary of Ralph Josselin*, 415.

42. J. Sharp, *The Midwives Book* (London, 1671), 372–4; J. Maubray, *The Female Physician* (London, 1724), 327; Bracken, *The Midwife's Companion*, 207–8.

43. See *OED*, 'bed' (noun, 2b, 6c); 'bring' (8c); 'cry' (verb, 21c); 'crying' (noun, 2); 'straw' (noun, 2b); 'month' (3f, 6).

44. LPL, Shrewsbury and Talbot papers, MS 3205, f. 151 (Anne, Countess of Arundel to George, Earl of Shrewsbury, August 1608, undated but after 21 August). I owe this example to Linda Pollock. See also Willughby, *Observations*, 211–13; Cooke, *Melleficium Chirurgiae*, 1685 edn, 167.

45. Sharp, *The Midwives Book*, 229; C. E. Fox, 'Pregnancy, childbirth and early infancy in Anglo-American culture: 1675–1800', unpub. Ph. D. thesis, University of Pennsylvania, 1966, 187–91.

46. See notes 44, above, and 47, below; Fox, 'Pregnancy', 203; Macfarlane, *Diary of Ralph Josselin*, 465–6, 415–19.

47. Trumbach, *The Rise of the Egalitarian Family*, 184; *OED*, 'upsitting' (1).

48. Macfarlane, *Diary of Ralph Josselin*, 167; Fox, 'Pregnancy', 204–5.

49. Trumbach, *The Rise of the Egalitarian Family*, 184–5. But compare S. Richardson, *Pamela; or, Virtue Rewarded* (first pub. 1740; ed. P. Sabor, Harmondsworth, 1980), 500–1: 'I had intended to make her a visit, as soon as her month was up.'

50. Matthews and Latham, *Diary of Samuel Pepys*, vol. 8, 177, 200 (courtesy Linda Pollock).

51. Aveling, *The Chamberlens*, 141; R. Barret, *A Companion for Midwives, Childbearing Women, and Nurses* (London, 1699); R. Gough, *The History of Myddle* ed. D. Hey, (Harmondsworth, 1981), 207.

52. *OED*, 'monthly' (4); for the quotation from Penelope Mordaunt see Pollock (ed.), *A Lasting Relationship*, 28.

53. Macfarlane, *Diary of Ralph Josselin*, 503; and see note 46, above.

54. M. Spufford, *Contrasting Communities: English Villagers in the Sixteenth and Seventeenth Centuries* (Cambridge, 1974), 254–5.

55. Sharp, *The Midwives Book*, 211–12; Blundell quoted in Trumbach, *The Rise of the Egalitarian Family*, 178.

56. The quoted phrases are from Macfarlane, *Diary of Ralph Josselin*, 118. Only for another four deliveries did Josselin record the date of his wife's first attendance at church after delivery; these were at intervals of 32, 36, 38, and 45 days after the birth, which suggests that the present case (36 days) was typical. See ibid., 165–9, 415–19, 465–6, 502–3.

57. F. Procter and W. H. Frere, *A New History of the Book of Common Prayer, with a Rationale of its Offices* (London, 1905), 638–9.

58. W. P. M. Kennedy, *Elizabethan Episcopal Administration* (3 vols, London, 1924), vol. 3, 149–50; P. Cunnington and C. Lucas, *Costume for Births, Marriages and Deaths* (London, 1972), 18.

59. 'In Herefordshire it was not considered "correct" for the husband to appear in church on the day of his wife's churching, at all events in the same pew with her.' J. E. Vaux, *Church Folk-lore*

(2nd edn, London 1902), 112. Contrast the case from the 1630s in note 105, below.

60. W. M. Campion and W. J. Beaumont (eds), *The Prayer Book Interleaved with Historical Illustrations* (10th edn, London, 1880), 219.

61. Ibid., *Notes and Queries*, 9th series, 2 (1898), 5, 212, 255; *OED*, 'uprising' (noun, 2c). (The 116th Psalm was slightly edited in its churching version, to render it specifically female in reference.)

62. Tate, *The Parish Chest*, 131.

63. Thomas, *Religion and the Decline of Magic*, 40–1.

64. See the case of Jane Minors, cited in note 104, below.

65. Matthews and Latham, *Diary of Samuel Pepys*, vol. 8, 201 (courtesy Linda Pollock; cf. note 50 above). See also Macfarlane, *Diary of Ralph Josselin*, 12, 327, 415, 503.

66. Campion and Beaumont, *The Prayer Book Interleaved*, 219; *OED*, 'chrisom' (2, 4); Tate, *The Parish Chest*, 59–60; Thomas, *Religion and the Decline of Magic*, 41, 63, 86.

67. Tate, *The Parish Chest*, 104. For tips to the nurse and midwife at baptism, see also Donnison, *Midwives and Medical Men*, 10, 29.

68. A significant exception to the all-female birth ritual was the specific case of Royal births, where male witnesses were always present. This was presumably because of the dynastic importance of the delivery, famously illustrated by the Whigs' promotion of the 'warming-pan' story concerning Mary of Modena's delivery in 1687.

69. The shortened 'month' is discussed in note 96, below. For the use of the bed as a lying-in space, see White, *Management of Pregnant and Lying-in Women* (2nd edn, 1777), Appendix, 58. Deliveries (and therefore lying-in) away from home are found, for instance, in Willughby, *Observations*, 120, and Laslett et al. (eds), *Bastardy*, 145.

70. See M. St Clare Byrne (ed.), *The Lisle Letters* (6 vols, Chicago, 1981), vol.1, 517; vol.3, 526; vol.4, 119,122; J. J. Cartwright (ed.), *Wentworth Papers 1705–39* (London, 1883), 325; C. E. Doble et al. (eds), *Remarks and Collections of Thomas Hearne* (11 vols, Oxford, 1885–1921), 6, 261.

71. Donnison, *Midwives and Medical Men*, 52–4 (though see also ibid., 110, 113).

72. N. St André, *A Short Narrative of an Extraordinary Delivery of Rabbits* (London, 1726), 25, 36. Mary Toft's experience and its wider significance have been explored by G. Hudson, 'The politics of credulity – the Mary Toft case', unpub. M.Phil. thesis, University of Cambridge, 1986.

73. A Warne, *Church and Society in Eighteenth-century Devon* (Newton Abbot, 1969), 156, quoting from accounts of overseers of the poor for either Kenton or West Alvington, n.d.

74. D. Davies, *The Case of the Labourers in Husbandry Stated and Considered* (London, 1795), 16.

75. Additional, indirect evidence to the same effect comes from the age profile of foundling children, which shows a marked bulge at ages of 30–39 days. The only plausible explanation for this pattern

is that it reflects the 'uprising' of mothers – in which case the children brought to the Foundling Hospital at younger ages (the great majority) would have been taken there not by the mothers but by someone else. See Wilson, 'Illegitimacy and its implications', section VI and Figure 3.

76. Macfarlane, *Diary of Ralph Josselin*, 12, 14–15, 50, 111–119, 165–9, 257–9, 324–7, 415–19, 465–6, 502–3. For Fleming see note 29, above.

77. Willughby, *Observations*, 305; see also ibid., 38.

78. Willughby, *Observations*, 213.

79. See also Cooke, *Melleficium Chirurgiae*, 1648 edn, 247–57; 1685 edn, 165–78; cf. John Locke's advice to Henry Fletcher, in Pollock (ed.), *A Lasting Relationship*, 33–4.

80. See A. Fraser, *The Weaker Vessel: Woman's Lot in Seventeen Century England* (2nd edn, London, 1985), 511–12.

81. Quoted in M. Roberts, '"Words they are women, and deeds they are men": images of work and gender in early modern England', in L. Charles and L. Duffin (eds), *Women and Work in Pre-industrial England* (London, 1985), 154–5.

82. This will be further explored in A. Wilson, *A Safe Deliverance: Ritual and Conflict in English Childbirth, 1660–1750* (Cambridge, forthcoming).

83. W. Cobbett, *Advice to Young Men* (repr. Oxford, 1980), 203 (Letter IV, 'Advice to a husband', para. 211).

84. A. van Gennep, *The Rites of Passage*, trans. M. B. Vizedom and G. L. Caffee (London, 1960; French original pub. 1906), 10–11, 46.

85. J. H. Miller, '"Temple and sewer": childbirth, prudery and Victoria Regina', in A. Wohl (ed.), *The Victorian Family: Structure and Stresses* (London, 1978), 27.

86. A. Wilson, 'Participant or patient? Seventeenth century childbirth from the mother's point of view', in R. Porter (ed.), *Patients and Practitioners: Lay Perceptions of Medicine in Pre-industrial Society* (Cambridge, 1985), 135.

87. Thomas, *Religion and the Decline of Magic*, 42–3 (cf. note 101, below.)

88. K. Thomas, 'Women and the Civil War sects', *P&P*, 13 (1958), 43.

89. N.Z. Davis, 'Women on top', in her *Society and Culture in Early-modern France* (London, 1975), 124–51. The quoted passages are from 145, 313.

90. For the deploying of conjugal power as an ideological resource, see P. Higgins, 'The reactions of women, with special reference to the women petitioners', in B. Manning (ed.), *Politics, Religion and the English Civil War* (London, 1973), 179–222, esp. 179–82, 203, 211–13; S. M. Okin, 'Women and the making of the sentimental family', *Phil. Pub. Aff.*, 11 (1982), 65–88; S.D. Amussen, 'Gender, family and the social order, 1560–1725', in J. Stevenson and A. Fletcher (eds), *Order and Disorder in Early Modern England* (Cambridge, 1985), 196–217, esp. 197–205.

91. Campion and Beaumont, *The Prayer Book Interleaved*, 203–7.

The ceremony of childbirth

92. See Baker, *An Introduction to English Legal History,* Crawford, 'From the woman's view' (note 8, above); K. Thomas, 'The double standard', *J. Hist. Ideas,* 20 (1959), 195–216, esp. 210–16.

93. The particular issue was that Elizabeth had written a memoir which, in Samuel's own words, was 'so piquant, and wrote in English and most of it true, of the retiredness of her life and how unpleasant it was, that being . . . in danger of being . . . read by others, I was vexed at it and desired her and then commanded her to tear it.' Matthews and Latham, *Diary of Samuel Pepys,* vol.4, 9, quoted in S. H. Mendelson, 'Stuart women's diaries and occasional memoirs', in M. Prior, (ed.), *Women in English Society 1500–1800* (London, 1985), 184.

94. This point has been elegantly developed by K. Hodgkin, 'The diary of Lady Anne Clifford: a study of class and gender in the seventeenth century', *Hist. Workshop J.,* 19 (1985), 148–61, esp. 150–1, 153–4.

95. C. Hill, *Economic Problems of the Church from Archbishop Whitgift to the Long Parliament* (Oxford, 1956), 168. The parish Poor Law officers might pay on the mother's behalf: Tate, *The Parish Chest,* 206. In Wakefield, Yorkshire, the custom had obtained that *every* householder with children would pay the vicar 10d at any churching. This was successfully challenged in law in 1558: see R. Burn, *Ecclesiastical Law* (2 vols, London, 1763), vol.1, 229–30.

96. See J. Boulton, *Neighbourhood and Society: A London Suburb in the Seventeenth Century* (Cambridge, 1987), 276–9. Most mothers were churched 14–27 days after the child's baptism, that is, probably 25–31 days after the birth. However, some were churched at longer intervals after the baptism, and a few (23 out of 671 churchings) within 0–13 days of the baptism. (These numbers pertain to a total of 732 baptisms, including seven where the mother is known to have died in childbirth.)

97. E. Gibson, *Codex Juris Ecclesiasticae Anglicani* (2nd edn, 2 vols, Oxford, 1761), vol. 2, 1468–9.

98. J. Cox, *The English Churches in a Secular Society: Lambeth, 1870–1930* (Oxford, 1982), 88–9, writes that 'it was to the parish church that working-class mothers regularly went for churching', citing Booth's survey material from St Mary, Lambeth, and St Philip's, Kennington. Hugh McLeod (pers. comm. 1985) has kindly passed on to me some more precise figures, from the same source, pertaining to East End parishes in the 1890s: 'The vicar of St Barnabas, Bethnal Green, said that he had conducted 150 baptisms and 200 churchings in the previous year . . . The vicar of St Paul, Virginia Row, said he had done 119 baptisms and 119 churchings.' Thus, churching was as popular as, or more popular than, baptism.

99. M. Young and P. Willmott, *Family and Kinship in East London* (3rd edn, Harmondsworth, 1986), 57.

100. The first anecdote I owe to Hugh McLeod (per. comm. 1984); my second informant wishes to remain anonymous.

101. Young and Willmott, *Family and Kinship,* 57. (It is worth noting that the authors' gloss – 'The idea still lingers on that

The ceremony of childbirth

childbirth has in some way made the mother unclean' – has no
support within the interview material they quote.)

102. Quoted in Thomas, *Religion and the Decline of Magic*, 68–9.

103. W. H. Hale, *A Series of Precedents and Proceedings in Criminal
Causes, Extending from the Year 1475 to 1640, Extracted from Act-books of
Ecclesiastical Courts in the Diocese of London* (London, 1847), 506; F. G.
Emmison, *Elizabethan Life: Morals and the Church Courts, Mainly from
Essex Archidiaconal Records* (Chelmsford, 1973), 160.

104. Hale, *Precedents and Proceedings*, 634; Emmison, *Elizabethan
Life*, 159.

105. J. Bruce (ed.), *Calendar of State Papers, Domestic Series, of the
Reign of Charles I, 1637–8* (London, 1869), 382. For a further
example from the 1630s, in similar vein, see Spufford, *Contrasting
Communities*, 236.

106. C. W. Foster, *The State of the Church in the Reigns of Elizabeth
and James I as Illustrated by Documents Relating to the Diocese of Lincoln*
(Horncastle, Lincs, 1926), 1, p.xxxix. See also Emmison, *Elizabethan
Life*, 160: in 1586 Edmund Fanninge was accused of having been 'a
hindrance to his wife in giving thanks'.

107. Compare A. Wilson, 'Inferring attitudes from behavior',
Hist. Meth., 14 (1981), 143–4. Nowadays I am inclined to doubt the
assumption that there exists a generalized 'popular attitude', either
in the past or in the present, which could meaningfully be
reconstructed.

108. After the suppression of the Book of Common Prayer, and
the substituting of the Directory for Public Worship, in 1645,
churching was sometimes performed at home: see, for instance, E. S.
De Beer (ed.), *The Diary of John Evelyn* (London, 1959), 325, 333.
The Directory did not include any churching service; however,
under the discretion permitted to ministers, it was entirely possible
for churching to continue in the traditional way. See J. W. Packer,
*The Transformation of Anglicanism 1643–1660, with Special Reference to
Henry Hammond* (Manchester, 1969), 13, 140.

109. Thomas, *Religion and the Decline of Magic*, 42–3; T. Comber,
The Occasional Offices Explained (London, 1679), 510.

110. Burn, *Ecclesiastical Law*, vol. 1, 229; *Second Report of the
Commissioners Appointed to Inquire into the Rubric, Orders, and Directions
for Regulating the Course and Conduct of Public Worship, etc.* (London,
1868), Appendix, 165.

111. E. L. Lipton, A. Steinschrader, and J. B. Richmond,
'Swaddling, a child care practice: historical, cultural and
experimental observations', *Paediatrics*, Suppl., 35 (1965), 519–67.

112. F. Loux, *Le Jeune Enfant et son Corps dans la Médecine
Traditionelle* (Paris, 1978).

113. The presence of the husband during the birth is attested for
Germany and for some parts of France. See L. Heister, *A General
System of Surgery in Three Parts*, transl. anon., Innys et al., (London,
1743), 207; E. Shorter, *A History of Women's Bodies* (London, 1982),
55; Loux, *Le Jeune Enfant*, 100–2. (Yet Mireille Laget suggests that the
French father was absent, though represented symbolically in some

66

localities by his shirt or hat: *Naissances: l'Accouchement avant l'Âge
de la clinique* (Paris, 1982), 135–7.) On the modern hospital ritual
see P. Lomas, 'An interpretation of modern obstetric practice',
in S. Kitzinger and J. Davis (eds), *The Place of Birth* (Oxford, 1978),
174–84. The process of historical transformation has been explored
for the case of North America by J. W. Leavitt, *Brought to Bed,
Birthing Women and Their Physicians in America 1750–1950*
(Oxford, 1987). A wealth of comparative material is available
in G. J. Witkowski, *Histoire des Accouchements Chez Tous les Peuples*
(Paris, 1887).

114. K. E. Paige and J. M. Paige, *The Politics of Reproductive Ritual*
(Berkeley, 1981), 43.

115. Ibid., 54. In sharp contrast, Diane Bell has recently stressed
that Australian aboriginal women's rituals are constructed and
chosen by the women themselves: *Daughters of the Dreaming*
(Melbourne, 1983). I am grateful to Gill Hudson for this reference.
For an open-ended exploration, written by women anthropologists
and nurses, see M. A. Kay (ed.), *Anthropology of Human Birth*
(Philadelphia, 1982). This collection contains some twenty new
ethnographic reports, produced under the guidance of the editor,
and also includes an invaluable critique of earlier approaches: C.
McClain, 'Toward a comparative framework for the study of
childbirth: a review of the literature', ibid., 25–59.

116. V. Fildes, *Breasts, Bottles and Babies: A History of Infant Feeding*
(Edinburgh, 1986); D. McLaren, 'Marital fertility and lactation
1570–1720' in Prior (ed.), *Women in English Society*, 22–53; and their
other studies listed in the bibliography to this volume.

117. Donnison, *Midwives and Medical Men*; Eccles, *Obstetrics and
Gynaecology* (note 10, above).

118. S. M. Okin, 'Patriarchy and married women's property in
England: questions on some current views', *Eighteenth-Cent. Stud.*, 17
(1983), 121–38; R. Mitchison, 'Man and wife', *Lond. Rev. Books*, 22
May 1986, 9–10; L. Pollock, '"An action like a stratagem": courtship
and marriage from the Middle Ages to the twentieth century', *Hist.
J.*, 30 (1987) 483–98.

119. S. Alexander, 'Women, class and sexual differences in the
1830s and 1840s: some reflections on the writing of a feminist
history', *Hist. Workshop J.*, 17 (1984), 125–49; L. Gordon, 'What's new
in women's history', in T. de Lauretis, (ed.), *Feminist Studies/Critical
Studies* (Bloomington, 1986), 20–30.

120. Mendelson, 'Stuart women's diaries'; P. Crawford,
'Women's published writings 1600–1700', in Prior (ed.), *Women in
English Society*, 211–82 (both including invaluable lists of such
sources).

121. For example, Okin in 'Women and the making of the
sentimental family' has shown that conjugal relations were treated,
in distinctive ways, by all major classical political theorists. Again,
Estelle Cohen has demonstrated that gender relations strongly
impinged upon learned theories of generation – and has found a
tradition of contest within this literature. See her 'Medical debates

on women's "nature" in England around 1700', *Bull. Soc. Soc. Hist. Med.*, 39 (1986), 7–11.

122. See T. G. Ashplant and A. Wilson, 'Present-centred history and the problem of historical knowledge', *Hist. J.*, 31 (1988).

123. The term 'counter-power' has been used with similar meaning, though in the different context of factory struggles, by Michelle Perrot, in a conversation with Jean-Pierre Barou and Michel Foucault. See M. Foucault, *Power/Knowledge: Selected Interviews and Other Writings 1972–1977*, ed. C. Gordon (Brighton, 1980), 163. For Elizabeth Pepys's resistance see note 93, above; other examples can be found in, for instance, Crawford's essay (note 8, above); Hodgkin's study (note 94, above); P. Mack, 'Women as prophets during the English Civil War', *Fem. Stud.*, 8 (1982), 19–45. Compare Macfarlane's perceptive summary: 'The kind of tension of identity and opposition that one finds in any system of hierarchy . . . was central to the marriage relationship as well' (*Marriage and Love*, 290). For some examples of collective struggles see Higgins, 'The reactions of women'; Clark (ed.), *The Life and Times of Anthony Wood*, vol. 1, 250–1; BL, Sloane MS 529, fols 1–19 (paginated 1–35), 'Domini Willoughbaei Derbiensis de puerperio tractatus', 14,22 (cf. Willughby, *Observations*, 99–101, 125).

124. On such a methodological strategy, compare Foucault: 'I would like to suggest another way to go further towards a new economy of power relations . . . . It consists of taking the forms of resistance against different forms of power as a starting point . . . . To use another metaphor, it consists of using this resistance as a chemical catalyst so as to bring to light power relations, locate their position, find out their point of application and the methods used' ('Afterword', 210–11, in H. L. Dreyfus and P. Rabinow, *Michel Foucault: Beyond Structuralism and Hermeneutics* (2nd edn, Chicago, 1983). The scope for a 'dissection' of patriarchal power is well illustrated by Middleton's pioneering exploration of this theme (based on a different methodological strategy) for the medieval period. See C. Middleton, 'Peasants, patriarchy, and the feudal mode of production in England: a Marxist appraisal', *Soc. Rev.*, 29 (1981), 105–35, 137–54.

125. I hope to explore these themes in a future paper, provisionally entitled 'Patriarchal power and women's resistance in early-modern England'.

126. See Chaytor, 'Household and kinship', esp. 48–9.

127. S. D. Amussen, 'Féminin/masculin: le genre dans l'Angleterre de lépoque moderne', *Annales ESC*, 40 (1985), 269–87; and *idem*, 'Gender, family and the social order'.

128. Ann Hess has suggested such a role for midwives in New England, drawing on court depositions: 'The New England midwife: women's work and culture in seventeenth-century America and England', unpub. dissertation, Yale University, 1987.

III

A MEMORIAL OF ELEANOR WILLUGHBY, A SEVENTEENTH-CENTURY MIDWIFE

The biographeme suspends narrative time and the *telos* that only such time can insure. Its ethos has affinities with . . . memory. Those who have lost their nearest and dearest do not recall their departed in the manner of the monumental biographer, but through discrete images, a love of cats and flowers, a liking for particular cakes, watery eyes like Ignatius of Loyola.

Sean Burke[1]

1 INTRODUCTION

Through the pages of Percival Willughby's *Observations in Midwifery*[2] – the classic source on childbirth in seventeenth-century England – there flits intermittently a daughter of Willughby's who practised as a midwife, both in tandem with her father and in her own right. She is unnamed in the treatise, but can be identified with the aid of further documentation as Eleanor Willughby, later Eleanor Hurt.[3] I shall suggest: (a) that the contours of Eleanor's practice are recoverable, even though her work is accessible only through her father's writings; (b) that while her connection with her father made her very different from most midwives, her practice helps to illuminate the activities of other midwives; (c) that the style of her midwifery practice reciprocally sheds light on that of her father; and (d) that Eleanor's presence in the *Observations* is wider and deeper than at first appears. We shall be attempting, then, to recover the agency of a woman from the writings of a man. The attendant hermeneutic problem is by no means confined to the case of Eleanor Willughby; for, ironically enough, the very fact that seventeenth-century childbirth was a collective female event is known to us chiefly from male documentary sources.[4] As we proceed, therefore, it will be appropriate to attend to the premises of our exercise – so far as we can identify those premises, for we may presume that no reading can in fact attain that transparency which (so it would seem) every reading tends to claim or to seek.[5]

Our enterprise raises a further issue, which is registered in the epigraph I have taken from Sean Burke, namely the tension between memory and biography. If a 'memorial' is to succeed in its aim, if it is to create a memory, it should offer what Roland Barthes called 'biographemes': that is (so Burke explains) flashing glimpses, detached images, linked with each other not through the medium of time but on the contrary in rigorously atemporal juxtapositions.[6] As I take it, this is precisely how the 'biographeme' mimics memory – establishing as it does a connection between its subject and ourselves whose very form defies the flow and the ravages of time. A memorial to Eleanor Willughby, then, ought rightly to present such biographemes. Yet we are constrained to proceed towards this *telos* in a starkly contrasting way, that is, in something like the ponderous 'manner of the monumental biographer', which Burke rightly depicts as the very antithesis of memory. For although we are already supplied with discrete glimpses and images of Eleanor, each and every one of these images was constructed by her father – which means that in order to build up our own biographemes of Eleanor, we have first to examine and to dismantle the images which her father constructed. Indeed, it may be doubted whether it is actually possible to free Eleanor from the circle of her father's representations; whether, in a case such as this, it is meaningful to posit a *hors-texte*; in short, whether our intended memorial can be made at all. But rather than debating the possibility in abstract terms, I shall proceed on the wager that this can be done. It will be up to the reader to decide whether that wager has been justified.

Having made this apology, I shall begin with a brief overview of what we know and can surmise of Eleanor's life – seen, inevitably, in reciprocal connection with that of her father. It will then be necessary to consider the form and content of her father's *Observations in Midwifery*; and his text will also serve as a lens through which to examine the world of practice from which it emanated, namely the contrasting roles of midwife and male practitioner in the management of seventeenth-century childbirth. In due course, as we turn to Eleanor herself, it will emerge that it was precisely this contrast which structured her practice as a midwife – in so far as we can reconstruct that practice from those surviving fragments which we will be taking as evidence.

The developing professional relationship between father and daughter can be divided, schematically, into three phases. Firstly, in about 1654, at the tender age of fifteen or sixteen, Eleanor embarked on the practice of midwifery – probably at her father's behest, and perhaps to augment the family's income in the wake of their recent move from Derby to Stafford. Working in cooperation with him, she practised as a midwife for five or six years, first in Stafford and then in London; and she helped her father with at least one delivery after the family's return to Derby in late 1659. Soon after this time, her father began to write his *Observations* – a midwifery treatise, designed chiefly for 'young country midwives', illustrated with 'observations' (that is, case histories) from his past and present practice. Secondly, by the time of her marriage to Thomas Hurt in 1662 Eleanor had stopped practising midwifery; and she now embarked on her own childbearing career. During the next ten years or so, while Eleanor Hurt was giving birth to the

140

first six of her nine children, her father was working intermittently on his book – particularly after the death of his wife, Eleanor's mother, in February 1667. He added more and more illustrative case histories from his continuing practice 'in the midwife's bed'; in 1668, he produced a finished version of the work and tried to get this published (though without success), and eventually in 1671–2 he wrote a complementary 'little work' or *Opusculum*. During these years Eleanor's life was entwined with her father's in a new way; for she called on his help in at least two of her own pregnancies and lyings-in, and she may even have used him in place of a midwife for all her deliveries. Thirdly, in 1672, Percival asked someone – we do not know whom – to edit his now unwieldy manuscripts for publication; and he duly entrusted to this intended editor the 'Opusculum' and his master copy of the 'Observations'. So far as we know, this unidentified individual did not succeed in the task of editing the texts, but she or he produced at least two verbatim transcripts of these works. And there are grounds for suspecting that this copyist was none other than Eleanor Hurt. If this surmise is correct, then Willughby's writings were chiefly delivered to posterity by his daughter's hand.

2 THE FORM AND CONTENT OF THE RECORD

We must first of all consider Willughby's *Observations* and the midwifery practices to which that work attests. Since no summary can do justice to a complex text of some ninety thousand words (for such was the length that the book had attained by 1672), let us instead start as Willughby himself often did: that is, from a particular case history. This will serve to exemplify the form of his 'observations' and, no less so, the complexities entailed in our own attempts to interpret such a story. For this was precisely a story, a story with an autobiographical element:

> Grace Beechcraft, the wife of Joseph, in St Peter's parish in Derby, being in labour several days, and having suffered much sorrow, desired my help. The child came with the head first, but it was great. Her midwife, with herself, desired my assistance, for that she could not deliver her. For her condition Divines were consulted, and in their opinions they were divided. Several women frowned upon some of these Divines, and upon the women's dislikes, they turned their coats and changed their opinions. I would not use the crotchet, for fear the child should be alive, but turned the head and brought it forth by the feet, after the way afore mentioned. The child was dead, but the woman's life was saved, and she recovered very well after this delivery.[7]

Willughby indicated the date of this particular case only obliquely (he was writing it down from recall), but we can locate the delivery at the end of September 1655.[8] His highly compressed account reveals that Grace Beechcraft's delivery was a complex drama, which involved at least five different agents or parties – mother, midwife, several women, divines, Willughby himself. Further, the divines were certainly of different minds, at least initially, and the women were probably divided as well;[9] so the number of distinct view points involved in the management of the case was at least six and very likely seven. What is more, reference to the other extant version of the 'Observations'[10] would add another one or two such view points – for Willughby there framed and told the story in a slightly different way. This underlines a point which is obvious enough, but deserves to be mentioned explicitly: Willughby's 'record' of the case was highly partial, in the double sense of being told very much from his own point of view and of being, like any narrative, incomplete. For instance, Willughby was living in Stafford at the time of this delivery, and so must have been called all the way from Stafford to Derby to deliver Grace Beechcraft; yet this circumstance, which he recorded for another Derby delivery around this time, was not included in his account of this particular case.[11]

In some respects this case description or 'observation' is typical of those in the *Observations* – utterly so in the fact that 'several women' were involved, in addition to the mother and her midwife, and very largely so in the fact that Grace had been in labour for some days by the time Willughby was called. Yet certain aspects of the case, or of Willughby's account of it, were atypical: for instance, his call to the delivery seldom came from the midwife, for midwives often resented his intrusion, and only occasionally did he report that 'Divines were consulted'. And some features of the story were unique: in no other case did he mention divisions of opinion among such ministers of religion, nor the pressure which women exerted upon them in Grace Beechcraft's case. If we partition the story along these lines, we arrive at the schema shown in Table 7.1, where the progress of the delivery is represented downwards line by line.

Table 7.1 Willughby's report of Grace Beechcraft's delivery, broken down into typical/untypical elements

Typical	Semi-typical	Unusual	Unique
several women present			
	birth by the head[a]		
	in labour several days[b]		
	only one midwife present[c]		
		called by mother+midwife[d]	
	child dead[e]		
		diagnosis uncertain[f]	
		Divines consulted[g]	
			Divines divided
			women frowned
			Divines turned
	delivered by the feet[h]		

142

ᵃ In about half of Willughby's reported deliveries the child presented by the head.

ᵇ This was typical of 'emergency' calls (Willughby's primary practice), as distinct from 'advance calls' and 'onset calls' (Willughby's secondary practice); these distinctions are explained below.

ᶜ In about one-third of Willughby's emergency calls two or more midwives were present before he was called (see further below).

ᵈ The 'calling agents' were specified in about half the cases; mothers, fathers, midwives and the mother's attending friends all participated in this process, in various combinations. Calls by mother and midwife combined were unusual (as were calls by the midwife alone).

ᵉ In the great majority of emergency calls, though not in all, the child was dead before Willughby was called.

ᶠ Usually Willughby was confident in his judgement as to whether or not the child was alive, though there were a few other cases where the diagnosis was uncertain.

ᵍ Such consultations were reported in only a handful of cases.

ʰ Willughby usually delivered obstructed head presentations by craniotomy with the sharp hook or crotchet; but sometimes, as in this case, he turned the child to the feet instead.

It so happens that the more or less typical themes appear in the early stages of this particular 'observation'. Other cases reveal a different pattern in this regard, as we shall see;[12] but the fact that the case history offers an admixture of the typical and the atypical was itself the norm. Indeed, the typical and the atypical in Willughby's case descriptions were mutually enfolded in complex ways. For instance, although the 'frowning' of the women was attested in this case alone, we can be confident that Willughby was always operating in a political field of force within which women were the dominant agents: for it was women who ran childbirth, and who were responsible for summoning him to the delivery.[13] Hence the fact that fathers-to-be are largely absent from his 'observations' – though, as will emerge in due course, this rule also had its exceptions.[14]

The case history we are considering reported both bodily events ('the child came with the head first') and social events ('her midwife, with herself, desired my assistance'); and the same was true of Willughby's 'observations' in general, including his descriptions of his daughter's cases. This interweaving of the bodily and the social was not merely a rhetorical device: on the contrary, it reflected the concrete experience of Willughby himself and (as we shall see) of Eleanor as well. Thus, in order to understand Willughby's practical choices in this case ('I would not use the crotchet . . . but turned the head, and brought it forth by the feet'), we must consider first the bodily processes of childbirth and then the various paths by which different practitioners were called to deliveries.

Largely following Willughby's categories[15] (though also drawing selectively on later obstetric knowledge), and leaving aside various rarities and complexities,[16] we may classify births into three broad types according to the way that the child presented.[17] By far the commonest occurrence was for the birth to present by the head; less often the child could present by the breech; and on rare occasions, perhaps one birth in 250, the child came by the shoulder or arm. Between these three categories, happily enough, difficulty corresponded to rarity. At one extreme, almost all births by the head delivered spontaneously, though a tiny minority of these became obstructed. At the opposite extreme, virtually every case of arm presentation was obstructed. And births by the breech, which were of intermediate frequency, were also intermediate in difficulty: most of them delivered spontaneously, though often with more trouble than births by the head, but a few of them became obstructed, and the incidence of such obstruction was greater than for births by the head. To some extent, this association between rarity and difficulty also obtained at the finer level which we are suppressing from consideration here: thus among breech births, one unusual variety was presentation by the feet or knees, and there is reason to suspect that these were more difficult than other forms of breech presentation.[18] Overall, about 1.5 per cent of births were obstructed. In addition, a small number of births – perhaps 0.4 per cent – were associated with serious difficulty due to other causes, notably 'flooding' (haemorrhage, in today's categories) and 'convulsion fits' (nowadays called eclampsia).

All births were managed by a well-developed and consistent popular ritual which was run by women collectively. But one woman in particular – the midwife – presided over both the social arrangements and the bodily management of birth: indeed, the midwife's authority was one of the central features of the ritual itself.[19] If difficulty arose, and if the midwife could not deliver the mother, there were two possible recourses. On the one hand a male practitioner could be called, as Willughby was in Grace Beechcraft's case. On the other hand, a second midwife might be summoned, and indeed sometimes a third or even a fourth midwife, as is shown by a number of cases where none of these midwives could deliver the mother, so that Willughby's services were finally required. (The practice of sending for a second midwife in such difficult births was required in some versions of the oath which midwives had to swear before receiving a licence from the Church; in this respect, as in some others, the oath probably reflected popular custom.)[20] Thus midwives were called to births not only in a *primary* capacity but also as *secondary* attendants, specifically for difficult births. Yet even if we make a generous allowance for this practice,[21] it is clear that the midwife's experience was overwhelmingly concentrated upon normal births. This point is illustrated in Table 7.2, which offers an educated guess as to the profile of a typical midwife's experiences over a ten-year period. Here it is assumed that the typical midwife's primary case load was twenty births per year; this figure, though derived from independent evidence, is consistent with the plausible expectation that most midwives practised over a small territory of one or two villages. The notion of such a typical midwife is of course a hypothetical abstraction, for some midwives – particularly those living in the larger towns –

tore it hee cannot be turned otherwife with the
hand conveyed in, the labouring-woman is to
be brought to her bed, where, if fhe fhall be faint
and feeble, fhe muft be refrefhed and comforted with convenient meats, and now fhee muft
proceed in the manner often fpoken of before,
untill the forme of a more convenient birth
fhall come.

CAHP. X.

Of the tenth forme and cure of it.

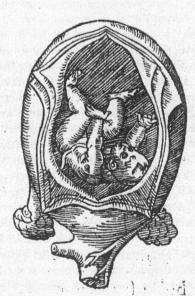

IT cómeth fome-
time to paffe that
the birth appea-
reth with the necke
turned awry, the
fhoulders bending
forward to the
birth, but the head
turned backeward,
and the feete with
the hands lifted up-
ward. In that cafe,
the Midwife fhall
remove the fhoulders of the childe backward,
that

A page from Jacob Rüff's *The Expert Midwife*, translated in 1637.

practised at much higher rates and were of more than local repute.[22] Nevertheless, Table 7.2 probably presents a reasonably reliable picture of the norm around which midwives' practical experiences revolved. Indeed, 'rural' case loads (of the order of twenty births per year) could be found at this time even in towns, up to and including London.[23]

Table 7.2 Estimate of a typical midwife's experience in 10 years

	Head	Breech	Arm	Total
	Numbers of births (rounded to nearest whole numbers) presenting by:			
Primary attendance:				
normal births	190	6	–	196
difficult births	3	–	1	4
total deliveries	193	6	1	200
Secondary attendance:				
normal births	–	–	–	–
difficult births	5	–	2	7
total deliveries	5	–	2	7
Total attendance:				
normal births	190	6	–	196
difficult births	8	–	3	11
total deliveries	198	6	3	207

Assumptions: (a) The typical midwife attended 20 births per year in a primary capacity. (b) The incidence of different presentations, and their associated rates of obstruction, were as follows: births by the head 966 per 1,000, of which 1 per cent were obstructed; breech births 30 per 1,000, of which 2 per cent were obstructed; arm presentations 4 per 1,000, all of which were obstructed. (c) An additional 4 births per 1,000 involved serious complications ('flooding', i.e. haemorrhage, or convulsions, corresponding to the modern eclampsia); the incidence of such complications was independent of presentation type (which means in practice that the few such cases all presented by the head). (d) All difficult births (i.e. cases of obstruction or serious complications) were attended by two additional midwives before a male practitioner such as Willughby was called. (e) Such secondary attendances were evenly shared among all midwives. (The latter two assumptions are generous: see note 21 to the text.)

Although the numbers suggested here are only approximations, we can be confident that some 95 per cent of the midwife's cases consisted of normal births – even including those where her attendance was in a secondary capacity. Correspondingly, midwives probably accumulated very little experience of

146

difficult deliveries. To take the case of arm presentations, our case load estimate of twenty births per year implies that the typical midwife saw such a birth only once in ten years in her primary practice, and another twice during that time in a secondary capacity. In all, therefore, she would encounter such a case about once every three years or so – indeed, more likely only once every four years.[24] And while our estimate of the average case load is only a guess, much the same implications would follow even if we doubled this to an implausibly high forty births per year. We may therefore venture the preliminary assessment that most midwives were unable to deliver these unusual and difficult cases.[25]

Percival Willughby's experiences 'in the midwife's bed' – very different from those of the midwife – were structured by the specific ways he was called to deliveries. Simplifying somewhat, we may distinguish in his practice three main 'paths to childbirth', which I term advance calls, onset calls and emergency calls. In an advance call he was summoned to reside in the mother's house in advance of the delivery; onset calls required him to attend from the onset of labour; and emergency calls, like that to deliver Grace Beechcraft, were occasioned by difficulty during the birth.[26] His advance and onset calls (which came only from wealthy mothers) resembled the primary practice of the midwife – but with this major difference, that he usually attended only as an adjunct to the midwife; his emergency calls (which took him to deliveries of all social ranks) corresponded to the midwife's secondary practice. Willughby's *Observations* supply various indications of his case loads in both primary and secondary midwifery; using these clues and some guesswork, we can estimate the profile of his practice over ten years as shown in Table 7.3. Here the key point is that emergency calls (Willughby's form of secondary attendance) comprised his chief form of practice.

This picture of Willughby's practice confirms our preliminary inference that most midwives were unable to deliver obstructed births and cases involving serious complications. For it was precisely these births that comprised the principal niche of practice for Willughby himself; and in view of the size of his catchment area and the incidence of difficult births, he would scarcely have had an emergency midwifery practice at all if midwives had been able to manage such cases.[27] Indeed, we can be more specific: Willughby's usual task was to deliver a dead child, in an obstructed birth by the head, in order to save the mother's life. Among his reported cases, over half the births which he actually delivered – as distinct from those he merely attended as an adjunct to the midwife – were of this kind; and as Table 7.3 implies, the proportion was probably higher still in his practice as a whole.

Schematic though they are, the numbers in Tables 7.2 and 7.3 probably offer a fair guide to the experiences of a midwife on the one hand and of Willughby on the other. As it happened, Willughby's overall case load was probably very similar to that of the typical midwife, at around twenty births per year; but the profile of his practical experience was very different indeed from hers. We can identify four

Table 7.3 Estimate of Willughby's experience in 10 years (based on his cases from the 1660s)

| | Numbers of births presenting by: | | | |
	Head	Breech	Arm	Total
Primary attendance:				
normal births	57	2	–	59
difficult births	1	–	–	1
total deliveries	58	2	–	60
Secondary attendance:				
normal births	–	–	–	–
difficult births	117	6	40	163
total deliveries	117	6	40	163
Total attendance:				
normal births	57	2	–	59
difficult births	118	6	40	164
total deliveries	175	8	40	223

Assumptions: (a) Willughby's primary practice (i.e. 'advance' and 'onset' calls) amounted to 6 cases per year. (b) The catchment area for Willughby's secondary (emergency) practice comprised 1,000 births per year. (c) Within this catchment area, Willughby was called to all obstructed births by the arm and breech, to 2/3 of obstructed births by the head, and to ½ of the births involving serious complications. (NB Excluded are cases of retained placenta.)

main contrasts. In the first place, the midwife's deliveries were concentrated on normal births, whereas Willughby's work centred on difficult deliveries. Indeed, this contrast was even more marked than our tables suggest; for in his primary practice, Willughby left the delivery to the midwife if the birth proved normal, as of course it almost always did. Thus difficult births made up not just 73 per cent of his total experience (the proportion suggested by the balance between his primary and secondary forms of practice), but probably well over 90 per cent; and this was the precise inverse of the midwife's experience. Secondly, and correspondingly, their expected roles were precisely complementary. The task of the midwife was to deliver a *living* baby – whence the fact that midwives were adept at reviving a weakly child[28] – and also to supervise the social arrangements for the birth. In contrast, what was chiefly expected of Willughby was to deliver a *dead* child, and he had little if any influence over the childbirth ritual.[29] Thirdly, Willughby saw a very different balance of presentation types from that which a midwife encountered – particularly with regard to malpresentations. In the midwife's experience, births by the breech far outnumbered births by the arm, particularly in her primary practice; but in Willughby's practice, 'the birth by the arm' was much more common than what he called 'the birth by the buttocks'. Finally, the midwife and Willughby had sharply differing experiences of one particular type of delivery, namely 'the birth by the buttocks'. In a ten-year period, they saw similar numbers of such births; but whereas all of the midwife's breech cases delivered spontaneously,[30] most of those which Willughby encountered were obstructed. This was, of course, an artefact of Willughby's particular 'paths to childbirth'. Much the same was true of births by the head – but in these cases Willughby had the countervailing experience arising from his primary practice, thanks to which he was well aware that births by the head could deliver by the natural powers. With respect to breech births, in contrast, his experience only rarely offered this practical lesson. As we shall see, Willughby's proclaimed views on the management of such births are intelligible in this light.

We are now in a position to appreciate the practical methods which Willughby mentioned as possible choices in Grace Beechcraft's delivery: the 'crotchet' on the one hand, turning to the feet on the other.[31] The crotchet or sharp hook was used to deliver a dead child in an obstructed birth by the head: it enabled the operator to exert traction, and was very effective for this purpose, but it could of course not be used on a living child. Devices of this kind, which took various forms, represented a standard part of the surgeon's armamentarium – which is one of the reasons for believing that Willughby's practice in midwifery was typical of its day. The crotchet was Willughby's preferred instrument for this purpose, and was also favoured by most other English male practitioners of the seventeenth century. The practice of turning to the feet[32] could be used on either a living child or a dead one; the point of the manoeuvre was that it enabled the surgeon or midwife to exert traction. This was the master-method advocated throughout Willughby's 'Observations' and 'Opusculum'. Although the technique had been introduced in the sixteenth century by Ambroise Paré, it was only slowly adopted in midwifery treatises; in endorsing turning, Willughby was out of line with most of the published advice of his time, and more in tune with the subsequent writings of Mauriceau and Deventer, who were to be the chief practical obstetric authorities of the early eighteenth century. Willughby had picked up this method in about 1646, that is to say after more than fifteen years of practice.[33] Once he had mastered the technique, he applied it in a variety of circumstances: for malpresentations such as the breech or arm;[34] for cases of 'flooding'; and sometimes for obstructed births by the head – particularly if the child was still alive, or was thought by some parties present to be alive. Hence the decision which Willughby took in Grace Beechcraft's case: 'I would not use the crotchet, for fear the child should be alive, but turned the head, and brought it forth by the feet.'

Indeed, it was one of the central messages of the *Observations* that turning to the

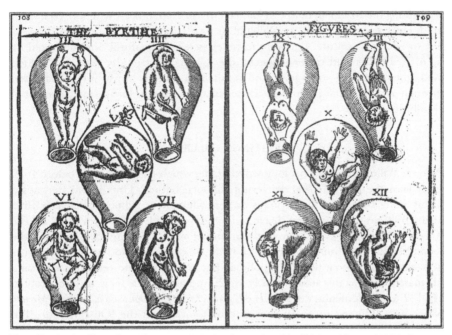

From Eucharius Rösselin, *The Byrth of Mankynde* translated by Richard Jonas (1626, first published, 1540).

feet was the master-method for delivering 'all difficult and unnatural cross births'.[35] Yet there was also another message: that if the birth was natural, no interference was required; on the contrary, the birth was best left to 'Dame Nature, Eve's midwife'. The critical question, then, was whether any given birth was to be regarded as difficult or natural – a question to which 'Nature' herself did not always offer a clear answer. In practice, Willughby's encounter with nature was of course mediated by the social paths which brought him to childbirth; and it was this conjuncture of the bodily and the social which governed his practical choices. And the 'birth by the buttocks', discussed above, nicely illustrates this issue and the way Willughby resolved it.[36] On the one hand, as will emerge below,[37] Willughby was well aware that breech births, unlike certain other malpresentations such as births by the shoulder or arm, could deliver spontaneously. On the other hand, as we saw in Table 7.3, most of the (few) breech births which he encountered were obstructed. And this predisposed him to treat such births as 'unnatural', and accordingly to deliver them by turning the child and drawing by the feet. Indeed, it so happened that his very first recorded use of turning to the feet, or at least his first recorded success in attempting the manoeuvre (on 14 January 1646/7), had been with a breech birth in an emergency call.[38] Hence Willughby's proclaimed advice: breech births were not to be left to nature, but were to be classed as 'unnatural' and delivered by turning. In this and other respects, the lessons of 'friendly Nature'[39] which Willughby imbibed so eagerly and retailed so lavishly were in fact refracted through culture – that is, through the social arrangements for the management of childbirth.

3 WRITINGS STILLBORN

Percival Willughby spent his long working life, which extended from before 1630 to at least the early 1670s, delivering stillborn babies. Thus it was perhaps a fitting irony that all of his writings on midwifery were stillborn. Between 1661 and 1672 he produced at least two and probably three versions of the 'Observations': the first, very likely an initial version, completed in 1662; the second certainly a finished version of 1668, which he sent to medical colleagues in London; and also a third, less polished but more complete version, comprising his master copy as this stood in early 1672. And as we have seen, he also wrote in 1671–2 a supplementary work, *The Country Midwife's Opusculum, or Vade-Mecum*, which was designed to accompany and to complement the 'Observations'. But despite Willughby's hopes, none of this literary output found its way into print: during this time, then, he produced two stillborn books, one of them at least twice and probably three times over. In contrast, his daughter Eleanor, the former midwife, was meanwhile giving birth to six living children (and also, as we shall see, to one stillborn child). The counterpoint between the activities of father and daughter was here at its sharpest.

Yet although they remained unpublished during his lifetime, most of Willughby's writings were preserved in manuscript after his own death in 1685. Of the (probable) initial version of the 'Observations' no copy is known to survive; its very existence is conjectural.[40] But we do have copies of the version of 1668 (this first surviving recension we may call the 'London version'), and also of the text of 1672 (which I term the 'Derby version'), the latter accompanied by the 'Opusculum'.[41] In fact the survival of these manuscripts was to occasion a further irony. For Willughby's hopes of publication were eventually realized – but not until long after his death, when most of his advice was out of date, and for very different audiences from the 'country midwives' for whom he had been writing. The 'London version' of the 'Observations' was published in 1754, some eighty-six years after it had been written – in a Dutch translation, intended for male obstetric surgeons, and merely as an appendix to a book on the newly publicized midwifery vectis (an instrument of which Willughby had been unaware). And after another nine decades (that is, in 1863) the 'Derby version', together with the accompanying 'Opusculum', was printed in English, in a limited edition produced by Henry Blenkinsop of Warwick. By this time, of course, the interest of these works was purely historical, and in any case Blenkinsop failed to sell out the 100 copies of his edition. A century later, in 1972, the two books again saw the light of day, in a facsimile reprint of Blenkinsop's edition. Once again their publication was not much of a success, for the facsimile edition was remaindered within a few years. Still, this edition has at long last supplied Willughby with an attentive audience – in the form of late twentieth-century historians of medicine.

Indeed, such ironies extend back to Willughby's own purposes and didactic methods. Willughby wanted to argue that practical experience was the only effective teacher; yet his medium contradicted his message, for he was using the written word. He sought to advise midwives on the delivery of normal births; yet his own experience was almost entirely restricted to difficult deliveries. He repeatedly criticized 'young midwives' and extolled the benefits of long experience; yet at the same time he vaunted the abilities of his daughter, who was less than seventeen years old when she embarked upon practice. He argued that all difficult births could be managed by a single method, namely turning to the feet; yet he also asserted that every case was different, and indeed the very cases which he used to illustrate his message also exemplify this bewildering variety, thereby distracting attention from Willughby's main argument. But perhaps the supreme paradox pertains to the use which Willughby made of William Harvey's essay 'De Partu', the concluding section of Harvey's *De Generatione* (which had been published in 1651, and translated into English in 1653). As it happened, Willughby had been personally acquainted with Harvey: indeed, in 1642, on the eve of the battle of Edgehill, Harvey, who was then attending Charles I, rode across to Derby to visit Willughby. Their conversation at this time concerned 'several infirmities incident to the womb'; Willughby's account gives no hint that they also discussed methods of delivery.[42] Nevertheless it came about that their subsequently recorded views on delivery showed certain similarities – and Willughby vastly exaggerated these resemblances. More precisely, when writing on midwifery in the 1660s he presented himself as following in the footsteps of Harvey (who had died in 1657); and since he also depicted his daughter's practice in the same light, our own purposes require us to notice this rhetorical framing on Willughby's part.

Harvey's discussion of birth was chiefly theoretical in intent; yet it had certain practical implications.[43] His argument was that birth was due to the joint efforts of (a) the foetus and (b) the entire body of the mother – not just of her uterus.[44] Both 'the woman in travail' and 'the foetus that is to be born' had to be 'ready for the business'; otherwise, 'the birth will scarcely ever follow with success, for it must occur at the hour that fits their joint maturity'. It followed, Harvey explained, that midwives should not attempt to 'accelerate and facilitate' the delivery by such practices as 'distending the parts' and 'offering medicinal draughts', for such efforts 'rather retard and prevent the delivery'. Harvey's argument neatly accounted for the fact that a normal birth proceeds head first: 'the foetus itself, *with its head turned downwards*, approaches the gates of the womb and opens them by its own strength and struggles out into the light'. But Harvey went on to explain that different considerations prevailed in difficult births:

> Nevertheless in an abortion and where the foetus is dead, or where otherwise the delivery would be difficult and hands would have to be used in the business, the more convenient way of coming forth is feet first, for by that means the narrows of the womb are opened more easily as if by driving in a wedge. Wherefore when the chief hope of giving birth lies in the *foetus* as being strong and lively, *there must be a striving to produce it head first*, but if the business depend chiefly on the *uterus*, then *its arrival feet first must be procured*.[45]

The point of turning the child to the feet was that its feet served as a wedge; what drove the wedge and thereby opened the 'narrows of the womb' was the action of the uterus.[46] In a normal birth, the foetus opened the 'narrows of the womb' with its head; turning to the feet, by producing a 'wedge', enabled the action of the uterus to substitute for the action of the child.

Willughby took this passage as a talisman, despite the vast gulf which separated Harvey's philosophical interest in birth from his own practical obstetric concerns. As he portrayed the matter, Harvey had produced a practical account of the methods of delivery, an account which precisely accorded with his own approach. Normal births were to be left to nature; difficult births were to be delivered by the feet. As Willughby put it (but with emphases added):

> Dr Harvey's learned observations about the birth ought be esteemed for their worth and goodness. The *oft reading* of them, with a due observation of his method, will be sufficient to make a midwife to understand her calling.

So much for the need for practical experience! Willughby went on:

> He showeth, in the first place, what to observe and how to deliver a woman labouring in a natural birth. And in difficult births, and abortive births, and where the foetus is dead, he maketh mention how to perform the work by the child's feet. In his works, he wishes midwives not to be too busy at the first approaching of labour, by striving to hasten or promote a sudden or quick birth; but willeth them patiently to wait on nature, to observe her ways, and not to disquiet her, for that it is the sole and only work of nature.[47]

Here Willughby, in characteristic fashion, inserted a case history – one which we shall have occasion to consider in due course.[48] Having completed the story, he returned to its practical moral:

I know none but Dr Harvey's directions and method, the which I wish all midwives to observe and follow, and oft to read over and over again; and in so doing, they will better observe, understand and remember the sayings and doings of that most worthy, good and learned Dr., whose memory ought to be had for ever in great esteem with midwives and child-bearing women.

Elsewhere Willughby stressed that midwifery was not to be learnt from books;[49] yet when it came to Harvey, he insisted on precisely the opposite message. But this was only one of the contradictions surrounding his claim to have followed 'Dr Harvey's directions and method'. For although Willughby's expectant approach to the management of normal births was precisely in line with Harvey's proclaimed views, his approach to *difficult* births was far removed from Harvey's – and this in several respects.

In the first place, we have seen Harvey advising that 'when the chief hope of giving birth lies in the foetus as being strong and lively, there must be a striving to produce it head first'; yet Willughby repeatedly argued against this technique.[50]

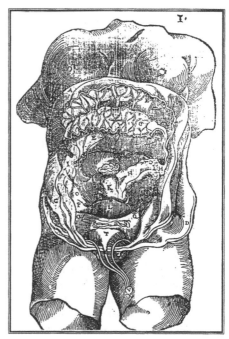

Secondly, the whole burden of Harvey's account was that the child should be delivered by the feet 'if the business depend chiefly on the uterus'; yet Willughby stressed, on the contrary, that by turning the child to the feet, 'the woman may be laid without throes', that is, without any action on the part of the uterus. To put this another way, Harvey simply did not consider the case where neither the foetus nor the uterus could accomplish the birth, that is, when the foetus was dead and the powers of the uterus were extinct – yet this was precisely what Willughby encountered in his routine practice. Thirdly, and correspondingly, Harvey depicted manual delivery by the feet as purely passive in intent – whereas Willughby turned the child to the feet *in order to exert traction*.[51] Finally, Willughby's own case histories demonstrated, as we shall see in due course,[52] that births which presented by the feet were even more difficult

A page from Eucharius Rösslin's *The Byrth of Mankynde*, translated by Richard Jonas (1626, first published, 1540).

154

than the 'birth by the buttocks': thus if, as Willughby believed, the unaided powers of the uterus could not be relied upon to deliver breech births, still less so could the uterus bring about a delivery which presented by the feet. Hence the efficacy of turning to the feet depended not on substituting for the action of the foetus, as Harvey claimed, but on the contrary on augmenting or replacing the powers of the uterus. In short, although Willughby was doubtless sincere in asserting that 'I know none but Dr Harvey's directions and method', that remark is not to be taken at face value. On the contrary, his use of Harvey was strictly rhetorical: it represented a rather strained attempt to give textual and learned support to his own argument in favour of delivering difficult births by the feet.

If the ironies associated with the *Observations* 'extend back', as I have been suggesting, to Willughby's very purposes, they also stretch forward to our own enterprise. For the very act of using Willughby's *Observations* as a historical source is inescapably fraught with contradictions. The book was a condensation of Willughby's experience; we want to reconstruct (as far as we can) the wider field of action from which he condensed it; thus to use the book as a source entails a necessary violation of Willughby's purposes; and yet this also requires us to attend to those very purposes. In particular, we are hoping to disentangle Eleanor Willughby and her practice from her father's presentation of her; yet as we shall now see, her very identity as a midwife was intimately bound up with her father's practice and indeed with his rhetoric.

4 ELEANOR WILLUGHBY'S PRACTICE IN STAFFORD

Of the 190-odd case histories described in the *Observations*, Eleanor is mentioned in just eight – but this small number becomes more impressive when we notice that it includes seven of the thirty-one cases from the five years or so when she and her father were living in Stafford (for no more than two years, between 1654 and 1656) and London (from May 1656 until late 1659). Let us now examine these cases one by one, beginning with the four Stafford cases. One of these was an emergency summons of Percival himself, but Eleanor accompanied him:

> I was sent for from Stafford, to come to a lady beyond Congerton [i.e. Congleton, Cheshire]. Her midwife had kept her several days in labour. I took my daughter with me. We travelled all night, and we were wetted with much rain to skins. We came, by break of day, to the place. But this Lady was dead, undelivered, before our coming. I much desired to see her corpse, but the midwife would not permit it. I knew this midwife not to be very judicious in her profession, and I believe that she was ashamed that her work should be seen Anno 1655. This midwife was gentle in habit of clothes, but ignorant in the ways of practice of midwifery.[53]

This case is chiefly of interest for the fact that Willughby took Eleanor with him. Although this is the only such instance mentioned in the *Observations*, we may surely presume that he was training her in midwifery – perhaps to augment the family income, for Willughby's own practice must have been disrupted by his move to Stafford. Other aspects of the case display the same mixture of the typical and the untypical that we encountered in Grace Beechcraft's case from the same year, 1655.[54] The very late call ('several days in labour') is characteristic of Willughby's emergency cases; so, too, is Willughby's claim that the midwife was 'ignorant'. The long journey was semi-typical: such calls came from a wide catchment area, with a radius of 10 miles or so, but seldom from the distance of over 20 miles which separated Congleton from Stafford. But the fact that the mother died undelivered before Willughby could arrive was unusual, and the description of the midwife as 'gentle in habit of clothes' is unique. Notice, finally, the authority of the midwife: she was in a position to prohibit Willughby from seeing the body of the deceased mother. Although this particular prohibition is unique, the authority which it reflects was probably typical, as we have seen.[55]

Eleanor's other three documented Stafford cases were births which she herself delivered; there is no hint that her father was present at these occasions, or indeed that he was involved in any way at all. Strikingly, all three were examples of 'the birth by the buttocks', and Willughby presented them together. In the light of our earlier guesses as to the structure of his practice (Table 7.3), it is not difficult to see why he resorted to Eleanor's practice for this purpose: in all probability, he had relatively few experiences of his own to draw upon when it came to breech births, in contrast with births by the head or by the arm. His argument in this passage – largely embedded in the case histories themselves – was that although breech births sometimes delivered spontaneously, prompt turning to the feet was the best method to adopt in such cases. And the first of these three case histories made it clear that this was Eleanor's own preferred practice, as will be seen from the phrase I have emphasized:

An inn-keeper's wife in Stafford desired my daughter's assistance for her delivery. Her labour was quick. The child followed the flowing of the waters, sitting in the birth with the buttocks. The birth was so speedy, that it would afford *no time to turn the child*. The mother, with the child, lived, and did very well after this birth.[56]

Willughby immediately commented, referring also to another similar case,[57] perhaps of his own: 'But one swallow, or two, doth not make a summer.' That is, these particular lessons from his alleged teacher, 'friendly Nature',[58] were *not* to be heeded: instead, breech births were to be treated as difficult deliveries from the outset, and were therefore to be delivered by the feet. It was just this argument which Eleanor's remaining two cases were meant to convey. The next

156

case was clearly a secondary attendance, for Eleanor was the fourth midwife called to the birth:

> In Staffordshire, nigh to Newcastle, Anno 1656, my daughter quickly laid this birth, according to the foresaid way, by the feet, where, otherwise, three old midwives had let the woman perish, taking the buttocks for the head. They knew not how to help her, until she showed them the way of delivery of this birth by the child's feet.[59]

The remaining case was described only briefly, with no explicit indication as to whether it involved a primary or a secondary attendance:

> She laid a barber's wife in Stafford of the same birth, after the same way. She, and her child, be living.

Observe that this little case history adds nothing new; it is merely another example. The impression this conveys is that Willughby has now recounted *all* of his daughter's breech deliveries from her time in Stafford; we may take this as our preliminary, working assumption.

Despite their brevity, these case descriptions bring several different themes into play. In addition to the mother herself – who she was (for instance, a barber's wife), how she fared after the delivery – Willughby mentioned the place, the course of the birth and how his daughter managed it; and we can also infer the timing of the call. As it turns out, these features of the three cases were interconnected, as emerges in Table 7.4.

Table 7.4 Structure of Eleanor Willughby's three Stafford cases

Place	Mode of attendance	Course of the birth	How E.W. delivered
1 Stafford	primary	delivered naturally	no time to turn to feet
2 near Newcastle-under-Lyme	secondary	obstructed	by the feet
3 Stafford	?	?	by the feet

The first two cases were of complementary kinds. Case 1 was a primary attendance, and it was typical of such cases in that the birth delivered spontaneously. In contrast, Case 2 was secondary in type; correspondingly, this was an obstructed breech which, if Willughby is to be believed, would not have been delivered without Eleanor's help. This is precisely in accordance with the different locations of these two cases. Eleanor's primary attendance (Case 1) took place in the town where she lived – which is as we should expect, for the midwife had to be on hand as soon as the mother fell into labour, and indeed this very case illustrates how quickly a spontaneous birth could proceed, even if it presented by the breech. But Eleanor's secondary attendance (Case 2) was located perhaps 14 miles away, and this is intelligible enough. In Stafford itself, we would not expect any obstructed breech births to have taken place during Eleanor's short stay;[60] but in the larger pool of births from the surrounding area such a case could plausibly have arisen even in this brief span of time.[61] And these considerations help us to interpret Case 3: it becomes well-nigh certain that this was a primary attendance (like Case 1), rather than a secondary one (like Case 2). In Case 3 there was evidently time to turn the child to the feet, suggesting that the labour proceeded more slowly (as indeed we would expect with a breech presentation); but otherwise this delivery resembled Case 1, for it took place in Stafford itself and no other midwives were present.

Within a period of some two years, then, Eleanor attended at least two breech births in a primary capacity, both of them in the town of Stafford. If we refer back to Table 7.2, it becomes apparent that she probably practised at something like the same rate as the typical midwife, perhaps indeed at a slightly higher rate. And this implies that the three breech cases which her father later included in his 'Observations' represented just a small sample of her total practice at this time. Thus, *in all probability, Eleanor delivered many other births in Stafford during her brief stay in the town* – though none of these was reported in her father's 'Observations'. Just how many births she managed in a primary capacity we can only guess, but we can be confident that she delivered more than ten mothers in this time,[62] and our best guess would be some sixty or so deliveries[63] – that is, about half of all the births in Stafford during the short time that she was there.[64] It would appear, then, that Eleanor Willughby was one of those urban midwives whose case load was rather higher than the twenty or so births per year of the typical midwife. For a girl of fifteen to sixteen years, newly arrived in the town, this was a remarkable achievement; and we may observe that in this short time she probably acquired more experience of normal births than her father accumulated in a lifetime's practice. Furthermore, her expertise was by no means confined to the management of normal birth. Perhaps the most impressive feature of her secondary attendance (Case 2) is the distance from which the call came: her reputation had extended – rightly, as it turned out – over 10 miles afield. To put this another way, we may observe that a typical midwife would be called in this way to an obstructed breech birth no more than once in twenty years or more,[65] and yet Eleanor received such a call within her first two years of practice. This in turn is consistent with our inference that her practice in Stafford itself was more extensive than that of most midwives. Notice in addition that our earlier working

158

assumption was probably correct: it appears that all Eleanor's breech cases from her time in Stafford were indeed included in her father's 'Observations'.[66] For during the two years (or less) which she spent there, probably only about three or four normal breech births took place in the town itself,[67] and just a single obstructed breech in the surrounding hinterland.

Even if her rate of primary practice was similar to that of midwives in general (which is difficult to assess), Eleanor Willughby was in other respects a most unusual midwife. Not only was she single, whereas most midwives were married or widowed;[68] she was also extraordinarily young when she embarked on practice. Further, she had been taught by a male practitioner, namely her father, whereas few if any other midwives embarked on practice in this way;[69] and correspondingly, she delivered breech births by turning the child to the feet, a method which most midwives probably did not use. It is also noteworthy that she applied this technique for breech births not only if these became obstructed but also, if there was time, in the early stages of labour – in effect, as a prophylactic method.

5 ELEANOR AND HER FATHER IN LONDON

In May 1656, Eleanor Willughby's practice in Stafford was cut short – for her father moved to London, 'there to live', as he later explained in his *Observations*, 'for the better education of my children'. With the help of 'an apothecary that formerly had lived in Stafford', he 'quickly had some practice in midwifery, among the meaner sort of women'.[70] What about Eleanor's practice in London? Again we have just three case descriptions to go on; as we shall see, their import is very different from that of the Stafford cases.

The first of Eleanor's three recorded London cases was another 'birth of the buttocks' – specifically, a secondary attendance. Although Willughby left this 'observation' undated, we can infer that the birth took place some substantial time after he moved to London; for by the time of this delivery, he had established there not only a reputation in midwifery, but also a circle of friends. His account of this case immediately followed Cases 2 and 3 from Stafford:

> She laid the same birth of the buttocks by the feet in Shoe lane, at London, where an ancient midwife knew not how to do it. I was send for to this woman, and, finding the birth to come by the buttocks, I sent for my daughter, and willed her to go to the woman, and to give me an account of the birth, sitting all the while with Mrs Joanna Mullins.

> She came from the travailing woman to us, and said that the birth came by the buttocks, the which the old midwife took for the head. Before Mrs Mullins the wife of old Mr. Edward Mullins the chirurgion, I asked her what hopes she had of laying this woman. She answered that she doubted not but that,

through God's assistance, she could quickly deliver her. So with the former old midwife's permission, the work was soon performed by the feet.[71]

Thus it was not only for the edification of his readers that Willughby invoked his daughter as the expert in breech births; he had also done so in actual practice, for he referred this particular birth to his daughter *because* it 'came by the buttocks'. Once again Eleanor succeeded in the task: although she reported the condition of the birth to her father, she delivered the child – as usual, by turning to the feet – without his help.

In two respects this case differed markedly from Eleanor's Stafford cases. In the first place, Eleanor gained access to this birth by way of her father – whereas in Stafford she had been practising independently of him. Secondly, when it came to the delivery itself, she secured 'the old midwife's permission' before delivering the child by the feet – whereas such 'permission' was not mentioned in her comparable case from near Newcastle-under-Lyme.[72] We shall return to these points a little later, when reviewing Eleanor's London practice as a whole.

The next case we must consider took place in 1657, and concerned one Mrs Wolaston. We have already encountered the rhetorical context of this story; for this was the very 'observation' which Willughby used to illustrate his encomium to William Harvey.[73] Thus the moral of Mrs Wolaston's delivery – or, rather, two deliveries – would be Willughby's endorsement of what he depicted as 'Dr Harvey's directions and method'. Like the unnamed mother in Shoe Lane, Mrs Wolaston first sought Willughby's services in an emergency:

My assistance was desired by Mrs Wolaston, a watchmaker's wife, of Threadneedle Street near the Old Exchange. When the midwife perceived that I was sent for, she resolved to hasten her work. She caused several women perforce to hold her by the middle, whilst that she, with others, pulled the child by the limbs one way, and the women [pulled] her body the other way. Thus, at the last, the child, by violence, was drawn from her, and made at the separation (as she told me) a report as though a pistol had been discharged.

A little while after this tugging and struggling usage I came, and found this woman faint and weak, but through God's mercy, with cordials she was restored. Her midwife's enforcements had made such deep remembrance in her senses, that she resolved to forsake her; at which time she pitched her affections on me, making a request unto me, if that she should have any more children, that I would be pleased to deliver her.[74]

This was a truly remarkable request, for very few women ever asked Willughby, or any other male practitioner, to act in lieu of a midwife.[75] Willughby declined – for he believed that normal birth was the province of the midwife, not of the male practitioner[76] – and made a different suggestion:

160

I desired her to spare me, and rather to engage my daughter, the which thing she was contented to do, so that in her extremity, I would not be far from her.

Thus *father and daughter were practising as a team*. Eleanor would deliver the mother; if difficulty arose, Percival 'would not be far'. This intended arrangement echoed what we have seen in the Shoe Lane case, where Eleanor, while taking responsibility for the delivery, reported the state of the case to her father before proceeding.

In due course Mrs Wolaston acted on this suggestion: that is, for her next delivery she engaged Eleanor as her midwife. For as Willughby went on to explain:

Being with child afterward, and my daughter with her, when the time of her delivery was come, and that the waters issued, a sharp throw accompanied the birth, and the child speedily followed the waters.

Then she began to grieve and complain (not imagining that the child was born), and to say, now I shall fall into my old pains and sufferings, and [I] perceive that it will be no better with me. My daughter, smiling, asked her what she meant, and whether she had two children, for one was born. She scarcely believed it, until that she heard the child to cry. The after-birth being fetched, and she laid in bed, she took my daughter by the hand and said to her, Surely you have art in these fingers, otherwise so quickly and happily I should not have been delivered.[77]

Doubtless the birth came by the head, though Willughby's account does not explicitly say so. This is the only such case of Eleanor's given in the *Observations*: all the others were breech births. Mrs Wolaston's two deliveries perfectly fitted the rhetorical setting in which Willughby placed her story, that is, the picture of normal birth which Harvey had sketched in his *De Generatione*. In the previous birth, the midwife's interference had inflicted unnecessary pain and suffering on the mother – bearing out Harvey's criticisms of 'officious' midwives. But in Eleanor's hands the birth proceeded naturally and easily, doubtless because Eleanor had waited for 'the time of her delivery', that is, for the moment when both mother and foetus were (as Harvey had put it) 'ready for the business'. As we have seen, Willughby immediately observed: 'I know none but Dr Harvey's directions and method'.[78] And in the London version of the 'Observations' he added: 'the which she always observed'.[79] That is, as Willughby depicted the matter, his daughter had been following Harvey's 'directions and method'.

Notice again the contrast with Eleanor's Stafford practice: she had gained access to Mrs Wolaston, just as she had to the mother in Shoe Lane, only by way of her father. Notice, too, that in each of these two London cases, Willughby was on hand should difficulty arise, though his services were not required in either case. This teamwork between daughter and father was also evident, albeit in a slightly different way, in Eleanor's remaining London delivery.

This final case of Eleanor's illustrates once again the complex intertwining of the typical and the atypical in Willughby's cases. In the first place, the delivery was typical of Eleanor's recorded cases in being yet another breech birth. Secondly, however, this was in other respects a remarkable delivery, and Willughby's description of the case has several unique features. Yet, thirdly, even the unusual aspects of the case (if not of Willughby's account of it) turn out to exemplify themes which were characteristic of his practice and indeed of seventeenth-century midwifery in general.

The delivery took place in 1658; Willughby located it not in London but in 'Middlesex' – that is, doubtless in the country house of the family in question. Willughby identified the mother cryptically (in the Derby version only) as 'Sir Tennebs Evanks lady': this was a code for someone with the surname Bennet – the key being 'Evank', i.e. 'Knave' reversed, which indicates what Willughby thought of the father.[80] It is almost certain that 'Sir Tennebs Evank' was Gervase Bennet – an irascible Puritan, who was (as Willughby described him in the London version) 'one of Oliver's creatures', that is, a client of Cromwell's, and who was active both in London (where he had a minor government post) and in Derby (where he served for a time as an alderman).[81] Bennet's first wife had died in 1655; this must have been either the first or the second delivery of his second wife. Willughby's account gives no indication of how Eleanor was chosen as midwife; but it is safe to assume that the choice had been made by Mrs Bennet herself (not by her husband), and it seems likely that she knew of Eleanor and/or of Percival not through London contacts but rather via some Midlands connection. Willughby's account of the birth began as follows:

In Middlesex anno 1658 my daughter, with my assistance, delivered Sir Tennebs Evanks lady of a living daughter.

All the morning my daughter was much troubled, and told me that she feared that the birth would come by the buttocks, and that she foresaw the same by the falling down of her belly.

About seven a clock that night labour approached. At my daughter's request, unknown to the Lady, I crept into the chamber upon my hands and knees, and returned, and it was not perceived by the Lady. My daughter followed me, and I – being deceived through haste to go away – said that it was the head. But she affirmed the contrary, however, if it should prove the buttocks, that she knew how to deliver her.

Her husband's greatness and oliverian power, with some rash expressions that he uttered flowing too unhandsomely from his mouth, dismayed my daughter.[82]

162

From the other recension of the *Observations* we learn what these 'rash expressions' were: 'Her husband, standing by us, said, what luck had he to be deluded by children and fools.' The word 'children', of course, referred to Eleanor's tender age (she was now nineteen or twenty years old); 'fools', to her father's ungainly crawling in and out of the lying-in chamber. We may picture Bennet as the anxious father outside the door – perhaps all the more anxious because he had lost his previous wife three years earlier, and forced to wait outside for the simple reason that husbands were always excluded from childbirth at this time. Indeed, the fact that the father is mentioned at all is one of the many unusual aspects of this particular 'observation'.[83] Willughby's account proceeded:

> She could not be quieted, until I crept privately again the second time into the chamber, and then I found her words true.
>
> I willed her to bring down a foot, the which she soon did. But being much disquieted with fear of ensuing danger, she prayed me to carry on the rest of the work.
>
> The Lady was safely laid of a living daughter by the feet. The child cried strongly and loudly, and was spriteful and very lively.
>
> Had this birth come by the head, I believe that it would have proved difficult, and more troublesome to the Lady, not without some disgraceful reflection upon me and my daughter.
>
> For the child's head, with the breast, was great. It would have slid very difficultly through the bones, and so the midwife could not have helped more than by anointing the body, and, with patience, waiting and expecting when that nature's force with the throes would have driven forth the child.
>
> But, when the birth cometh by the feet, the woman may be laid without throes – as hath formerly been said, and showed by several examples.[84]

There is much of interest in this remarkable story. In the first place, we see that Eleanor was better able than her father to diagnose the presentation; indeed, she correctly predicted, even before 'labour approached', that the birth would come 'by the buttocks'. This suggests that she had acquired significant experience not only of breech-births but also, for comparison, of births by the head – in line with our earlier inference as to her practice in Stafford. Secondly, and conversely, her father's misdiagnosis, which he explained as the result of his 'haste to go away' (that is, his concern to remain undetected by the mother), is also intelligible in the light of his limited experience of such cases, particularly in their early stages. Indeed, this may well have been the first time he had ever encountered a breech birth so early in the labour. Thirdly, it will be observed that Willughby's concluding remark – 'the woman may be laid without throes' – puts paid to Harvey's interpretation of the efficacy of delivery by the feet. The point of the manoeuvre was not, as Harvey had claimed, to assist the efforts of the uterus but, on the contrary, to replace those efforts.[85] Had Eleanor and her father literally been following 'Dr. Harvey's directions and method' when turning the birth to the feet, they would thereupon have left the delivery to the powers of the uterus; in fact, of course, they did the very opposite, for they turned the child to the feet in order to exert traction. This confirms that, as was observed earlier, Willughby's use of Harvey was rhetorical rather than literal.

Finally, the most striking aspect of the case is the fact that Willughby crept in and out of the lying-in room on his hands and knees – something unique among his case histories. The point of this deception, surely, was simple enough. The arrival of the male practitioner signalled that the birth was difficult; thus Willughby concealed his presence so as to avoid disquieting the mother. And what made this possible was the fact that the midwife was his own daughter; for the deception absolutely required the midwife's collusion, and there was no other midwife with whom Willughby enjoyed the necessary relation of mutual trust. In its very uniqueness, then, this feature of the story reflected entirely typical themes: the association of the male practitioner with difficulty and danger, and the fact that Willughby's relations with midwives were fraught with tension.

Equally significant is the sequel to the delivery – for this probably explains why Willughby included the case in his 'Observations'. Reverting again to the London version of the text, we find the following account:

He sent me home; I came several days after, but was scarce made to drink . . . [and was] never thanked for the care that I had of his wife.[86] [Here 'never thanked' means never paid.] About the 3rd or 4th day I asked him whether he had a nurse; he replied me, No, and said that he scorned that his child should suck any pocky whore. The child was fed with unfitting slip-slop nourishment; about the 7th day a nurse was procured, that would have given it the breast, but the infant had forgotten how to suck. Presently after the red-gum appeared, and for want of help, the child died.[87]

Now came the point:

Within a few days after, he endeavoured to blacken my daughter's practice, saying that she had made a hollowness in his child's head. Had his little worship known that all children have loose disjointed bones, with hollowness in the head, when they are born, his poor judgment would have been silent – seeing that every woman can assure him that without this hollowness and loose bones, a child will not be born. Had he had a nurse in fitting time, doubtless the child might have lived.

Bennet's vindictive efforts did not stop at his attempt to 'blacken' Eleanor's reputation in and about London, for as we shall see in a moment, he also put

164

about in Derby a story against Eleanor's father. We may guess that Bennet had not omitted to tell the hands-and-knees story, for Willughby could thus be ridiculed.

There can be little doubt that Willughby's account of the case was written in riposte to the rumours which Gervase Bennet was putting about. This becomes still more clear from a postscript which he added to the text a few years later, that is, after Bennet's death in 1670. With regard to Bennet's remark that 'he scorned that his child should suck any pocky nurse in or about London',[88] Willughby now commented: 'He well knew many unworthy women in that, and other places' – and posed a rhetorical question: 'And was he free from the lues venerea when he died?' Thereupon Willughby went on to assert that

> He loved variety of places, and several pastures. He reported about Derby, to disgrace me, that I would not come near to help his wife before that he had given me a hundred pieces [100 sovereigns – a very large sum]. He was never so worthy as to give or offer me the worth of a penny. And *if ever it be found out what his true name was*, and where he lived and died, let this postscript affirm, that he would not let me come near his wife after her delivery. And although I came several times, yet he did not afford me so much civility as to offer me a cup of ale or beer, or that ever he did give me the worth of a brass farthing for my oft visiting her afore her delivery; or for my being with her in her labour, and helping of her; or for my several visits after her delivery [emphasis mine].[89]

Plainly Willughby intended that his readers should be able to identify 'Sir Tennebs Evank' – but since this version of the 'Observations' languished in manuscript, this hope went unrealized.

Taken as a group, Eleanor's London cases suggest a very different profile of practice from that which she had enjoyed in Stafford. If, as is plausible, Willughby included all of her breech cases in his 'Observations', it is suspicious that although she spent nearly twice as long in London as she had in Stafford, we find only one instance of her acting in a primary capacity at a breech birth from London (namely the case of 'Sir Tennebs Evanks lady'), as against two from Stafford. This might, of course, be a random effect, yet *prima facie* it suggests a much lower rate of practice;[90] and other considerations point in the same direction. We have seen that Eleanor gained access to two of her three recorded London cases – the primary delivery of Mrs Wolaston and her secondary attendance on the mother in Shoe Lane – through her father. And her remaining recorded London case, namely the delivery of 'Sir Tennebs Evanks lady', had a Midlands connection: thus there is every possibility that 'Sir Tennebs Evanks lady' was aware of Eleanor through some Staffordshire link, rather than from any

London reputation of Eleanor's. What is more, this case, too, may have come Eleanor's way thanks to her father – for it will be observed that Percival himself had (if his postscript is to be believed) been attending the mother before the delivery. In short, there is strong reason to suspect that Eleanor was unable to achieve in London the success she had attained in Stafford in recruiting a clientele. In Stafford she had arrived as an unknown girl, yet had rapidly secured a remarkable reputation; but in London this eluded her, despite the experience she had by now acquired. Yet, meanwhile, her father's experience had been quite different, for as we have seen, on moving to London he had 'quickly had some practice in midwifery, among the meaner sort of women', thanks to 'an apothecary that formerly had lived in Stafford'. This double contrast with her own Stafford practice and with her father's achievements in London underlines the puzzle that has now arisen: why did Eleanor experience such difficulty in establishing herself as a midwife in London?

The explanation is probably to be sought in a set of arrangements which Willughby himself attested in a separate context, and which are also known from various other sources.[91] 'The young midwives in London', Willughby wrote, 'be trained seven years first under the old midwives, before they be allowed to practice for themselves.'[92] That is, in London – uniquely – a midwife was expected to begin practice as a deputy to an already established midwife: this custom was well established long before this date, for it was attested in the midwife's oath for the diocese of London as early as 1588.[93] This arrangement, which was evidently created by the midwives themselves, effectively constructed a guild system; yet it managed to achieve this without the institutional apparatus of enforcement usually associated with guilds. Notably, the deputy system *antedated* the various seventeenth-century attempts to create a London incorporation or college of midwives;[94] and whereas all these initiatives came to naught, the deputy system lasted for a century or more. Just how this system interacted with ecclesiastical licensing is unclear, and is indeed a matter of contention among historians.[95] But when the Willughby family was in London, that is, in the late 1650s, the deputy system certainly did not depend on church licensing – for that licensing had been a dead letter for fifteen years or more, with the suspension of the church courts after 1641. According to the later testimony of Mrs Elizabeth Cellier, London midwives were subject at this very time to licensing by the Company of Barbers and Surgeons;[96] thus if Mrs Cellier's picture is to be trusted, there was perhaps a form of institutional backing for the deputy system in the 1640s and '50s. But Mrs Cellier was a highly interested party (in 1687, when she recounted this story, she was trying to create a 'college of midwives' with herself at its head) and an unreliable witness, and there is no other evidence to indicate that any such arrangement in fact obtained.[97] In short, it appears that the deputy system was constructed and maintained by the midwives themselves, without the help of any institutional sanctions at all.

The various fragments of evidence which attest to the existence of the deputy system do not make clear how effective the system was in practice. But Eleanor Willughby's experience offers us an indication of this – for in view of her limited practice in London, it is plausible to infer that the system was highly successful. That is to say, *Eleanor was largely excluded from primary practice in London because she had not been trained as a deputy there.* Correspondingly, in the London secondary case which she obtained thanks to her father, she required 'the old midwife's permission' before delivering a child by the feet,[98] whereas no such permission was mentioned in her secondary case from Staffordshire. This authority of the older midwife, which was specific to London, becomes intelligible in the light of the deputy system, and again indicates that the system was functioning effectively at this time. Furthermore, Willughby's 'Observations' supply yet another reason for believing that the deputy system actually worked. For that system should have raised the standards of practice, by enabling midwives to pool their experience across the generations; and sure enough, we find that Willughby held a much higher opinion of London midwives than he did of their Midlands counterparts.[99] In short, there is every reason to believe that the London deputy system was thriving in the 1650s, and doubtless long before that time.

The very existence of the deputy system represented a remarkable achievement on the part of the London midwives. That achievement becomes truly astonishing if the system actually succeeded along the lines I have been suggesting. Yet there seems to be no other way of accounting for the remarkable disparity between Eleanor Willughby's meagre practice in London and the substantial practice she had sustained in Stafford.

6 ELEANOR AND HER FATHER IN DERBY

Towards the end of 1659 the Willughby family moved yet again, this time back to their starting-point in Derby. This move, which probably reflected a change in the political climate in Derby, seems to have curtailed Eleanor's midwifery practice, for no further cases of hers are recorded in the *Observations*. Nevertheless, we find her assisting her father in one case, and an important one at that: a delivery of Mrs Jane Molyneux of Woodcoats, Nottinghamshire. This was a case which Willughby recorded in immense and almost unparalleled detail, and with good reason. The mother's previous obstetric history supported his own views on the ignorance of midwives; her delivery gave him direct access to a birth from the onset of labour; the outcome was a happy one; and last but not least, the case occurred while he was beginning to write his 'Observations'.

Mrs Molyneux sought Willughby out for her delivery, and came to stay in his house for the last month of her pregnancy. She had been driven to this highly unusual course of action – using Willughby in lieu of a midwife – by losing no less than four children, under four different midwives, all in footling births.[100] (We may presume that she had some particular predisposition, for footling presentations were very rare.) When she fell into labour the birth came yet again 'by the knees doubled'; Willughby delivered her with the combined help of his daughter and one of the attending women – a 'threefold united force' – and Mrs Molyneux gave birth to a living child, a girl baptized Mary. Not surprisingly, this won her confidence for the future: she subsequently came to Derby again for three further deliveries, two of them after her remarriage in 1666 to Mr Thomas Wildbore.[101] These cases, too, Willughby wrote up in his 'Observations', one of them in lavish detail. But what we must notice is that when first helping Mrs Molyneux, Willughby involved his daughter as his equal in the procedure of the delivery even though it was to him not to Eleanor that Mrs Molyneux had come in the first place.[102] For this there was a simple but telling reason, which was mentioned in passing when we considered the case of Mrs Wolaston.[103] Just as very few mothers asked him to play the role of midwife, so too Willughby himself – for all his criticisms of practising midwives – believed that the female midwife, not a male practitioner such as himself, was the proper person to manage childbirth.[104] This ingrained assumption on Willughby's part reflected the conceptual horizon imposed by the fact that the male practitioner's task was to deliver a dead child, not a living baby.[105]

By this time, as we have seen, Eleanor Willughby seems to have stopped practising midwifery; perhaps she was now caught up in her impending marriage to Thomas Hurt, which took place in 1662, and which took her away from Derby (I have not ascertained precisely where the Hurts lived, but this was at some distance).[106] Notably, her father did not involve her in the subsequent deliveries of Mrs Molyneux/Wildbore in 1665, 1667 and 1669: indeed in the delivery of 1669 he was forced to entrust Mrs Wildbore to a Derby midwife, since he himself was already engaged elsewhere, and yet Eleanor did not play this role. This is hardly surprising, for at this time (November 1669) Eleanor had three young children of her own and was six months pregnant.[107] But meanwhile she had acquired a new connection with her father in the sphere of midwifery – for she called on his help in the management of at least two of her deliveries and lyings-in, and Willughby included these two cases in his 'Observations'. Although her father identified her in the text only as 'a young gentlewoman', not mentioning her in this context as his daughter, his marginalia and index name the patient as 'El. Hurt',[108] and it is well-nigh certain that 'El. Hurt' was indeed his daughter Eleanor.[109] Indeed, we shall see that Eleanor may even have taken the remarkable step of using her father in lieu of a midwife for all her deliveries, though this is a matter of conjecture.

After one of her first three deliveries (that is, in 1663, 1665 or 1666),[110] Eleanor was bleeding with clots for some seven weeks. Accordingly, she called on her father's help: after trying two prescriptions without success, he administered 'the powder of an unripe gall', which 'in thrice taking . . . quite stopped the flux'.

168

A few years later, during her seventh pregnancy (in late 1671), she experienced a different problem: the baby had ceased to move in the womb. She asked her father 'to come and stay with her'; after ten days, she fell into labour and he delivered her of a dead child, which came naturally and did not need to be turned to the feet.[111] Early in the 'Observations', Willughby stated: 'I have delivered, through God's gracious permission, a gentlewoman of several children'[112] – implying that this particular mother had used him in lieu of a midwife, for a whole sequence of deliveries, and apparently without any precipitating reason of the kind which had driven Mrs Molyneux to call on his services.[113] And it does indeed seem that he had acted as a midwife for this mother, for he had had something of a say in the social arrangements for these births: 'I . . . desired her, in the time of her travail, not to have her chamber thronged with much company.' This form of involvement was unique in the cases described in the 'Observations' precisely because even in Willughby's 'advance calls' it was not he but the midwife who presided over the social arrangements, just as it was the midwife who managed the birth as a bodily event. Thus this particular mother reposed a special trust in him, using him as she did in the role of a midwife. Who might this have been? There is no way of knowing, for Willughby completely concealed this gentlewoman's identity; but conceivably this too was Eleanor Hurt. If so, it would appear that she chose her father, in place of a midwife, from the outset of her childbearing career.

By early 1672, Percival Willughby's still-unpublished writings on midwifery had attained a paradoxical form, arising from the inevitable tension between systematic advice and its empirical exemplification, and from his changing handling of this problem. Originally, that is to say in the early 1660s, his 'Observations' had fused these two elements, using only a few selected case histories and subordinating these to a larger didactic frame. But since that time he had interpolated dozens of new cases into the text; and this additional illustrative material had come to obscure the structure of the work. Thus when three new popular books on midwifery were published in 1671,[114] he was spurred to re-state his argument in a new text, systematic in form and devoid of case histories. Accordingly he swiftly penned a new treatise, which he called 'The Country Midwife's Opusculum, or Vade-Mecum' – emphasizing by its very title that this was, in contrast with the now unwieldy 'Observations', a 'little work'. Yet he still wanted to support his claims with empirical proofs – 'de facto, what I have really performed'[115] – and he now recruited the 'Observations' for this purpose. His plan, then, was to publish the two works together so that they complemented each other: the 'Opusculum' would set out his advice systematically, while the 'Observations' would supply the illustrative case histories. Accordingly the 'Opusculum' referred explicitly to the 'Observations',[116] and Willughby also supplied some less explicit cross-references in the other direction.[117]

of Children. 113

cause him to sucke a Goate ; which I haue caused some to doe.

A Treacle water for the little child.

℞. *Theriac. veter.* ℥ *i. Cons. Rosar. anthos. Borag. Buglos. an.* ℥ *ij. Rasur. interior. lign. Indi.* ℥ *i. Rad. sarsæ par Chinæan.* ℥ *ss. Rad. scorzoner.* ℥ *vi. flor. Cordial. Calendul. Genist. an. m. ij. Aquar Cardui Benedict. Scabios. Borag. Buglos. Melissæ an. lib. 3. ponantur omnia in Alembico vitreo, postea macerentur spatio xxiiij. horar. deinde fiat destillatio, vt artis est.*   *Aqua Theriacalis.*

Let the child take a spoonfull of this water, three times a day, in the morning, at noone and at night, adding thereto a little suger Candy or sirup of Limons. The nurses may also take two ounces of it in the morning.   *The vse.*

And because the true Antidote against this disease, is Quickfiluer, therefore will it be very fit to annoint the childs pustules with some such Ointment, not bringing him to a fluxe of the mouth.

℞. *Vng. Rosat. Mes.* ℥ *iiij. Hydrargiri cum succo limonum extincti* ℥ *s. misce, fiat vng. pro litu.*   *The Ointment.*

If the child bee elder, let him bee purged twice with a little *Sene*; and sirup of Cichory, with *Rubarb*, neither will it be amisse (if hee be bigger and stronger) to open a veine, and take away a saucer full of bloud : He may also vse the foresaid decoction, and Opiate some eight or ten daies : onely diminishing the dofes of the Ingredients.

Bbb   *of*

A page from Jacques Guillemeau's *Child Birth or the Happy Deliverie of Women*, translated in 1612.

170

Had the 'Observations' consisted solely of case histories, Willughby would thus have arrived at precisely the literary form that was to be adopted a little later by François Mauriceau and again in the eighteenth century by William Smellie: that is, the textual separation of obstetric system on the one hand and its concrete exemplification on the other. But Willughby's pair of texts represented only an imperfect approximation to this solution, for the 'Observations', which were meant to supply the empirical component, still contained systematic advice as well. Further, the two works were structured in different ways, making it no easy matter for the reader to move between them as Willughby's new plan required.

Well aware of such problems, Willughby now placed the two texts in the hands of someone who was to act as editor; and he inserted some marginal instructions which recognized the unwieldy nature of the 'Observations' and gave this intended editor a free hand to revise the text as she or he saw fit.[118] In all probability, it was this individual who produced the two copies of the 'Observations' and 'Opusculum' which have come down to posterity. We do not know who this individual was; but there are grounds for suspecting that this was none other than Willughby's daughter Eleanor Hurt, the former midwife. Certainly the copyist was someone close to Willughby and indeed devoted to him. She or he copied out the whole text a second time for the sole purpose of incorporating 'The Index of the Auctor' (that is, Willughby's index of personal names). Further, this copyist also compiled 'An Additional Table' – to wit, a detailed subject-index, something which Willughby himself had not supplied.[119] With its 284 headings and 460 page-entries this table was remarkably complete, including as it did such headings as 'This book contains chiefly the Auctor's own ways in midwifery'; 'How a London midw: made' (referring to the deputy system); and 'When the Auctor left Stafford'.[120] Yet, strikingly, this copyist made no reference in the index to the 'Auctor's' daughter and her practice. The 'Additional Table' *did* cite Eleanor's cases – but merely under the headings 'Belly, back, buttocks'[121] and 'Dr. Harvey commended'.[122] It would appear, then, that this copyist deliberately refrained from including in the index the fact that the 'Auctor's' daughter was a midwife. And I suggest that the most plausible explanation of this omission is that the copyist was Eleanor herself.

This is, of course, only a conjecture; I have not been able to test it, for nothing has so far come to light which is known to have been written in the hand of Eleanor Hurt neé Willughby. But the conjecture is attractive – for it would mean that the *Observations*, in the physical form of their larger extant version, are themselves a memorial to Eleanor Willughby.

Notes

1 Sean Burke, *The Death and Return of the Author* (1992), p. 39.

2 Percival Willughby, *Observations in Midwifery. As also the country midwife's opusculum or vade mecum* (1863; facsimile reprint 1972); cited hereafter as *Observations*. This printing is based on the manuscript

as it stood in 1672, and includes the accompanying 'Opusculum', discussed below. An earlier recension, produced by Willughby in 1668, is BL, Sloane MS 529, ff. 1–19; this has never been published in English, though the Dutch printing of 1754 was based on essentially the same text. I refer to this 1668 recension as the 'London version' of the 'Observations' (cf. below, at note 41); a transcript is given in Appendix B of Adrian Wilson, 'Childbirth in Seventeenth- and Eighteenth-Century England' (D. Phil. thesis, University of Sussex, 1982). On the various MSS and editions, see Ch. 8 of the latter thesis, and also John L. Thornton's introduction to the 1972 reprint.

3 Percival Willughby and his wife Elizabeth (née Coke), who were married in 1631, had two daughters: Eleanor, baptized as Hellena on 10 February 1638/9, and Dorothy, baptized on 15 June 1642 (both at St Peter's, Derby). The midwife-daughter was practising in 1655; this surely rules out Dorothy, since she was only thirteen years old at this time. See further Wilson (1982) 'Childbirth', Appendix E.

4 Thus we learn more about the routine management of childbirth from Ralph Josselin's diary and from Willughby's *Observations* than we do from Alice Thornton's retrospective account of her deliveries. See Thornton (1873), pp. 84–98, 123–7, 139–51, 164–7; Josselin (1976), pp. 37–50, 101–11, 145–65, 231–57, 313–25, 399–415, 453–65, 496–502; *Observations, passim.*

5 Cf. Paul de Man (1983), particularly the essay 'The rhetoric of blindness: Jacques Derrida's Reading of Rousseau' (pp. 102–41).

6 Burke (1992), pp. 38–9.

7 *Observations,* p. 125; this case will be discussed in detail in my *A Safe Deliverance: childbirth in sevententh-century England* (London, UCL Press, forthcoming). In this and most other extended quotations I have modified Willughby's punctuation.

8 Willughby's account suggested that the delivery took place a 'few years' before Grace Beechcraft was buried (after another difficult birth) on 24 September 1657. In fact the case he delivered occurred only two years before her burial, for the stillbirth he delivered can certainly be identified with a (double) entry in the register of St Peter's, Derby, referring to the burial of an 'infant filia Joseph Beechcraft' on 1 October and 30 September 1655: see Wilson (1982), 'Childbirth', Appendix C (p. 4).

9 Had the women been united in this respect, Willughby would probably have written that 'the women' frowned upon some of these divines; but in fact he wrote only that '*several women*' did so.

10 'Observations', London version, p. 22. On the extant versions, cf. below, at note 41.

11 *Observations,* p. 94 (the case of Clare Pearson). Similarly, it is quite possible that he took his daughter to Grace Beechcraft's delivery (as he did in another case around this time: below, at note 53), even though this is not mentioned in his account of the case.

12 Above, at pp. 161 and 166–7 (Mrs Bennett, Mrs Molyneux).

13 See my essays 'The ceremony of childbirth and its interpretation', in Fildes (1990) and 'William Hunter and the varieties of man-midwifery', in Bynum and Porter (1985).

14 Above, p. 162.

15 In the case of births by the head, what is nowadays regarded as most important is the *orientation* of the foetal head. But Willughby never reported this; in his eyes, what counted was the *size* of the child's head. In fact these aspects were probably related: cf. A. Wilson (1995).

16 Particularly compound presentation (hand and foot). These can probably be regarded as a

172

variant of arm-presentation; including these would make little difference to the picture presented below.

17 Cf. A. Wilson (1995), pp. 11–15.

18 Incidence: Galabin (1904). Difficulty: below, at note 100.

19 See 'The ceremony of childbirth and its interpretation', Fildes (1990).

20 See for instance Hitchcock (1967); the origins of the various clauses of the oath will be considered in A. Wilson (forthcoming).

21 This allowance is achieved by assumptions (d) and (e) in Table 7.2, each of which probably overstates the case. As to assumption (d), only in about a third of Willughby's emergency cases was more than one midwife present (though, admittedly, the number was sometimes as high as four, or 'several'). As to assumption (e), certain individual midwives were probably favoured in calls of this kind, and these particular midwives must have received a disproportionate share of the total. For some justification of the first three assumptions, see A. Wilson (forthcoming), chs 2 and 3.

22 Thus Willughby referred to one midwife 'that was accounted the prime midwife of Staffordshire': 'Observations', London version, p. 33.

23 Thus in Derby, where Willughby was based for most of his working life, there were three midwives in a single parish in the 1680s. See further A. Wilson (1995), pp. 33–5, and Wilson (1982), Table 5.3.1.

24 The incidence of arm presentations has been inflated by rounding. The estimate of 1 such primary case in ten years has been rounded up from 0.8; the estimate of 2 such 'secondary' cases in ten years has been rounded up from 1.6. A more accurate estimate of the total number would thus be 2.4 in ten years, i.e. about one such case every four years.

25 As Bernice and Jeffrey Boss have correctly observed, systematic training could have conferred the requisite experience, even with low prevailing case loads: Boss and Boss (1983). But there was no such system of training in seventeenth-century England – with the important exception of London (p. 165, above).

26 For further details and illustrative cases, see my 'William Hunter and the varieties of man-midwifery' in Bynum and Porter (1985).

27 As presented here, this reasoning appears to be circular, since Table 7.3 has assumed (for convenience) that Willughby was called to most of the difficult births in his catchment area. But, in fact, this assumption is itself derived from an analysis of his recorded cases, to be presented in A. Wilson (forthcoming).

28 Revival of the child: *Observations*, pp. 40, 66, 82 (but contrast p. 186); A. Wilson (1995), p. 36.

29 But if he was called to act in lieu of a midwife, he did take an interest in such matters: cf. below, after note 108.

30 In Table 7.2 this is an artefact of rounding; the estimated incidence of such cases, according to the assumptions used in constructing the table, was in fact 0.37 obstructed breech births in ten years (0.12 in a midwife's 'primary' practice, plus 0.25 in her 'secondary' practice). That is, in a ten-year period about one in every three midwives would encounter a case of breech obstruction. Further, most midwives probably saw no obstructed breech births at all in their 'primary' practices – since even in thirty years of practice (a generous assessment of the typical midwife's working life), the expected number of such cases was only 0.36.

31 For a fuller discussion of what follows see A. Wilson (1995), pp. 19–22.

32 In later technical jargon: internal podalic version with traction.

33 This relative lateness of his arriving at the method was well concealed in the *Observations* – for good reasons, which will be discussed in A. Wilson (forthcoming). Cf. notes 38, 50, 57 below.

34 'Let midwives therefore be persuaded, that as oft as they perceive the child to be coming forth in an evil posture, either with his belly or back forward, or as it were doubled, in a crooked posture, or with his hands and feet together, or with his head forward and one of his hands stretched over his head, or with the buttocks, that they ought to turn the birth, and to draw it out by the feet' (*Observations*, p. 56).

35 'Observations', London version, p. 35. In practice Willughby was remarkably equivocal about using turning for obstructed births by the head: see A. Wilson (1982), pp. 282–9, and A. Wilson (forthcoming). For 'Dame Nature' (below) see *Observations*, pp. 10, 234.

36 Precisely the same tension was manifested by twin births, by the management of the placenta, and in births by the head where the child was still alive. On the placenta and twins see A. Wilson (1995), pp. 162–3; a more detailed discussion of Willughby's experiences will be included in A. Wilson (forthcoming).

37 'I have known some children coming by the buttocks, and so born' (*Observations*, p. 56); below, at note 57.

38 *Observations*, pp. 132–3 (John Plimer's wife). Note that in the case of 'Tab's wife', from 1632 (p. 130), Willughby had *not* turned the child to the feet, but instead had 'alter[ed] the posture' in some unspecified way. He left unclear in the 'Observations' just what this earlier technique was – because he no longer followed the method. Cf. notes 33 above, 50 and 57 below.

39 *Observations*, p. 6.

40 On the postulated initial version of 1662, cf. A. Wilson (1982), pp. 171–3 and Appendix D.

41 On these MSS, and also on the printed editions discussed below, see John L. Thornton, 'Introduction' to *Observations*, and A. Wilson (1982), Ch. 8.

42 *Observations*, p. 257.

43 William Harvey, *Disputations*, tr. Gweneth Whitteridge (1981), pp. 393–419, quoted from pp. 403–4; my emphases in the following quotations.

44 Yet cf. note 46 below.

45 Harvey (1981), pp. 405–6.

46 At this point Harvey was curiously eliding his own argument that it is not just the uterus but the whole of the mother's body which accomplishes the delivery.

47 *Observations*, p. 118.

48 Above, p. 159.

49 *Observations*, pp. 12, 151, 191; cf. also pp. 73, 156, 158, 206, 310, 324 and 342, where Willughby asserted the need for practical experience.

50 *Ibid., passim*, esp. pp. 324, 326 (this passage is part of the 'Opusculum'). In fact, Willughby had followed this method in his early practice, as we discover fortuitously from a case of 1633 which he 'inserted' for other reasons: see *Observations*, pp. 97–8 (Goodwife Osborn). Cf. notes 33, 38 above, 57 below.

51 Cf. above, p. 149.

174

52 See above, p. 166; also *Observations*, p. 126 (case of Mrs Okeover).

53 *Ibid.*, p. 158.

54 Above, at Table 7.1.

55 Above, p. 145. On the midwife's authority, cf. above, pp. 159, 165.

56 *Observations*, p. 130.

57 *Ibid.*, 'One Mrs Staynes, a chirurgion's wife in Derby, was delivered of a child in such a posture, in the year 1630, the child coming double, sitting with his buttocks in the womb. She did very well after her delivery, and her child lived.' Willughby left it unclear whether he had actually carried out this delivery, doubtless because he now wanted to distance himself from this expectant approach. Cf. notes 33, 38, 50 above.

58 *Observations*, p. 6; cf. above, p. 150.

59 *Ibid.*, pp. 134–5.

60 No more than 75 births were taking place each year in Stafford at this time, and probably fewer: see note 64 below. If there were 75 births per year, an obstructed breech birth would take place there only once in twenty years, on the assumptions of Table 7.2.

61 If the catchment area accounted for 1,000 births per year, we find (again applying the assumptions of Table 7.2) that one such case would take place every twenty months, which is just enough to account for this one such case of Eleanor's.

62 If the incidence of breech births was 1 in 30, and Eleanor saw 2 breech births from the onset of labour, then the odds are more than 20 to 1 against her rate of practice being as low as 10 cases per year. This result is reached by binomial probability, for which see Spiegel (1975), p. 108.

63 This from the fact that breech births were about 1 in 30 of all births (1 in 33 on the assumptions of Table 7.2). Precision is impossible because the occurrence of rare events (in this case, breech births) is subject to massive random variation. Even a very low case load cannot be ruled out absolutely (cf. the previous note); conversely, a high case load is also possible (for instance, if Eleanor attended as many as 100 deliveries, there would still be a better than 1 in 3 chance that she saw as *few* as two breech cases or less).

64 The population of Stafford at this time was probably somewhere between 1,400 and 1,800. Assuming that the birth rate was in the range 30 to 40 per 1,000, the annual numbers of births fell somewhere between 42 and 72. A best guess might be a population of 1,600, a birth rate of 35 per 1,000, and thus some 56 births per year. See *Victoria County History Staffordshire*, vol. 6 (1979), p. 186; Whiteman and Clapinson (1986), pp. 438, 454; Wrigley and Schofield (1981). In view of the figures from the town survey of 1622 and from the 1666 Hearth Tax returns (*VCH Staffs*, vol. 6), it would appear that the Compton census return for 'Stafford' included the whole town (as Whiteman assumes at p. 438), rather than the parish of St Mary alone (as Whiteman suggests at p. 454, note 219).

65 Even if each obstructed breech birth drew in as many as four midwives in a 'secondary' capacity, a typical midwife would have been called to just one such case every twenty years (on the assumptions of Table 7.2). If such cases drew in three 'secondary' midwives (as obtained in Eleanor's Case 2), this becomes almost twenty-eight years; if they drew in just two 'secondary' midwives, it would take over forty years for the typical midwife to receive such a call.

66 Above, p. 156, after note 59.

67 Even if as many as 75 births took place each year in Stafford, this would only yield 4.5 breech

births in two years; the more plausible estimate of 60 births per year implies 3.6 breech births in two years (cf. note 64 above).

68 Harley (1993).

69 I have come across no examples of this in some dozens of Norwich testimonials for ecclesiastical licences c. 1700: Norfolk and Norwich Record Office, Norwich diocesan records, TES/8, file i.

70 Observations, p. 238.

71 Ibid., p. 135.

72 Cf. above, at note 55, and see further below, at note 98.

73 Above, p. 153.

74 Observations, pp. 118–19.

75 When Alice Thornton was disappointed by her midwife, she found another midwife rather than securing the services of a male practitioner. Again, when the wife of an eminent apothecary in Newark (Notts) 'resolved never more to make use of the midwife's assistance', she did not resort to a male practitioner but instead gave birth unassisted, alone in her bedroom. Further, Willughby's cases include only a few mothers who used his services in lieu of a midwife, and in such cases special circumstances prevailed. See Thornton (1873), pp. 123–7; Observations, pp. 40–2, 240–1; note 113 below.

76 Cf. p. 167.

77 Observations, p. 119.

78 Above, p. 153.

79 'Observations', London version, p. 10.

80 Willughby also used 'evank' for 'knave' to refer to two other individuals: Observations, pp. 31, 249.

81 I owe this identification to Gerald Aylmer; detailed supporting reasons and further biographical details are given in A. Wilson (1982), Ch. 9, notes 76 and 77.

82 Observations, pp. 135–7.

83 Cf. above, p. 142.

84 Observations, p.136.

85 Cf. above, p. 153.

86 I have modified the wording here; in the MS this reads as follows: 'I came several days after, but was scarce made to drink; however never thanked for the care that I had of his wife.'

87 Observations, p. 21.

88 Notice that in this, the Derby version, Willughby slightly reworded the quotation from Bennet: e.g. 'pocky nurse' for 'pocky whore'.

89 Observations, p. 137

90 It will be recalled that in Stafford, her case load was probably well over 10 births a year (cf. note 62 above). In London, by contrast, a best guess would be less than 10 births a year, for she had one breech case which she had attended from the onset of labour, suggesting a total practice of 30 cases in a period of three and a half years.

91 Cf. Aveling (1882), p. 37, and other references cited below.

92 Observations, p. 73.

93 Hitchcock (1967).

176

94 Two such attempts were made by members of the Chamberlen family in 1617 and 1634: see Aveling (1882). A final such initiative came from Mrs Elizabeth Cellier in 1687; see King (1993), pp. 115–30, and cf. below.

95 Doreen Evenden suggests that ecclesiastical licensing worked to support the deputy system; I have argued that the efforts of the Church worked in the long run to undermine the deputy system. See Evenden (1993), pp. 9–26; A. Wilson (1995), p. 33.

96 Elizabeth Celleor (*sic*) (1688), p. 6, quoted in Aveling (1872), p. 89.

97 Cf. King, 'The politick midwife', p. 122. For Mrs Cellier, including her earlier stormy political career, see also *DNB*; Donnison (1977), pp. 18–20; Aveling (1872), pp. 63–85; Fraser (1984; 1985), pp. 513–22.

98 Above, p. 159.

99 *Observations*, pp. 45, 239, 240 (though cf. also pp. 22–4, and of course the cases of Mrs Wolaston and the Shoe Lane mother, pp. 118–19, 135, discussed above).

100 *Ibid.*, pp. 138–40.

101 *Ibid.*, pp. 140–6; see also pp. 22, 330.

102 As it happened, Willughby was to act as midwife to another mother (Lady Byron) just a few months later, in August 1661 (*ibid.*, pp. 40–2). Surprisingly, Eleanor was not involved on this occasion; perhaps this was because this particular engagement involved Willughby's staying in the mother's house.

103 Above, pp. 158–9.

104 Hence the fact that several of his uses of the word 'man-midwife' were scornful and associated with what he saw as malpractice: *Observations*, pp. 22, 88, 248 (though for neutral references see pp. 17, 340).

105 Cf. A. Wilson (1995), Ch. 4.

106 The marriage took place on 23 October 1662 (the year is given as '1663' in A. Wilson (1982), Appendix E, p. (1), but this is a typographical error). Although the family lived at some distance (as we know from the case discussed above, p. 168), Eleanor's children were all baptized in Derby (see note 107 below).

107 Dates of her children's baptisms (and burials), from the bishop's transcripts for St Peter's, Derby (Lichfield Joint Record Office): 6.8.63; 9.6.65 [bur. 4.12.67]; 25.9.66; 8.10.67 [bur. 18.1.71/2]; 21.12.68 [bur. 20.2.68/9]; 15.2.69/70; 11.2.72/3; 1.9.74; 23.12.80.

108 Marginalia: 'El. Hu.' (*Observations*, p. 179), 'El. Hurt' (*ibid.*, p. 254). Index: 'El. H. El. H.' (*sic*, p. 281, citing both the former entries).

109 The date of her stillbirth (6 December 1671) falls within a three-year gap in the sequence of recorded baptisms for Eleanor Hurt's children (i.e. between 15 February 1669/70 and 11 February 1672/3): cf. note 107 above and see A. Wilson (1982), Appendix E, p. 4.

110 The fact that this case was included in the London version dates it to before April 1668, thus restricting it to Eleanor's first four deliveries; the fact that the case was undated probably rules out her fourth delivery, since at this time (October 1667) Willughby was giving exact dates to all the cases he included in the 'Observations'. (Cases which occurred during the years 1663–6 were mostly written down later, from recall, and were thus left undated, as in this instance, or were dated only approximately: A. Wilson (1982), Appendix C.) *Observations*, p. 179; London version, p. 32.

111 Willughby inserted the case as an illustration of a technical point from Harvey: that when the foetus has died yet the delivery proceeds naturally, 'the water is the cause of the delivery . . . in that by its corruption and acrimony, it doth extimulate the uterus to relieve itself', *Observations*, pp. 254–5.

112 *Ibid.*, p. 38.

113 The few other women who resorted to Willughby in lieu of a midwife did so either because they had previously had difficult births (Mrs Wolaston in London, Mrs Molyneux in the Midlands) or through 'great fears' of giving birth (Lady Byron: *Observations*, pp. 40–2). In contrast, Willughby's account of the deliveries of this unnamed 'gentlewoman' include no mention of any expected difficulty in the birth.

114 Sermon (1671), Sharp (1671), Wolveridge (1671).

115 *Observations*, p. 210. This remark is not from the 'Opusculum' itself; but for words to similar effect from the latter, cf. *Observations*, pp. 311–12.

116 *Ibid.*, pp. 304, 315, 318 (margin), 324, 326.

117 *Ibid.*, pp. 101, 164, 166 ('See the schemes', etc.).

118 See *ibid.*, pp. 93, 99 (marginalia).

119 It appears that the copyist first proceeded without attending to pagination; that on encountering Willughby's index, she or he realized that this created a problem of collation; and that she or he accordingly produced a second copy which followed Willughby's pagination. See A. Wilson (1982), Appendix D.9.

120 *Observations*, pp. 296, 296, 298 respectively.

121 *Ibid.*, p. 277, referring to pp. 91, 120, 129, 130 'etc.', i.e. 130ff.

122 *Ibid.*, p. 294, referring to pp. 118–19.

BIBLIOGRAPHY

PRIMARY SOURCES

Cellier, E. (1688) *A Letter to Dr. —— An Answer to his Queries, concerning the Colledg of Midwives; Together with the Scheme for a Cradle Hospital, for Exposed Children.* [London].

Galabin, A.L. (1904). *A Manual of Midwifery.* 6th edn. London: Churchill.

Harvey, William (1981). *Disputations Touching the Generation of Animals,* tr. Gweneth Whitteridge. Oxford: Basil Blackwell.

Josselin, Ralph (1976). *The Diary of Ralph Josselin 1616–1683,* ed. A. MacFarlane. *British Academy Records of Social and Economic History,* New Series, 3.

Sermon, William (1671). *The Ladies Companion or the English Midwife.* London.

Sharp, Jane (1671). *The Midwives Book. Or the whole art of midwifry.* London: Simon Miller.

Thornton, Alice (1873). *The Autobiography of Mrs. Alice Thornton, of East Newton, C. York,* ed. C. Jackson. Surtees Society Publications, vol. 62.

Willughby, Percival (1863). *Observations in Midwifery. As also the country midwife's opusculum or vade mecum,* ed. Henry Blenkinsop. Facsimile reprint, ed. John L. Thornton, Wakefield: S.R. Publishers, 1972.

Wolveridge, James (1671). *Speculum Matricis.* London.

SECONDARY SOURCES

Aveling, J.H. (1872). *English Midwives: Their History and Prospects.* London: Churchill.

—— (1882). *The Chamberlens and the Midwifery Forceps: Memorials of the Family and an Essay on the Invention of the Instrument.* London: Churchill.

Boss, Bernice and Boss, Jeffrey (1983). 'Ignorant Midwives – a Further Rejoinder', *Bulletin of the Society for the Social History of Medicine,* 33.

Burke, Sean (1992). *The Death and Return of the Author: Criticism and Subjectivity in Barthes, Foucault and Derrida.* Edinburgh: Edinburgh University Press.

Bynum, W.F. and Porter, R. (eds) (1985). *William Hunter and the Varieties of Man-Midwifery.* Cambridge: Cambridge University Press.

Donnison, Jean (1977). *Midwives and Medical Men: a History of Inter-Professional Rivalries and Women's Rights.* London: Heinemann.

Evenden, Doreen (1993). 'Mothers and their Midwives in Seventeenth-Century London' in Marland (ed.) (1993), pp. 9–26.

Fildes, Valerie (ed.) (1990). *Women as Mothers in Pre-Industrial England. Essays in Memory of Dorothy McLaren.* London: Routledge.

Fraser, Antonia (1984). *The Weaker Vessel: Woman's Lot in Seventeenth-century England.* London: Weidenfeld & Nicolson. (Pbk edn, London: Methuen, 1985.)

Harley, David N. (1993). 'Provincial Midwives in England: Lancashire and Cheshire, 1660-1760' in Marland (1993), pp. 27–48.

Hitchcock, James (1967). 'A Sixteenth-Century Midwife's License', *Bulletin of the History of Medicine,* 41, 75–6.

King, Helen, 'The politick midwife: models of midwifery in the work of Elizabeth Cellier', in Marland (ed.) (1993), pp. 115-130.

Man, Paul de (1983). *Blindness and Insight: Essays in the Rhetoric of Contemporary Criticism.* Minneapolis, MN: Minnesota University Press. (First published 1971.)

Marland, Hilary (ed.) (1993). *The Art of Midwifery: Early Modern Midwives in Europe.* London: Routledge.

Spiegel, Murray R. (1975), *Theory and Problems of Probability and Statistics* (New York: McGraw-Hill.)

Whiteman, Anne with Clapinson, Mary (1986). *The Compton Census of 1676: a Critical Edition.* London: British Academy, and Oxford: Oxford University Press.

Wilson, Adrian (1982). 'Childbirth in Seventeenth- and Eighteenth-Century England', unpublished D.Phil. thesis, University of Sussex.

—— (1995). *The Making of Man-Midwifery: Childbirth in England, 1660-1770.* London: UCL Press.

—— (forthcoming). *A Safe Deliverance: Childbirth in Seventeenth-Century England.* London: UCL Press.

Wrigley, E.A. and R.S. Schofield (1981). *The Population History of England 1541–1871.* London: Edward Arnold.

IV

The politics of medical improvement in early Hanoverian London

EIGHTEENTH-CENTURY 'IMPROVEMENT' AND MEDICINE

How does medical history fit into history at large – into 'general' or 'political' or 'social' history? The history disciplines themselves both imply and construct an answer: the relationship is the non-relationship of parallel stories, linked only by the fact that they inhabit the dimension of time. We have a sub-discipline called medical history, with its own sources, methods, topics, problems and concerns; this is more or less walled off from that series of other sub-disciplines which together comprise mainstream academic history – political, social and economic history. These in turn are to some extent sealed off from each other; so too a similar hermetic quality is to be found in all the sub-disciplines, such as ecclesiastical history, history of art, history of science. Worst of all, perhaps, is the fate of the study of what is deemed literature: hived off into an entirely separate discipline. What historians have sundered, let no woman or man put together again: there are

Editors' note. The term 'whig' and its derivatives are used in this chapter in two senses. One (whig, whiggery), to refer to the Whig political party and its values; this is to be contrasted with 'Tory'. Two (whig, whiggish), to refer to a certain kind of history-writing in which the criteria for deciding what counts as 'interesting' and what constituted 'success' or 'progress' in the past, are drawn from the criteria of what counts as 'interesting', 'success' or 'progress' *in the present*; on this usage see Herbert Butterfield, *The Whig Interpretation of History* (London, 1931).

Acknowledgements: The research for this paper was supported by the generosity of the Wellcome Trust. Manuscript and printed sources were consulted in the Greater London Record Office; the British Library; the Wellcome Institute Library; and Cambridge University Library. I am grateful to the staffs of all these institutions for their help. From 1983 to 1986 I was fortunate to have the opportunity to teach on these topics in the Wellcome Unit for the History of Medicine, Cambridge. Participants in the discussion at the 1987 conference, especially David Harley, offered valuable comments. For detailed advice I wish to thank Jonathan Clark, Mark Goldie, Gill Hudson, Robert Kilpatrick and Julian Martin. Craig Rose and Simon Schaffer have given me extended help in the course of many valuable discussions. Finally, I am particularly grateful to Andrew Cunningham for several years of generous encouragement, stimulation and advice in the exploration of the themes treated in this paper.

many individual examples of the transcending of these barriers, yet these remain isolated examples which have little or no effect on the structure of the discipline. Thus even when eighteenth-century English history is hotted up by recent fierce debate, the battle has been conducted largely on the traditional high-ground of political history, with only occasional side-glances elsewhere.[1]

Most of my own research concerns early-eighteenth-century England. One of the striking characteristics of that society was the vast and profound influence exercised by its capital, the metropolis of London, a concentration of population which when set against its hinterland had no parallel or precedent in European history. (Paris had more inhabitants, but could not compare with London's astonishing share of its nation's population – something approaching 10 per cent.) The complex threads of trade, migration, politics and propaganda tied even the remotest parts of the kingdom to London. The social history of London in the eighteenth century, then, must comprise a very important part of English, indeed British, history at large.

Historiographically, one work has now towered over this field for over sixty years: Dorothy George's *London Life in the Eighteenth Century*.[2] Published in 1925, that book was to prove the most enduring and successful monument to the labours of the remarkable 'first wave' of English women historians – the circle including Eileen Power and Alice Clark, and centring around the influence of the redoubtable Olive Schreiner.[3] George's study was an extraordinary *tour de force*, a commanding survey of many aspects of eighteenth-century London life (from the family to the economy) and, no less so, of the vast pamphlet literature of the period. To this day no challenge has been mounted to George's synthesis, and it is not difficult to see why: the terrain she covered remains dauntingly vast. I doubt whether any historian since has read a tenth of the materials she covered: the Old Bailey Sessions Papers (almost her sole manuscript source); the Bills of Mortality; the writings of Hanway, Fielding, Place, Colquhoun, and a host of less eminent reformers, projectors and improvers; and dozens

---

[1] I refer to the debate opened up by J. C. D. Clark, *English Society 1688–1832: Ideology, Social Structure and Political Practice during the Ancien Régime* (Cambridge, 1985). For a discussion of the implications of what has been called 'tunnel history' see T. G. Ashplant and Adrian Wilson, 'Present-Centred History and the Problem of Historical Knowledge', *The Historical Journal* 31 (1988), pp. 253–74.

[2] M. Dorothy George, *London Life in the Eighteenth Century* (London, 1925; Harmondsworth, 1966).

[3] See the discussion by Jane Lewis in Miranda Chaytor and Jane Lewis, 'Introduction' to Alice Clark, *Working Life of Women in the Seventeenth Century* (London, 1982, reprint of 1919 first edition).

of tracts concerning the regulation of wages, the administration of the Poor Law, the constructing of hospitals, the managing of police – and even medicine. In its breadth and intensity, her study is reminiscent of the writings of her equally daunting predecessors, Sydney and Beatrice Webb. These days, few historians even consider tackling topics of this scale.

What place did medicine find in this remarkable synthesis? The answer can be given in a single word: *improvement*. In this respect medicine simply exemplified George's wider themes: the story she told was precisely one of 'improvement' across a vast social terrain: improvements in housing, in lighting, in hygiene, in the care of children, in policing, in prisons, in diet. Down to roughly the mid-century, conditions were squalid and crowded and probably worsening; thereafter, a series of schemes for improvement brought about a gradual, but eventually massive, amelioration. In some spheres of life there would be a temporary decline – for instance, an 'epidemic of gin-drinking' in the 1720s and 1730s, or the massive abandonment of children when the Foundling Hospital's doors were temporarily thrown open between 1756 and 1760. But each such instance brought about the appropriate response: the Gin Act of 1736 and the restriction of Foundling Hospital admissions in 1760. In some contexts there were schemes for improvement at an unusually early date – as, for instance, in the parish of St James Westminster, with its workhouse, infirmary and provision for lying-in women, all evident by 1732; other parishes lagged far behind, yet a variety of supra-parochial initiatives eventually spread such benefits across the capital. Thus the story of improvement was by no means simultaneous or geographically homogeneous. Yet that story was indeed the general pattern; and in broad terms, the mid-century marked a watershed. Most of George's central improving characters – Hanway, Fielding, Colquhoun and Howard – were active after 1750.

It would be going far beyond my present brief to offer that general critique of George's work which remains wanting from the historical profession as a whole. Not until we have become able to mount such a critique, I suggest, will we be able to move beyond George's achievement and thus to build constructively on the foundations she laid: as long as we remain mesmerised by her achievement, our horizons will remain defined by her problematic. Thus the task of appraising George's study cannot properly be attempted here. Nevertheless, if we are to move forward at all, we must make some attempt to characterise the boundaries of her approach, the limits of her problematic; and in this spirit three observations are in order. First, it is striking that for George, the process of 'improvement' she chronicled in such detail never posed an *explanatory* problem. The need for improvement, in her eyes, was self-evident: squalor itself begat the schemes for its abolition; the Hanways and the Fieldings emerged, so to speak, by spontaneous generation from the filth and disorder, the crime and the uncertainty, of London. Given Gin Lane, we have Hogarth, and given Hogarth, we have the Gin Act; a logical necessity generated ameliora-tion. Second, the towering absence in George's book is the sphere of *politics*. One would never have guessed from her study that eighteenth-century London was riven by political faction; that Jacobites plotted in coffee-houses; that the charity schools were the arena not only of education but also of faction; that this was the city where the cry 'Wilkes and Liberty' brought tens of thousands onto the streets in the 1760s; that here, a generation later, the first Corresponding Society came into being. This should begin to trouble us when we notice that some of these phenomena impinged directly on George's own themes. We see this at the beginning of the century with the charity schools, and at the end with the fact that Francis Place – George's most favoured observer – was heavily involved in the London Corresponding Society and in later schemes for electoral reform, culminating of course in Chartism. Strangely enough, George's idea of social history turns out to conform remarkably well to the definition offered by her near-contemporary G. M. Trevelyan: 'history with the politics left out'.[4] Is it not curious that we now remember Trevelyan's description only with amusement, yet we continue to be held in thrall by George's study, which in fact embodies that very definition at work?

A third observation concerns George's source materials. I am not suggesting that the historian is the passive prisoner of her or his sources: on the contrary, the historian constitutes the sources, above all by selecting them. And George's selection, as we have already noticed in passing, was overwhelmingly concentrated upon printed materials. Now these materials – the pamphlets and accounts which George used on such a massive scale – have this in common: they were *appeals* for public support. The printed pamphlet was an intervention in a market-place: what was at stake was support, both political and financial, for the given scheme of improvement, whether it be the raising of a tax on spirituous liquors, or the marshalling of a more effective police force, or the preservation of the lives of parish children.

---

[4] G. M. Trevelyan, *English Social History* (London, 1944), p. vii.

Any such scheme for improvement began as the plan or dream of a small and select group – sometimes, indeed, of a single individual – and then had to mobilise wider support. The pamphlet literature was precisely the means by which that mobilisation was brought about. Now in order to achieve this, the pamphleteer was subject to one cardinal rule: he or she (it was usually he) had to present the given scheme as having universal benefits or, to be more precise, benefits universal amongst the intended audience, that is, the politically and financially active class. And this had two general effects. First, there was a rigorous suppression of any *particular* interest which lay behind the given scheme. The key to success was precisely presenting interests as general: thus, for instance, in propounding a Tory scheme for a workhouse, the pamphleteer would carefully conceal the party provenance of the initiative. Secondly, and relatedly, there was developed a specific rhetoric for such appeals: the rhetoric of 'improvement'. It was the concept of improvement which permitted the eighteenth-century projector or reformer to couch his (or, rarely, her) scheme in a language of potentially universal appeal. 'Improvement' seized the moral high ground: opponents could appear as the obstructors of progress. Thus the medium of print and the market-place for support inexorably pulled the language of the pamphlets in the direction of 'improvement'.

These three aspects of George's work were inextricably bound together. The vocabulary of improvement gave her an instant rapport with a certain set of source materials – for that vocabulary, taken up and developed by nineteenth-century progressives, remained in force for George's own generation and precisely for her own intellectual circle. George's own indifference to party-political themes found ample confirmation in the pamphlets' concealment of the particular interests which had given rise to their various schemes. And this happy collusion between the historian and her materials was what excluded explanatory questions from the historiographic agenda: identification, such as George's identification with Hanway or Fielding, does not breed the curiosity which alone can provoke the search for a causal explanation. George's eighteenth-century London became an early-twentieth-century England writ onto an earlier canvas: a struggle for social improvements, not so much against the forces of reaction as against the forces of poverty. Amelioration was neither a class cause nor a party cause, but the cause of humanity itself; if there was a central enemy, this comprised not a specific political force or set of forces but rather a set of living conditions with their associated products of poverty, overcrowding, dirt and disease. Hence perhaps George's particular vision: a massive humanity deployed without a political cutting-edge.

The corollary of this analysis is that if we wish to discover the social causes of the process of 'improvement', we must dissolve the boundary between political and social history; and we must either turn to different sources from those George used, or else find a different way of reading such public appeals. The key, I suggest, is the identification of *interests*. Projects for 'improvement' may appear to the twentieth-century historian – of George's day or our own – to look forward to the future; yet their genesis lay in the past, in the specific constellations of interests which brought such projects into being. To specify the particular interests at work in any given case is to reinsert the scheme in question back into its original context. In this chapter I shall be attempting a series of exercises in this spirit.

As we have seen, medicine was one of the spheres of George's 'improvement': her first specific theme in fact was 'life and death in London', and the improvement in this sphere (evidenced from the Bills of Mortality) could be attributed not only to changes in living conditions but also to advances in medicine. Those advances, like most other aspects of improvement, were most marked after the mid-century; the early decades of the eighteenth century represented the more or less stagnant ground-level against which the post-1750 takeoff could be favourably compared. In this respect George's picture of eighteenth-century medicine anticipated a much later minor classic of whiggish medical history: Le Fanu's 1972 paper bearing the revealing title, 'The Lost Half-Century in English medicine, 1700–1750'.[5] If we were to take either George or, especially, Le Fanu as our guide, we would come to the conclusion that early-eighteenth-century English medicine was a vast lacuna between the heroic ages which preceded and succeeded the calm, not to say the tedium, of this so-called 'Augustan age'. Le Fanu's account is an edifice of negatives: Arbuthnot 'contributed no new knowledge'; he and Radcliffe were 'unprogressive physicians' who 'made almost no advance towards deeper understanding of disease and its treatment'; it was a 'quiescent period', a 'pause' in history; medical men 'made little effort to devise new techniques'; 'advanced medical teaching . . . was sadly wanting'; there was 'no interest in experimentation', and 'a similar neglect of instruments'; it was a 'barren age' marked by a general 'lack of urgency'. By the end of his paper Le Fanu's

---

[5] William R. Le Fanu, 'The Lost Half-Century in English Medicine, 1700–1750', *Bulletin of the History of Medicine* 46 (1972), pp. 319–48. I quote below from pp. 321, 322, 323, 330, 334, 335, 340, 343, 345 and 348.

rhetoric became even stronger: from 'almost no advance' it had shifted to 'no real advance'. Physicians, he concluded, like divines, 'wrote pietistic, tranquilising books'. In sum, this was 'an empty age'.

It is strange to reflect that it took Le Fanu some thousands of words merely to summarise the many non-events, as he saw them, of this 'lost half-century'. Stranger still is the fact that many of the post-1750 improvements which he (like George) recognised and celebrated, actually had well-known roots in pre-1750 developments. This chapter is devoted to three of these medical themes: the creation of voluntary hospitals; the adoption of inoculation for smallpox; and the rise of man-midwifery. In each of these cases, it is beyond dispute that crucial advances took place well before 1750. In each case, again, it is widely accepted that the given 'improvement' had major long-term consequences. Those consequences have attracted considerable historiographic interest; but to the best of my knowledge, no historian has ever seriously asked what were the *causes* of these three advances. It is precisely as we turn from effects to causes that we will begin to explore – that is, to *find* – the 'lost half-century' from 1700 to 1750. One of my purposes here will be to demonstrate that this period was not barren, but creative; not dull, but exciting; not an ocean of consensus but rather a whirlpool of conflict. In short, this will be an invitation to historians to investigate further what is probably the most neglected period in English medicine after 1600. The interest of that period is by no means confined to those spheres where we can demonstrate, by whiggish criteria, a permanent 'advance', a piece of 'improvement'. But against the historiographic background I have been outlining, it is surely best to start by putting this period on the map of what is whiggishly interesting. Hence the choice of the three particular case-studies to which I shall now turn.

VOLUNTARY HOSPITALS: THE ORIGINS OF THE WESTMINSTER INFIRMARY

The voluntary hospitals were amongst the most important permanent institutions produced by Hanoverian England. They comprised a new kind of philanthropy, financed by voluntary subscriptions (hence the term 'voluntary' to describe them); they constructed a new political space for the practice of medicine; and as a result they produced and fostered many new medical initiatives in the eighteenth century and afterwards. Through their impact on the French hospital reformer Jacques Tenon they may have contributed indirectly to the Paris 'birth of the clinic'; and they were certainly the site of an independent London medical revolution along similar lines.[6] Their founding is usually described as a 'movement', and it was certainly a large-scale development: by 1750 there were seventeen of them in England, when in 1718 there had been none. We can distinguish three types of voluntary hospital: London general hospitals (the first to be founded); provincial general hospitals (beginning with the Winchester County Hospital in 1736); and London specialist hospitals (such as the Lock Hospital for venereal disease and the Smallpox Inoculation Hospital, both founded in 1746).

In order to grasp the way these institutions operated, it is easiest to proceed from a particular example. The figure sets out the organisation of the Lying-in Hospital in Brownlow Street (established in 1749), some six or seven years after its foundation.[7] First, it is no accident that the people at the centre of the diagram are neither doctors nor patients, but rather the subscribers. It was these men and women – mostly men – who usually started the institution and who always maintained it by their annual donations, typically of a guinea or more. The subscribers appointed the medical staff; a committee of the subscribers supervised the running of the hospital; and last, but not least, the subscribers had the role of recommending prospective patients for admission. For a poor man or woman, the month or two spent in a voluntary hospital was a massive subsidy from his or her social superiors, and thus there was never any shortage of would-be patients. But in order to get admitted, the prospective patient had to be recommended by an individual subscriber; and thus this form of charity reinforced the power of the elite by enabling them to dispense

[6] For Tenon see C. C. Gillispie, *Science and Polity in France at the End of the Old Regime* (Princeton, 1980), pp. 254–7. On the transformation of the Paris hospitals and its effects, see Michel Foucault, *The Birth of the Clinic*, trans. A. M. Sheridan (London, 1973). London developments are discussed in Robert Kilpatrick's 1989 Cambridge Ph.D. thesis, entitled 'Nature's Schools: The Hunterian Revolution in London Hospital Medicine, 1780–1825'. The voluntary hospital movement as a whole has been reviewed by John Woodward, *To Do the Sick No Harm* (London, 1974); David E. Owen, *English Philanthropy 1660–1960* (Cambridge, MA, 1965), pp. 36–57; and A. Delbert Evans and L. G. Redmond Howard, *The Romance of the British Voluntary Hospital Movement* (London, n.d.). For brief but very perceptive comments see Charles Webster, 'The Crisis of the Hospitals During the Industrial Revolution' in E. G. Forbes (ed.), *Human Implications of Scientific Advance* (Edinburgh, 1978), pp. 214–23; and Roger French, 'Disease, Theory and Practice in a Voluntary Hospital' in F. M. Ricci (ed.), *A Social History of the Biomedical Sciences* (Milan, in press).

[7] The diagram is based on *An Account of the Rise, Progress and State of the British Lying-in Hospital for Married Women, Situated in Brownlow-Street, Long-Acre, from its Institution in November, 1749 to Lady-Day, 1756* (London, 1756). It was from this date that the hospital took the name 'British'. Details varied: thus this hospital's perpetual Presidency seems not to have been typical.

117

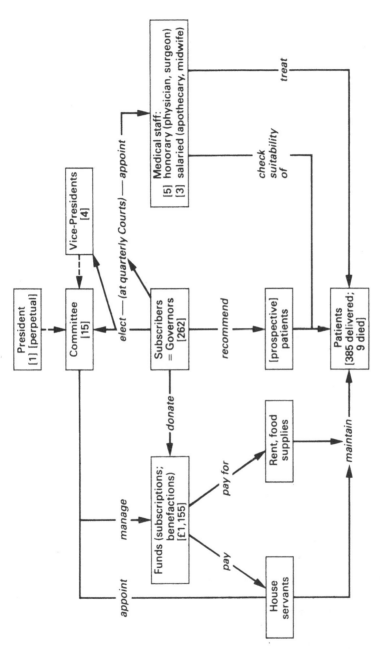

General structure of voluntary hospitals, illustrated by the particular case of the Lying-in Hospital, Brownlow Street, with [numbers] as for 1755–6

selectively a new form of largesse. The subscribers, then, were at the hub of the whole institution. The second important point which emerges from the figure is how *small* these institutions were. The Brownlow Street lying-in hospital was thriving, yet it had an annual budget of barely £1,000; it delivered fewer than 400 patients; and there were only 262 subscribers. Against this we have to remember that the potential number of subscribers in London at this time would have been comfortably of the order of 10,000.[8] This in turn has two important corollaries. For one thing, would-be founders did not need to convert a vast mass of people to their point of view; all that was required was to recruit a few hundred supporters. For another, despite the apparent popularity of the voluntary-hospital 'movement', the fact is that this was a *minority* activity amongst the London elite at this period. This becomes still more true if we focus not on the mass of subscribers but on the much smaller core of key activists who ran any given voluntary hospital, and who probably recruited many of their more passive fellow-subscribers. Each voluntary hospital was in practice the result of dedicated activity by a small and probably close-knit group of philanthropic individuals.

Against this background we can begin to open up the explanatory question as to why these institutions were founded. The voluntary hospitals resulted, not from the general interest of the elite, but rather from the particular interests of specific groups within that elite. The way forward in our understanding of these institutions must begin by identifying the interests involved. For the mass of subscribers this is no easy matter; but the leading individuals are often relatively easy to identify in standard sources, which enables each given institution to be located on the complex politico-religious map of interests in this period. Here is an attractive and important field for research; so far as I am aware, every one of these London voluntary hospitals still awaits study in these terms.

I have suggested that it was the subscribers who were the founders, as well as the managers, of these institutions. In fact the voluntary hospitals came into being in three distinct ways. Most usual was for a group of lay subscribers to get together and set up such an institution: such was the case with the very first of the voluntary hospitals, the Westminster Infirmary, as we shall see in a moment. But secondly,

---

[8] A guesstimate, based on a London population of over 500,000; assuming a household size of about 5, i.e., 100,000 families; allowing 10 per cent of these families to have the wealth required to subscribe to a voluntary hospital; and assuming only one subscriber per household. The latter two assumptions are almost certainly very conservative; relaxing these, we might estimate a pool of potential subscribers of the order of 20,000 or even more.

some such institutions arose by a process of splitting: a group of subscribers would secede from a hospital through some disagreement within the ranks. Such a process is illustrated by St George's, the second of the London voluntary hospitals, which split off from the Westminster in 1733. Thirdly, it sometimes happened that a medical man was the first initiator, such as John Harrison who set up the third such institution in London, the London Hospital, in 1740. He would of course have to mobilise a group of subscribers in order to achieve this, which reinforces the key role of subscribers; nevertheless this comprised a distinct style of foundation. The third route was subsequently responsible for two of the four London lying-in hospitals: the General (founded in 1752 by Felix Macdonogh) and the Westminster New Lying-in Hospital (set up by John Leake in 1767).[9]

Finally, in considering the character of these institutions, we must attend to the complex and specific *relations of power* which obtained within them. Here, although the role of the hospital's paid servants is also important, the key issue concerns the triangular relationship between subscribers, medical practitioners and patients. The medical practitioners served in two very different capacities. On the one hand, the physician (and in most cases the surgeon) gave his advice gratis; on the other hand, most hospitals had a salaried apothecary (rarely, a surgeon) who of course was part of the staff of servants. For the physician the rewards of the honorary post were considerable: not only would his name be printed in the published appeals of the hospital, thus instantly advertising his good charitable name to a prospective clientele of elite patients, but also the hospitals served increasingly as a site for teaching. Moreover, and this applied to the salaried apothecary as well, the hospital made it possible to experiment on the patients. Experimentation and teaching were both rooted in the same crucial fact, that voluntary hospitals created a new and distinctive political environment for medical practice. In the patronage-dominated world of eighteenth-century England, where one success or failure with an aristocratic patient had more implications than a dozen countervailing experiences with less affluent patients, the medical man was necessar-

[9] See, for St George's, G. C. Peachey, *The History of St. George's Hospital* (London, 1910–14); for the London, A. E. Clark-Kennedy, *The London: A Study in the Voluntary Hospital System* (London, 1962); for the General Lying-in Hospital, *An Account of the Rise, Progress, and State of the General Lying-in Hospital, the Corner of Quebec-Street, Oxford-Road* (London, 1768) and Jean Donnison, 'Note on the Foundation of Queen Charlotte's Hospital' *Medical History* 15 (1971), pp. 398–400 ('Queen Charlotte's' was the name later given to the General Lying-in Hospital). The Westminster New Lying-in Hospital is the subject of Philip Rhodes, *Doctor John Leake's Hospital* (London, 1977); confusingly, this became known as the 'General Lying-in Hospital'.

ily deferential towards his patients.[10] But in the voluntary hospitals the possibility was opened of far greater medical authority over the patient: hence the use of patients as raw material for experimentation and teaching. Nevertheless the subscribers could intervene to prohibit or to limit such practices; the medical man was not wholly free from the dictates of patronage. The voluntary hospital was not simply a medical space, nor merely a charitable space; rather, it comprised a *medico-charitable* space, whose interior practices and events were governed *both* by the lay subscribers *and* by medical men. The corollary is that throughout the history of the voluntary hospitals there ran a recurrent, though intermittent, theme of tension between medical men and lay subscribers. Each group wanted power; conflict between the two groups thus inevitably flared up from time to time. A simple instance of this is the fact that when a *minority* of the subscribers of the Westminster seceded in 1733 to form St George's, *all* the medical staff (both honorary and salaried) went off to the new institution, leaving the Westminster in the position of having to recruit an entirely new medical staff. Nor did this end the conflict: only a few years later, a struggle arose within St George's itself over the wish of some of the medical men to perform experiments on their patients.[11]

By now it should be clear that the founding of the Westminster Infirmary in 1719 was crucially important. Not only was this the first of the voluntary hospitals; it was also the parent of the second, since St George's was created in 1733 as a split-off from the Westminster. Thus in terms of London general hospitals, the voluntary-hospital 'movement' in its first two decades – from 1718 to 1739 – in fact consisted of the history of this single institution and, after 1733, its offspring. Thus the origins of the Westminster Infirmary command attention, not just as one case-study amongst the many that need to be carried out, but as the birth of the voluntary-hospital movement as a whole.

The origins of the Westminster Infirmary lay in the meetings of just four men, calling themselves 'the Charitable Society', between January and May 1716. The meetings lapsed thereafter for over three years, whereupon they suddenly resumed – with an enlarged and somewhat different personnel – in December 1719. From the latter date the

---

[10] See N. D. Jewson, 'Medical Knowledge and the Patronage System in Eighteenth-century England', *Sociology* 8 (1974), pp. 369–85. Recently Jewson's neglected argument has been taken up and developed in a highly fruitful way by Malcolm Nicolson, 'The Metastatic theory of Pathogenesis and the Professional Interests of the Eighteenth-Century Physician', *Medical History* 32 (1988), pp. 277–300.

[11] See Peachey, *History of St George's Hospital* and *HMC Egmont Diary*, vol. 2, *passim*.

society had a permanent existence, and it was at this stage that the actual Infirmary was created. But in order to grasp the origins of the institution, we must attend to both these two phases of founding. Table 1 tabulates the dates of all the 1716 meetings, and goes on to specify some highlights of the post-1719 phase, down to the 1735 move into premises which were to be kept for almost a century.[12]

The Charitable Society of 1716 was intended to be both the seed for wider developments, and the umbrella organisation which would oversee those developments. It was intended:

to establish particular societies in distant parts of this City . . . who may be mutually helpful and assistant to one another . . . all under the general direction of the Society.

There was no intention of setting up an infirmary. The purpose of the charity was to relieve the sick and needy *in their own homes*, both to supplement and to reinvigorate the Poor Law:

Notwithstanding the provision settled by our laws and the [assistance of voluntary collections] for the relief of the poor, it is obvious to anyone who walks the streets that [this] is [insufficient], to the great grief of all good men, and the no small reproach of our religion and country . . . How deplorable [then] must the condition be of such persons whose poverty is accompanied with sickness . . . it seems above the power of humane laws to remedy this evil. Nothing but the revival of the true Christian spirit of justice and charity in the persons employed to take care of the poor and the voluntary assistance of others acted by the same spirit . . . can effectually redress the grievances they [the poor] suffer and make their deplorable condition more tolerable and easy to them.

The aim, then, was to infuse a Christian and charitable spirit into the operation of the Poor Law, mainly by force of example. The means proposed for doing this were several, but did not include any mention of an infirmary or hospital. Five activities were put forward: (1) free medical advice for the sick; (2) lodging and nursing for lying-in women; (3) visitation and relief of sick prisoners; (4) the repatriation of sick and destitute foreigners; and lastly (5) 'to take care of the souls of those who are sick and needy as well as of their bodies'.

Conspicuous by its absence amongst these aims and methods is any mention of the 'improvement of physic'. Thus the usual claim, that this group was responding to the recent suggestions of John Bellers (1714),

---

[12] The following account is based on Greater London Record Office, Westminster Charitable Society/Infirmary, Minutes, vol. 1, *passim*. (The roll of early subscribers to the Society is held in the Westminster City Libraries; this document, which I have not examined systematically, suggests that Whig as well as Tory subscribers and benefactors were recruited in the course of the 1720s. I am grateful to Colin Brooks for drawing my attention to this source.)

Table 1. *Westminster Infirmary: select early chronology*

1716	January 14	Charitable Society meetings
	February 1, 26	– St Dunstan's Coffee-House,
	March 5, 12, 20, 26	the Strand
	April 3, 7, 14, 21, 28	(except April 7, at Revd
	May 5	Cockburn's house)
	January 14	Cockburn 'desired to draw up a scheme of this design';
		a messenger to be found;
		repositories for gifts-for-sick-poor to be sought.
	February 26	'In order to collect subscriptions some of the Proposals were ordered to be bound . . .'
	March 5	500 copies have been printed by Mr Downing (Hoare)
	20	Hoare declines to be Treasurer; Wogan 'was prevailed upon to accept the same for the first year . . .'
	April 3	Cash crisis; 'resolved to admit no more patients till the contributions come in; and that our principal care be confined to the sick and needy . . . of St Margarets Westminster until it shall please God that our stock increase.'
		Letter from Dr John Colbatch (to Mrs Frowde, here via Wogan): has seen the proposal, wishes to help, and notes that the City of London has 'several noble foundations to relieve the needy sick', but Westminster has none, 'which is a great reproach to it'.
	April 14	Mr Saville (apparently employed as apothecary) to buy drugs, utensils, a still;
		Society trying to get hold of Colbatch.
	April 28	Colbatch attends, 'and offered his service . . . gratis'.
	May 5	. . . routine meeting, no hint of discontinuing . . .
1719	December 2	refounding 'after long intermission'
1720	March 23 to April 20	Petty-France house taken (in-patients from 1 May)
1724	March to June 10	Chapel Street house taken instead
1733	June	. . . first moves towards 3rd infirmary . . .
1733	October to	
1734	January	. . . St George's Hospital splits off . . .
1734	January 8 to	
1735	February 24	St James's Street house taken (kept till 1834)

is refuted.[13] Whatever the stimulus for setting up the Charitable Society, this did not come from the Quaker Bellers.

Why did the Society lapse in 1716? One historian has suggested that there was strife between the four original founders, observing that two of them were no longer members when the Society was refounded in 1719.[14] Another possibility, not incompatible with this, is that conflict arose over the suggestion received in April from Dr John Colbatch (mentioned in table 1), which implied that a residential hospital should be set up, that is, a departure from the original aims. Thirdly, there may have been too little response to the public plea for subscriptions: this would certainly have discouraged the original founders. Some subscriptions came in – one of twenty guineas – but neither the number nor the total sums were very great. We shall return to this question later, after considering the political provenance of the Society.

In 1719 it 'pleased Almighty God to stir up the hearts of some persons to revive the charitable design of relieving the sick and needy'. Accordingly they met – at the same venue, St Dunstan's Coffee-House in the Strand – 'to consider of the most proper and effectual methods for putting the same in execution'. Now there were twelve founders – two out of the original group of four, and ten new ones. At this very first meeting of the new group, the Society resolved to set up an infirmary as the means to its charitable ends. Proposals were again published, and this time there was an immediate and sustained response. In the first year, subscriptions to the value of about £200 were received; after four years, income from this source stood at £400 per year. This was mostly made up of small subscriptions – one or two guineas per year – and, as this implies, there were over 100 subscribers by 1723. Meanwhile, the plan of founding an Infirmary had rapidly come to fruition: a house was leased in March 1720 (that is, within four months of the re-founding), and patients were admitted in May of that year. From this point on, the history of the Charitable Society becomes the history of the Westminster Infirmary.

Nevertheless some of the earlier themes persisted; three aspects of the group's activities should particularly be mentioned in this regard.

[13] Woodward, *To Do the Sick No Harm*, pp. 9–11, citing the anonymous study, 'The Origin and Evolution of the Eighteenth-Century Hospital Movement', *The Hospital* 55 (1913–14), pp. 290, 428, 485, 538, 596, 649 and 706. Bellers's idea resembled William Petty's much earlier concept of a 'nosocomium': see Charles Webster, *The Great Instauration: Science, Medicine and Reform in England, 1626–1660* (London, 1975), pp. 293–5.

[14] John Langdon-Davies, *Westminster Hospital: Two Centuries of Voluntary Service* (London, 1949), chapter 1. See also W. G. Spencer, *Westminster Hospital* (London, 1924) and J. G. Humble and Peter Hansell, *Westminster Hospital 1719–1966* (London, 1966).

(1) The Society continued to visit the sick and to give medical advice to non-resident sick and needy people. These were now described as 'out-patients', to distinguish them from those actually admitted to the Infirmary; and they were now expected to turn up at the Infirmary each week. Nonetheless this represents a continuation of what the Society had been doing before an Infirmary was ever mentioned. (2) The Society continued to operate at two levels, the parochial and the supra-parochial. Before the first house was taken, it was made clear (by a special order relating to persons from other parishes) that the infirmary was primarily designed to meet the needs of St Margaret's Westminster – the parish in which it was situated, and the same parish to which the Society had decided to confine its efforts in 1716 (see table 1). At the same time, the Infirmary did receive sick poor from other parishes, as both in- and out-patients. In such cases, the recommender of the patient was obliged 'to take care of the said person upon his recovery and return to his [own] parish'. It seems likely, in fact, that the Society's aim was to stimulate the creation of an entire network of parochial infirmaries, or of charitable societies, emulating its example across the metropolis. This, however, signally failed to occur. (3) The Society continued to be very much a *participatory* enterprise. It did not use committees: instead, all the subscribers were free to attend the weekly meetings, held on Wednesday nights, and it was at these meetings that all the important business took place, including the admission and discharge of patients. Thus all the subscribers could involve themselves fully, if they wished, in the running of the Society. This was a direct continuation of the initial aim, the 'revival of the true Christian spirit of justice and charity'.

All this was based on a specific model, namely *the charity-school movement* and its leading organisation, the SPCK (Society for the Promotion of Christian Knowledge).[15] The SPCK had begun in 1698 with just four founders – the same number as initiated the Charitable Society some eighteen years later. The SPCK had acted as an umbrella organisation, and had set up individual schools in dozens of parishes; again this was mirrored in the aims of the Charitable Society. Further, when the Charitable Society retreated from its wider goals and decided, in April 1716, 'that our principal care be confined to the sick and needy . . . of St Margaret's Westminster', it was now modelling itself on the individual charity school. These schools were parish-based; and they had always manifested the participatory methods which we have

---

[15] See M. G. Jones, *The Charity-School Movement: A Study of Eighteenth Century Puritanism in Action* (London, 1964).

seen were a conspicuous feature of the work of the Charitable Society. Of course the charity school had its salaried professional – the teacher – and so too did the Charitable Society, in the form of its apothecary. In each case, the status of the professional person involved neither professional autonomy, nor mere subservience. He was paid, but paid to exercise a trust; in the conduct of charitable affairs he and the trustees met as complementary equals. Finally, there were many direct links between the SPCK and the Charitable Society, links which appear at three levels. Two of the members of the Society, Henry Hoare (a member in both 1716 and 1719) and Samuel Wesley (1719 only), were members of the SPCK itself. Further, Hoare was for many years the chairman of the complementary umbrella organisation, the Grand Committee of London Charity Schools. Thirdly, there were tangible links with one specific charity school, namely the Grey Coat School (so named from the uniforms of its pupils), the largest, the most successful and the most famous of all the charity schools.[16] It had been founded in 1698, as the charity school of St Margaret's Westminster – that is, the same parish as the Charitable Society's later focus. Hoare and Wesley were both on its board, so was another 1719 Charitable Society member (Thomas Wisdom), and there were other individuals who were subscribers or benefactors of both the school and the Society. And in 1720, it was in the Grey Coat School that the Society held its weekly meetings – after their re-founding meeting at St Dunstan's Coffee-House, and until the first Infirmary building was fitted out.

To sum up: the Charitable Society, which created the Westminster Infirmary, was designed to extend into the care of the sick poor a form of charitable provision which had already worked effectively for the education of the children of the poor. It drew on the same personnel, the same methods and the same religious motive: the care of the sick was linked with their eternal salvation, just as the education of children was designed to this end. The trustees of the Charitable Society were not trying to lower the death-rate, any more than the trustees of the charity school were trying to raise the literacy-rate. *They were instead seeking actively to Christianise the society in which they lived.* They saw themselves as active instruments of a beneficent Providence; every new subscription was proof of God's approval of the design, and every patient was required, after receiving the help of the Society, to render thanks 'to God and to the Society'.

Why then was this initiative taken at this time? The SPCK dated

[16] For the Grey Coat School, see Elsie S. Day, *An Old Westminster Endowment* (London, 1902).

from 1698; it had flourished for eighteen years without any move into this new sphere of charitable activity. What led to this sudden extension of participatory philanthropy in 1716 and 1719? We can approach this question by considering who the founding fathers were; when they founded it; and, first of all, the changing political complexion of the SPCK. As the researches of Craig Rose demonstrate, the SPCK was created as a specifically Anglican missionary society, an attempt to revitalise the Christianity of the Church of England in the wake of the new flourishing of Dissent – and particularly of Dissenting education – resulting from the Toleration Act of 1689.[17] The Established Church was threatened by toleration with becoming merely one amongst many sects; the SPCK sought to strengthen the Church by catechising and educating the young. (The simplest way to grasp this objective is by analogy with the more familiar case of Methodism, a generation or so later. It is perhaps no accident that Samuel Wesley was prominent in the SPCK and that his sons were leaders of the Methodist movement for spiritual revival within the Anglican church.) In the political climate of the reign of Anne, this aim made for an inexorable drift of the SPCK away from its initial, rather eirenic Anglicanism towards a High-Church, Tory and even Jacobite orientation. Thus by the time the Charitable Society was founded – early in 1716 – the SPCK was firmly placed at the Tory end of the political spectrum.

We would therefore expect that the founding fathers of the Charitable Society were specifically Tories and High Churchmen. And in fact, wherever information as to their allegiance can be found, this does indeed turn out to have been the case. Table 2 sets out the names of the fourteen men involved; I have identified the allegiance of just six of these men, but the pattern is so clear for these six that we can be confident it extended to the whole group.[18] To mention only the four

[17] Craig Rose, personal communication, 1988, drawing on his forthcoming Cambridge Ph.D. dissertation on charities in London, c.1680–1720.

[18] For Cockburn, Hutton and Wesley, see the *Dictionary of National Biography*. Hoare belonged to the Goldsmiths' Company, Witham to the Vintners' Company, and these were two of 'the three great tory London guilds' (the other being the Grocers' Company): Linda Colley, *In Defiance of Oligarchy: The Tory Party, 1714–60* (Cambridge, 1982), p. 87. Both men voted Tory in 1713: see W. A. Speck and W. A. Gray (eds.), 'London Pollbooks 1713', in H. Horwitz (ed.), *London Politics 1713–1717* (London Record Society, vol. xvii, 1981), pp. 94 and 128. Finally Trebeck must have been at least a Tory and possibly a non-juror in June 1715, since a sermon of his was strongly approved by Thomas Hearne at that time: see D. W. Rannie (ed.), *Remarks and Collections of Thomas Hearne*, vol. 5 (Oxford, 1901), p. 67. (Trebeck, however, went over to the Court in the middle of the 1720s.) Note in addition that Wogan is probably to be identified with the man of that name in the DNB, whose precise allegiance at this time is unclear to me. Wesley's wider circle is discussed by Thomas E. Brigden, 'Samuel Wesley Junior, and His Circle, 1690–1739', *Proceedings of the Wesley Historical Society* 11 (1918), pp. 25–38, 97–102, 121–9 and 145–53.

Table 2. *Founders of the Westminster Charitable Society,*
1716 and 1719

1716 only	1716 and 1719	1719 only
Revd Patrick Cockburn	Henry Hoare	Revd Mr Fitzgerald
Robert Witham	William Wogan	Revd Pengrey Hayward
		Revd John Hutton
		Revd Dr. Alexander Innes
		Revd Richard Russell
		John Russell
		John Thornton
		Revd Andrew Trebeck
		Revd Samuel Wesley
		Thomas Wisdom

most prominent cases: *Henry Hoare* was a member of the Tory family of bankers and goldsmiths. *John Hutton* was a non-juring clergyman, who had lost his living and had supported himself by taking in boarders from Westminster School, itself a centre of high-flying Toryism. *Patrick Cockburn* was at this period technically a Jacobite, since he had been removed as curate of St Dunstan's, Fleet Street, for refusing to take the oath of abjuration on the accession of George I. (Later, in 1726, he became reconciled to the Hanoverian succession, took the oath and duly obtained a living.) *Samuel Wesley* was closely associated with Atterbury, was head usher at Westminster School and belonged to a substantial circle all of whose members were High Churchmen. Thus these four men were so far to the Tory end of the spectrum that it is difficult to imagine their working with colleagues who did not share their basic principles; we may safely infer that the whole group, both in 1716 and 1719, was of deeply Tory allegiance. The same conclusion is suggested by the simpler fact that so many of these founding fathers were clergymen; seven of the 1719 group of twelve were in holy orders. At this period almost all the lower clergy were of Tory persuasion, believing that under the Whigs the Church of England was 'in danger'.

In this context we can begin to grasp the significance of the date of founding. By January 1716, when the Charitable Society was set up, the Tories had witnessed in turn the accession of George I and the associated flight of Bolingbroke to France and the creation of a Whig ministry; a crushing defeat in the General Election which followed; and the abortive Jacobite uprising of 1715, which was now in the process of

being mopped up. They well knew that they were about to be consigned to the political wilderness; the only question was for how long.
The Whigs were already setting about purging Tories from a variety of
local offices, tightening their own grip on all levels of government and
creating a one-party State. As one instance amongst many, the Commission for Building Fifty New Churches, set up under Anne in 1711 as
a High Church initiative, was purged of Tories and filled with Whigs;
the date at which this took effect was 5 January 1716, that is, nine days
before the first meeting of the Charitable Society, and one of the
Commissioners purged was Henry Hoare.[19] A further move in the
same direction was the Close Vestries Bill, which came before Parliament at about this time; this was designed to wrest control of parish
vestries in London from Tories and to replace them with Whigs.[20] No
wonder that Henry Hoare and his colleagues began to feel that the
Poor Law was insufficient: it was now likely to be administered by
their political enemies, men whom they probably regarded as infidels.

The subsequent disbanding of the Society in May 1716, and its re-
founding in December 1719, may also be intelligible in this light. The
Close Vestries Bill was a key issue for the Tories, who put a major
effort into lobbying against it. Given their strong emphasis on the
parish as the unit of activity, Hoare and his associates may well have
diverted their efforts in this direction once the Bill came before the
House of Commons in April 1716. In the Commons such efforts were
unsuccessful; but the Tories won a famous victory in the Lords, where
the Bill was thrown out on 1 June. It is just conceivable that with this
success they lost the impetus which had fuelled the Charitable Society.
But why then did it 'please Almighty God to stir up the hearts of some
persons to revive this charitable design' in December 1719? All these
questions deserve to be explored through a study of vestry affairs in St
Margaret's Westminster; but it can be suggested that it was now
electoral politics which provided the crucial stimulus. The City of
Westminster, which sent two MPs to the House of Commons, was one
of the largest, the most democratic and the most keenly fought of all
electorates in the country. By reviving the Charitable Society in 1719,
Hoare and his associates may have been preparing for the General
Election of 1722. Charity was a means of securing respect, affection
and political leverage: this is amply shown by Rose's work on the City

[19] See M. H. Port (ed.), *The Commissions for Building Fifty New Churches: The Minute Books,
1717–27, a Calendar* (London, 1986), pp. xvi, xvii and 45.
[20] See John Oldmixon, *The History of England*, vol. 2 (London, 1735), p. 633; *House of Lords
Journal* 20 (1716), pp. 365–8 and 372.

hospitals, St Thomas's and St Bartholomew's, where the struggle for political control had been intense throughout the reigns of James II and William III.[21] If the underlying aim of the 1719 re-founding was indeed political, then this succeeded – for the Tories won both seats in the Westminster electorate in the 1722 election.

The two motives I have suggested – religious and political – were not at odds, nor was the one altruistic and the other interested. Politics and religion were different facets of the same set of issues: it had been over a religious question (the succession of a Catholic monarch) that the Whig/Tory split within the elite had developed in 1679, and while that split had evolved into new shapes after 1688, chiefly through the impact of war and the resulting problem of the National Debt, it nevertheless retained a fundamentally religious orientation. Thus, for the founders of the Charitable Society, to promote the Tory cause in politics and to work for a Christian revival in daily life were the same thing.

This case-study amply bears out the earlier contention, that behind the founding of any given voluntary hospital there lay not the general interests of the leisured classes but rather some particular set of interests within those classes. The chief sphere in which such interests were demarcated was, throughout our period, politico-religious. In the case of the Westminster Charitable Society, it was specifically the Tory interest which was at work. What prompted the founders to involve themselves in the care of the sick, and thus eventually to found the first voluntary hospital, was the new political conjuncture arising from the accession of George I and the creation of a Whig one-party State.

INOCULATION OF SMALLPOX

Smallpox inoculation is one of those forgotten medical practices which, while playing an immensely important historical role, must be distinguished from the later techniques which succeeded it.[22] The term 'inoculation' simply meant *engrafting*, and indeed it was this word which was first used to describe it: the language, then, was taken from horticultural botany. Purulous matter was taken from one of the many pustules on the body of a sufferer from smallpox. This matter was then

[21] Craig Rose, forthcoming Ph.D. and his paper on St Thomas's and St Bartholomew's in Lindsay Granshaw and Roy Porter (eds.), *Hospitals in History* (London, 1989).
[22] See Genevieve Miller, *The Adoption of Inoculation for Smallpox in England and France* (Philadelphia, 1957); Peter Razzell, *The Conquest of Smallpox* (Firle, 1977); Derrick Baxby, *Jenner's Smallpox Vaccine* (London, 1981); J. R. Smith, *The Speckled Monster: Smallpox in England, 1670–1970, With Particular Reference to Essex* (Chelmsford, 1987).

'prepared' in some way – for instance, by drying. Meanwhile the recipient individual, someone who had never had the disease, was also 'prepared' by manipulation of regimen. Finally the noxious matter was inserted into or under the skin of the recipient, again by any of a variety of techniques, chiefly through an incision (sometimes deep, sometimes shallow). The recipient then, within a few days, would develop a very mild form of smallpox – marked above all by the presence of far fewer pustules than were usually observed with the natural disease. In another week or so the pustules would fade away and the recipient would recover. The result, it was alleged by promoters of inoculation, was permanent immunity from the natural disease, an immunity just as effective as that acquired from a natural attack. The advantage of inoculation-conferred immunity was that the inoculated disease was far less lethal than the natural smallpox: not only did it produce far fewer pustules on the individual, but it also produced far fewer deaths amongst the mass. (The typical mortality seems to have been about one in seventy or eighty from inoculations, as against one in six or seven from smallpox itself.)

The long-term history, viewed in whiggish perspective, was to vindicate dramatically the claims of the inoculators. Inoculation was promoted by the Royal Society through the 1720s, and gradually came to prevail against a stubborn resistance mounted by various critics. From the middle decades of the eighteenth century it was more and more widely adopted, chiefly through the remarkable activities of the Suttons, who developed a cheaper and simpler technique. In a rural village there would be a 'mass inoculation' of the whole population as soon as an epidemic of smallpox threatened. Large towns, on the other hand, were more reluctant to adopt the practice, since here a universal inoculation was a practical and political impossibility, and it was widely feared that an *inoculated* person could transmit the *natural* and lethal disease to someone who had not been inoculated, thus starting an epidemic. It was to combat this fear and to promote inoculation in the towns that John Haygarth and his colleagues at Chester Infirmary created their new practice of inoculation-with-isolation, together with the accompanying rationale that infection obeyed an inverse-square law of diminishing effects with diminishing distance. Their success – much promoted by the Howard-Percival network of social reformers in the late eighteenth century – led by the 1790s to a campaign for the actual eradication of the disease in Britain.[23] It seems to have been this

---

[23] Francis M. Lobo, 'John Haygarth, Smallpox, and Religious Dissent in Eighteenth-Century England', this volume, pp. 217–53.

rival stimulus which prompted Edward Jenner to intensify his researches on the immunity to smallpox conferred by the diseases of cowpox in cows and 'grease' in horses. Hence Jenner's 1798 experiments and publication on what was soon to be called *vaccination* – the inoculation of cowpox (so called from the Latin *vacca*, a cow). Vaccination rapidly triumphed over inoculation (despite the sustained opposition of Burdett, Cobbett and other radicals), swiftly receiving military use and State backing.[24] In the nineteenth century a series of moves towards *compulsory* vaccination led to political campaigns against the practice; one of the monuments of this struggle was Creighton's massive *History of Epidemics*, animated by his opposition to vaccination.[25] Meanwhile Pasteur and Koch were extending the basic technique to other diseases; the word 'vaccination' lost its connection with cowpox and was used by Pasteur for the creation of artificial immunity in general. Thanks to all this and to the involvement of the laboratory in these researches and experiments, we have the scientific field of immunology and a vast range of 'vaccines' against specific diseases. It is in the promotion of inoculation for smallpox in the 1720s that this heroic story finds its real roots. Consequently, it is difficult to resist the basic assumption that the inoculators were 'right' and their opponents were 'wrong'.

Yet from the perspective of around 1720, the question appears in a very different light. Not only could the long-term results not be anticipated, but also the success of inoculation itself lay in the future. And inoculation was extraordinary, for it consisted in deliberately *giving a disease* to someone in health – the very inversion of the notional role of the physician. It is thus hardly surprising that inoculation was resisted; what requires explanation is not so much this resistance, as the very fact that the practice was promoted at all. We are fortunate to have the excellent study of Genevieve Miller – an important classic of medical history – on *how* inoculation was promoted. But Miller, proceeding from the modern perspective I have already outlined, was not concerned with the question as to *why* an important cadre of physicians set about promoting it.[26] As we shall see, an exploration of this question takes us again into the realm of early Hanoverian politics and religion.

We may approach the question of the 'why' by looking in some detail at the mechanics of the 'how'. The practice of inoculation arose chiefly in the Middle East, where it appears to have been a popular or

[24] See Paul Saunders, *Edward Jenner: The Cheltenham Years 1795–1823* (Hanover, New England and London, 1982).

[25] Dorothy Porter and Roy Porter, 'The Politics of Prevention: Anti-Vaccinationism and Public Health in Nineteenth-Century England', *Medical History* 32 (1988), pp. 231–52.

[26] Unless otherwise stated, my account here follows Miller, *Adoption of Inoculation*.

folk practice. (Thus here, just as with Jenner's later vaccination and much earlier with cinchona for malaria, Western medicine is indebted to popular or indigenous traditions for some of its most heroic achievements.) Reports of its success reached the Royal Society, chiefly through John Woodward, in 1714. But it was not until Lady Mary Wortley Montagu returned from her stint as wife of the ambassador to Constantinople that any campaign for inoculation was mounted. Lady Mary persuaded the apothecary Charles Maitland to inoculate her three-year-old daughter; since Maitland had been with the Montagues in Constantinople, he was familiar with the practice, yet it required some pressure from Lady Mary to convince him to perform the act. With remarkable speed the idea was taken up by Hans Sloane, who used the Royal Society to promote an investigation into the efficacy of inoculation. This may appear as an open-minded study, but all the evidence suggests that Sloane and his backers were convinced in advance that inoculation would work. The crucial moves were a series of experiments, carried out in the nine months from June 1721 to March 1722. Table 3 summarises their chronology and content. All these experiments deserve detailed study as pieces of public theatre, but I shall focus simply on the first of them, 'Experiment I' in my own terminology. Sloane and some of his colleagues – including opponents as well as supporters of inoculation – went down to Newgate prison and selected six prisoners, all condemned to death, all in good health, and offered them repeal from execution if they would submit to an experiment in inoculation. It was not difficult to get the prisoners to agree to this: certain death was exchanged for the uncertain. The six prisoners were duly inoculated: significantly, the inoculator was Charles Maitland, so that here as with other experimental innovations we see the necessity for physical and personal transfer of techniques from one context (Constantinople) into another (London). The inoculated prisoners were carefully observed, over the next few weeks, by the interested physicians of both the pro- and the anti-inoculation camps. In due course they developed pustules and other symptoms and then recovered. None of them died; the experiment had succeeded. On 6 September 1721 they were given a public pardon and release. For these six prisoners, then, inoculation certainly worked: it saved their lives.

The whiggish perspective, then, is that inoculation worked; and this, from a different point of view, was also the conclusion of the pro-inoculators. But the anti-inoculators interpreted the experiment quite differently. In the publications of William Wagstaffe on the one hand, and Charles Maitland on the other, we have two quite different

Table 3. *The promotion of smallpox inoculation by public experiments, 1721–2*

1721 April:	Lady Mary Wortley Montagu prevails on Charles Maitland to inoculate her 3-year-old daughter
June:	[Experiment I] already under way, probably at the initiative of Sir Hans Sloane
Aug 9:	[Experiment I]: Six condemned prisoners in Newgate prison inoculated in exchange for their lives. Inoculator: Chas Maitland In charge: Sloane and Dr John George Steigerthal
Sept 6:	Public pardon and release. [Expt I] complete.
Oct:	[Experiment II]: Performed by Maitland under direction of Sloane and Steigerthal, on a 19-year-old woman, one of the subjects of [Expt I). She is exposed, in 2 different ways, to natural smallpox; survives.
[Oct]:	[Experiment III]: Performed by Maitland, at Hertford: inoculated children pass the disease on.
1722 Feb to March	[Experiment IV]: Performed by Maitland, in London: six 'persons' inoculated, then displayed to the public. Announcement in the newspapers, etc.
March	[Experiment V]: Maitland inoculates a child with pus from a person with the inoculated disease.
March	[Experiment VI]: Five pauper children from the parish of St James's, Westminster inoculated and displayed to the public. (This expt had been publicly initiated, the previous November, by the Princess of Wales.)

accounts of the 'same' experiment. For Maitland, what had happened was that the prisoners had received a mild form of smallpox and had duly recovered: this was what a pro-inoculation person *saw* in the experiment. But an anti-inoculation physician, Wagstaffe, saw something quite different: some odd-looking pustules, not the same as the smallpox pustules; an inflammation surrounding the pustules, different from what was observed with smallpox; and a constellation of other, febrile symptoms, once again quite different from smallpox. Here we have an elegant example of the structuring of perception by the preconceptions of the observer. The result, of course, was that Wagstaffe was totally unconvinced of the alleged results of the experiment, whereas Maitland was confident that the inoculation had worked.[27]

[27] William Wagstaffe, *A Letter to Dr Freind; Showing the Danger and Uncertainty of Inoculating the Small Pox* (London, 1722); Charles Maitland, *An Account of Inoculating the Small-pox* (London, 1722; second edition, enlarged, 1723); *Mr Maitland's Account of Inoculating the Smallpox Vindicated from Dr Wagstaffe's Misrepresentations* (London, 1722). I owe the latter reference to the kindness of Robert Kilpatrick.

134

This pivotal experiment thus illustrates some basic principles of the historical sociology of science. But what should also command our attention is the political precondition of the experiment. In order for the experiment to be performed, Sloane and his allies had to be given the power of life and death over the six prisoners. *The State handed over to the Royal Society its control over six human lives.* Without this fundamental resource, the experiment could not have been carried out; and the availability of that resource was an extraordinary political fact, a quite remarkable donation from the State to a select group of its citizens. This can only mean that inoculation had prior support from the Crown and the ministry. And this was indeed the case. Inoculation was specifically a project of the Court Whigs; opposition to the practice came exclusively from Tories. This fundamental cleavage of attitudes to inoculation was to persist until at least the 1740s.

Table 4 sets out the association between political allegiance and attitudes to inoculation, between 1721 and the late 1740s, for those individuals who can be allocated a position in both spheres. There is a powerful connection between Whig allegiance and support for inoculation, and between Toryism and opposition to the practice; the odds against this being a chance association are 77 to 1.[28] Only two out of sixteen individuals go against the stream, and in each of these cases their departure from the main pattern is at least partly intelligible. *John Arbuthnot* was the only Tory supporter of the operation so far identified; and it is striking that he alone, of all the authors under discussion, published anonymously. What lay behind his support was apparently his interest in statistical questions, and perhaps also his involvement in the recent discussions leading up to the Quarantine Act for control of plague (discussed below).[29] *Sir Richard Blackmore* was the only known Whig opponent of inoculation, and in fact his opposition fits with other aspects of his eccentric career. He was a much older Whig than most of the supporters, having been knighted by William III. From about 1720 he was apparently moving rapidly away

[28] Using the Fisher exact-probability test, for which see Sidney Siegel, *Nonparametric Statistics for the Behavioural Sciences* (Tokyo, 1956), pp. 96–104. At least another twenty individuals with known attitudes to inoculation can be identified from Miller's study, split approximately evenly between supporters and opponents. This table includes only those of known politico-religious allegiance; the latter has been identified from standard sources, chiefly the *DNB*.
[29] For Arbuthnot, see Larry Stewart, 'The Edge of Utility: Slaves and Smallpox in the Early Eighteenth Century', *Medical History* 29 (1985), pp. 54–70, at pp. 55 and 65; Ian Hacking, *The Emergence of Probability* (Cambridge, 1975), pp. 166–71; and the entry for him in the *Dictionary of Scientific Biography*. Arbuthnot's approach is particularly intriguing in view of the otherwise Whig associations of the statistical approach to inoculation, discussed below. On the later ramifications of this statistical theme, see Leslie Bradley, *Smallpox Inoculation: An Eighteenth-Century Mathematical Controversy* (Nottingham, 1971).

Table 4. *Politico-religious allegiance and attitudes to inoculation, 1721–46*

Whigs/Dissenters/members of Royal household	Tories/Non-jurors
Supporters of inoculation	
Claude Amyand	
Dr Samuel Brady	
Ephraim Chambers	
Dr James Jurin	
Dr Richard Mead	
Lady Mary Wortley Montagu	
Rev Daniel Neal	
Dr Thomas Nettleton	
Sir Hans Sloane	
Dr John George Steigerthal	Dr John Arbuthnot
Opponents of inoculation	
Sir Richard Blackmore	Dr John Byrom
	Dr Peirce Dod
	Revd Edmund Massey
	Dr William Wagstaffe

from the Court; this was signalled by his various published attacks on 'modern Arians', that is, on the religious tendencies manifested by the new Court divines Samuel Clarke and William Whiston. He retired to the country in about 1722, and then began to publish medical works which argued against the monopolistic practices and pretensions of the Collegiate physicians. After his death in 1729 he was mentioned with affection and respect by two Tory medical writers. Blackmore, then, was fast becoming a 'Country' Whig at the time of the inoculation campaign.[30] The exceptions (Arbuthnot, Blackmore) are thus intelligible; and the main pattern has further evidence for its support. For one thing, the most sustained opposition to inoculation in the newspapers of the day came from *Applebee's Original Weekly Journal*, which was a Tory paper. For another, consider the following passage from Edmund Massey's *Letter to Mr Maitland* of 1722. Here, towards the end of his counter-attack against Maitland, Massey referred also to the the pro-inoculation (and anti-Massey) text of Samuel Brady of Portsmouth:

[30] For Blackmore, see his entry in the *DNB* and the various works of his cited there. The later respectful Tories were Edmund Chapman, *A Treatise on the Improvement of Midwifery, Chiefly With Regard to the Operation* (London, 1735), p. 101, and Henry Bracken, *The Midwife's Companion* (London, 1737), p. 186.

I had almost forgot to take notice, that amongst all the advantageous symptoms of inoculation, I do not remember any that are so squeamish as the following, viz., that it is a diagnostic of a man's affection or disaffection to the government; for, says your brother Brady, I wish the happy conduct of the Royal Family in this particular has not, out of an abundant respect, occasioned some people's zeal against the practice. I assure the Doctor, that I neither have, nor expect, place or pension under the government; and yet I . . . am certain, that I am as good a subject as some who have . . .

Thus Brady had insinuated that opponents of inoculation were Jacobites; and Massey, who was a Hanoverian Tory, found this smear deeply offensive ('squeamish').[31] Here we have a rare occasion on which the political connections of the contending medical interests actually become explicit.

It is not difficult to see why Tories were opposed to inoculation. As David Harley observes, the Tory doctrine of passive obedience to the monarch was naturally transferred into the realm of the supernatural as this impinged on the affairs of man.[32] Diseases were judgements of God; resistance to such judgements was impious. We can find something like this position elegantly articulated by John Byrom, in a poem he wrote against inoculation (emphasis added):

I heard two neighbours talk, the other night,
About this new distemper-giving plan,
Which some so wrong, and others think so right.
Short was the dialogue, and thus it ran:
– 'If I had twenty children of my own,
    I would inoculate them every one.'
– 'Aye, but should any of them die, what moan
    Would then be made for venturing thereupon!'
– 'No; I should think that I had done the best,
    And be resigned, whatever should befall.'
– 'But could you really be so quite at rest?'
– 'I could'. – '*Then why inoculate at all?*'
– 'Since, to resign a child to God, Who gave,
    Is full as easy, and as just a part,
    When sick and led by Nature to the grave,
    As when in health, and driv'n to it by Art'.

The very *possibility* of a fatality from inoculation, Byrom was arguing, refuted the practice. To inflict disease, and thus the possibility of death, was to usurp the role of God.[33]

[31] Edmund Massey, *A Letter to Mr Maitland, in Vindication of the Sermon Against Inoculation* (London, 1722), p. 22. (Brady was also mentioned at the beginning of the text, p. 2.)
[32] David Harley, comments in conference discussion, September, 1987. This interpretation is amply borne out by Massey's writings. See Edmund Massey, *A Sermon Against the Dangerous and Sinful Practice of Inoculation* (London, 1722), and his subsequent *Letter to Mr Maitland*, cited in the previous note. The *Sermon* must have been popular, for it ran to at least three editions in 1722.
[33] *Remains Historical and Literary Connected with the Palatine Counties of Lancaster and Chester*, new series, vol. 29 (Manchester, Chetham Society, 1894), pp. 204–5.

But what of the reasons for the Whig support for the 'new distemper-giving plan'? Part of the reason may lie in the fact that smallpox, already a subject of bitter contention amongst physicians as to the right method of treatment, was likely to become a concern of the State.[34] At the time when the first experiment was carried out (it started in June 1721), the ministry was recovering from the ravages of the South Sea Bubble, which had burst in 1720, and was dealing with the threat of the plague epidemic, raging in France and widely feared as imminent in England. The Bubble had brought to power the 'screen-master general', Walpole; the government response to the plague scare was the Quarantine Act of February 1721. (What with these upheavals, Atterbury's Jacobite plot of 1721–2, and the Black Act of 1722, the 'political stability' allegedly achieved by 1725 appears as a rather delicate equilibrium.)[35] Plague posed a passive threat not only to human life but also to trade and to public order; hence the draconian measures of the Quarantine Act. Since smallpox had recently assumed a new and more virulent form, there was reason to fear that another, different but scarcely less fatal plague was already developing – one which quarantine would be quite powerless to prevent. Against smallpox, what was needed was a pre-emptive strike; it can be seen as a blow struck, not just against the disease, but also against the *fear* of the disease. If smallpox could be depicted as preventable, the public could be massaged into a grateful tranquility. Hence its political importance.

On this reading, inoculation was backed by the Whigs simply because the Whigs were in power: it was they who held the reins of State, and thus they who had most to gain and to lose from the success or failure of the management of disease. Yet there are grounds for suspecting that a deeper predisposition was at work. The arguments deployed in favour of inoculation rested upon a distinctive morality, one which ran precisely counter to Byrom's views already described. For James Jurin, the most publicly active supporter of inoculation in the Royal Society, the question of the merits of inoculation was statistical. What was the death-rate from natural smallpox? What was the death-rate from inoculation? If the latter was lower than the former, then inoculation was justified. (This rested implicitly on the

[34] On the controversy of *c.*1718 over the treatment of smallpox, in which Freind and Mead were ranged against Woodward, see Miller, *Adoption of Inoculation*, p. 36; R. J. J. Martin, 'Explaining John Freind's *History of Physick*', *Studies in History and Philosophy of Science* 19 (1988), pp. 399–418; Joseph M. Levin, *Dr Woodward's Shield* (Berkeley, 1977), pp. 9–17. For the connection with plague, quarantine and the Bubble, see Stewart, 'Edge of Utility', *passim*.
[35] Compare J. H. Plumb, *The Growth of Political Stability in England, 1675–1725* (London, 1967), and E. P. Thompson, *Whigs and Hunters: The Origins of the Black Act* (London, 1975).

premise, which was probably false, that everyone caught smallpox at some stage in his or her life.) Here we see a concept of *utility*, a weighing of this good against that evil, in which individual life is an atomic entity to be viewed *de haut en bas*. Such a morality – some would see it as an anti-morality – had powerful Whig and Latitudinarian roots.[36] The corollory was that man did indeed have a God-like role: against disease there was a right of resistance. (Meanwhile the traditional Whig doctrine of a right of *political* resistance was fast becoming a forgotten shibboleth: by labelling Tories as Jacobites, by repealing Habeas Corpus and by passing the Septennial Act, Walpole and his colleagues rapidly constructed a new Whig compound of loyalty to the ministry and to the Hanoverian succession, with resistance consigned to the single moment of 1688.) It is tempting to see inoculation for smallpox as the Whig and Hanoverian equivalent of the Stuart practice of touching for scrofula, for the 'king's evil'.[37] In each case we have State action against a familiar and disfiguring disease. In each case this action was deployed with massive publicity in an orchestrated campaign. But whereas the Royal Touch mobilised divine powers, based on hereditary right, inoculation deployed natural powers harnessed by man, with the monarch as the benevolent onlooker rather than indispensable participant. This role for the sovereign – involved yet marginal – precisely fitted the Walpolian Whig political role assigned to George I, just as the thaumaturgical power of the Stuart monarchs corresponded to the Tory conception of the relationship between Crown and subject. The strongly theatrical character of the early inoculation experiments, together with the fact that relatively few actual inoculations were carried out in the 1720s, similarly suggests that inoculation was political massage as well as medical intervention.

These are only speculations as to the underlying motivations behind the inoculation campaign. Here, just as with the voluntary-hospital movement, we have a large and open field which invites further exploration. Inoculation remained controversial until at least the 1750s, and generated a variety of new initiatives, from the creation of

---

[36] The emerging concept of utility can be traced in different ways within Margaret Jacob, *The Newtonians and the English Revolution* (Ithaca, New York, 1976), and Lorraine C. Daston, 'Probabilistic Expectation and Rationality in Classical Probability Theory', *Historia Mathematica* 7 (1980), pp. 234–60.

[37] See Mark Bloch, *The Royal Touch: Sacred Monarchy and Scrofula in England and France*, trans. J. E. Anderson (London, 1973); Keith Thomas, *Religion and the Decline of Magic: Studies in Popular Beliefs in Sixteenth- and Seventeenth-Century England* (first published 1971; Harmondsworth, 1978), pp. 227–41; French, 'Disease, Theory and Practice'; W. E. Tate, *The Parish Chest* (Cambridge, 1946; third edition, 1969), pp. 157–61.

the London Smallpox-inoculation Hospital in 1746 to Haygarth's remarkable work at Chester in later decades. Larry Stewart has shown how inoculation was swiftly taken up by the slave-traders of the Africa Company, with the heavy involvement of Sloane, the Royal Society, and the Duke of Chandos;[38] similarly the subject can and should be pursued further in many local contexts. Once such research is carried out, it will no doubt become possible to develop a more nuanced and concrete account than I have been able to offer here. But it is already certain that this theme, like that of the voluntary-hospital movement, opens directly into the terrain of political and religious conflict and allegiance in early Hanoverian England.

CONCLUSION

My third case-study – on the rise of man-midwifery – will be considered only briefly; it has been discussed in detail elsewhere, and space permits only a summary here.[39] After outlining this third theme I shall reflect on the significance of the overall pattern.

The emergence of man-midwifery, which took place in London between about 1720 and 1750, was one of the most remarkable and consequential changes in English medicine at any point in the past. Down to the early eighteenth century, male involvement in childbirth was almost entirely restricted to difficult births: the typical form of male practice was the emergency call. A transition period, which we will examine in a moment, can be observed in the next few decades. Then, from about 1750, we find male practitioners acting *in lieu of a midwife*, delivering normal births – setting up a competition between the midwife and the man-midwife which was to continue, in a complex and unfolding struggle, until the beginning of the present century. The 1750 shift in the nature of male practice had effects on the scope of technical knowledge: thus William Hunter, the most successful exponent of the new form of male practice, brought the womb itself within the domain of male knowledge with his *Anatomy of the Gravid Uterus*, published in 1773 but based on researches started around 1750. The

[38] Stewart, 'Edge of Utility'.
[39] For a more detailed treatment, and for supporting references at greater length, see Adrian Wilson, *A Safe Deliverance: Ritual and Conflict in English Childbirth, 1600–1760* (Cambridge, in press), chapters 6–10. See also Herbert R. Spencer, *The History of British Midwifery from 1650 to 1800* (London, 1927); Jean Donnison, *Midwives and Medical Men: A History of Inter-Professional and Women's Rights* (London, 1977); and Margaret Connor Versluysen, 'Midwives, Medical Men and "Poor Women Labouring of Child": Lying-in Hospitals in Eighteenth-Century London' in Helen Roberts (ed.), *Women, Health and Reproduction* (London, 1981), pp. 18–49.

watershed of practice simultaneously generated a series of (largely ineffective) counter-attacks, starting in the 1750s, which criticised the new man-midwifery as immodest and interventionist and sought to raise the status and skills of midwives so that they could reverse the new trend. The transformation was most marked in the wealthier classes, that is, in the more lucrative sphere of practice. It has been variously seen as a heroic 'revolution in obstetrics' and as a tragic 'decline of the midwife', according to the viewpoint of the observer.[40] It embodied a new form of practice, not only by specialist *accoucheurs* such as Hunter, Smellie and Denman, but also amongst humbler surgeon-apothecaries, who now found that the management of normal birth was one of the standard tasks of their 'general practice'.[41] Its causes are baffling: it has usually been attributed to the dual influences of fashion and the midwifery forceps; yet the first of these explanations begs the question as to how the new 'fashion' got started, while the forceps was explicitly restricted to the small minority of difficult births.

It is on the phase of transition, from about 1720 to 1750, that I shall focus here. This was the period in which the midwifery forceps – one of the alleged causes of the 'revolution in obstetrics' – came into wider use (it had previously been a family secret amongst its inventors, the Chamberlen family), was published (in 1733–5), and was systematically taught to a new generation of male practitioners (by William Smellie in the 1740s).[42] With whiggish hindsight, the forceps seems to have played a critical role; and thus we have a story of a single, uncomplicated, unidirectional transition in this period. Yet, in fact, the forceps were *contested* from the outset. The crucial resource deployed against it was the suite of obstetric theories and techniques of the Dutch surgeon Hendrik van Deventer. Deventer's works, first published in 1701, were translated into English by Robert Samber in 1716; thereafter, a protracted struggle ensued between forceps practitioners on the one hand and the followers of Deventer on the other. The many and unprecedented public initiatives in midwifery in this period – the publication of treatises, systematic teaching, the creation of lying-in hospitals – were blows struck in a battle. That battle was not, as it appears with hindsight, between the old (midwives) and the new (men-

[40] J. H. Aveling, *English Midwives: Their History and Prospects* (London, 1872). p. 86; Donnison, *Midwives and Medical Men*, chapter 2.

[41] Irvine Loudon, *Medical Care and the General Practitioner* (Oxford, 1986), pp. 85–93.

[42] J. H. Aveling, *The Chamberlens and the Midwifery Forceps: Memorials of the Family and an Essay on the Invention of the Instrument* (London, 1882); Wilson, *A Safe Deliverance*, chapters 2, 8 and 9.

midwives); rather, it was between two parties of men-midwives, struggling for hegemony over practice and theory. Nor was the aim of this generation of men-midwives to replace the female midwife. Rather, their purpose was to gain much earlier access to difficult births; the midwife's role was intended to be circumscribed and defined, limited to managing easy natural labours, but there was no intention of displacing her. Earlier male access to difficult births meant the delivery of a living child, rather than a dead child; it meant a different social 'path' to the delivery-room;[43] and it made for substantially higher fees for the male practitioner. This was the domain of practice being contested between forceps practitioners and Deventerians. The struggle between the two groups has been obscured from historical vision by the fact that the forceps party eventually triumphed and Deventer's methods were forgotten. But this outcome was by no means inevitable; the struggle was keenly contested throughout this 'period of transition'.

The two parties of men-midwives were distinguished not just by obstetric allegiance but also in other ways. And amongst the *differentiae* between them was party-political allegiance. The early forceps practitioners, so far as their allegiance can be identified, were Tories; the followers of Deventer, by contrast, were Court Whigs. A shift took place in the 1740s, when the leading teacher of the forceps, William Smellie, was a Whig; but his was a Country rather than Court allegiance (signalled by his close association with Smollett), and meanwhile the Court Whig men-midwives continued to follow Deventer. The same battle still generated new initiatives: thus in 1746, when Smellie got one of his pupils to translate into English the earlier midwifery treatise of La Motte, this was a blow struck against Deventer's methods, while the Court Whig men-midwives who ran the lying-in wards of the Middlesex Hospital (1747) and who created the Brownlow Street Lying-in Hospital (1749) deployed Deventerian arguments and eschewed the forceps. Thus the teaching activities of Smellie and the creation of lying-in hospitals, which were seen by Dorothy George as a single movement, were in fact the visible effects of an underlying struggle and rivalry.[44]

The domain of man-midwifery thus illustrates yet again the role of party-political allegiance in the medical initiatives of the early Han-

[43] See Adrian Wilson, 'William Hunter and the Varieties of Man-Midwifery' in W. F. Bynum and Roy Porter (eds.), *William Hunter and the Eighteenth-Century Medical World* (Cambridge, 1985), pp. 343–69. In the terminology developed there, it was *onset calls with a midwife* which were now being sought.

[44] George, *London Life in the Eighteenth Century*, pp. 60–1.

overian period. The contest appears as a battle between Whig and Tory in the 1720s and '30s, and between Court and Country in the 1740s, with the Deventerians consistently on the Court Whig side, and forceps practitioners in the oppositional role. Whether this association between obstetric and party-political allegiances was a matter of accidents of patronage, or whether by contrast it reflected some deeper affinity between the two spheres, is a question for further research. But it is clear that there was such an association; that this helped to fuel the conflicts over technical obstetrics; and that each party of men-midwives had its lay supporters. The rise of man-midwifery can no more be grasped in isolation from the political history of the period than can the emergence of the first voluntary hospital or the campaign for smallpox inoculation.

We have examined three central instances of medical 'improvement' in early-eighteenth-century London: the creation of the first voluntary hospital; the campaign for smallpox inoculation; and the rise of man-midwifery in place of traditional obstetric surgery. Each of these developments turns out to have strong associations with political allegiance: the first was Tory, the second was Whig, and the third was a site of contest between the two parties. The concrete nature of the connections between medicine and politics remains to be explored, but at least we have established the existence of such connections in all three cases. It would be interesting to pursue a corresponding investigation for the other main site of practical medico-surgical innovation in this period, namely the treatment (both surgical and medical) of the excruciating and widespread complaint of stone in the bladder. Moreover the vast terrain of medical *theory* in this period awaits exploration along these lines. With the new resource of a listing of *Eighteenth Century Medics* – their book-subscriptions, education, apprenticeships – it is now becoming possible to locate medical practitioners within the complex and shifting networks of eighteenth-century patronage, thus vastly facilitating further explorations of the kind attempted here.[45] (If only the correspondence of Hans Sloane could be published, or at least calendared and indexed, the rich possibilities for further research would be still more handsomely demonstrated.) My aim has been both substantive and historiographic: not only to suggest some interpretations, but also to invite other scholars to engage in

---

[45] Peter J. V. Wallis, Ruth Wallis, Juanita Burnby and T. D. Wittet, *Eighteenth Century Medics (Subscriptions, Licences, Apprenticeships)* (Newcastle, 1985), and the associated lists of books published by subscription. New editions of these works, incorporating still more details, are now in press.

further exploration along these lines. As has repeatedly emerged, there is no shortage either of interesting topics or of source materials for investigation.

The central result of the findings outlined here is to insert medical history firmly within the matrix of the political history of the period. We began by observing the disciplinary phenomenon of 'tunnel history': the division of the past into separate zones such as political history, social history, ecclesiastical history, history of science. By now it should be clear that these divisions, applied to our period, have robbed the past of much of its meaning and interest. No doubt political historians who read *Applebee's* noticed its attacks on inoculation, but so far as I am aware, none of them thought this interesting or relevant to their own concerns. Similarly, historians of medicine have been well aware of party-political conflict in our period, without apparently noticing that this had medical implications. Similar arguments can be advanced against *all* the walls which modern sub-disciplines have erected within the past. Literature emerged from a social matrix; demographic phenomena were intertwined with economic matters and thus with politics; natural philosophy was a sphere of active contests which connected, for instance, with the critique of the stage.[46] It is precisely in their interconnectedness that the events and phenomena of the period can be understood and explained. Total history is the only viable approach, difficult though this may be to construct. What is required in the first instance is active collaboration between historians of different competences. Alas, institutional divisions make such collaboration very difficult to sustain.

If there is a single dramatic question which arises from the present findings, this concerns the *chronology* of the processes explored above. Strikingly, in all three spheres we have investigated, the crucial moment of conflict and initiative turns out to be the first five years or even less of the reign of George I. It was in 1714 that the first reports of smallpox inoculation were transmitted to the Royal Society; in 1716 that the Westminster Charitable Society was first set up; and in 1716, again, that Deventer's treatises were first translated into English. Yet party-political conflict – the explanatory resource I have deployed here – did not begin in 1714; on the contrary, it had begun, in the form of a Whig/Tory contest (though over different issues), well over a genera-

---

[46] See Simon Schaffer, 'Electricity, the People, and the Wrath of God: The Martin–Freke Debate', *Isis*, forthcoming; and compare Rosemary Bechler, '"Triall by what is Contrary": Samuel Richardson and Christian Dialectic' in Valerie Grosvenor Myer (ed.), *Samuel Richardson: Passion and Prudence* (London, 1986), pp. 93–113, at pp. 94–8.

tion before. Were the battles of the Exclusion Crisis (1679–81) and subsequent developments translated into medical initiatives? If so, what were those initiatives? If not, why not? It is precisely for the exploration of questions such as these that collaborative research is required.

The general claim that medical initiatives had politico-religious roots, while novel for the period, is of course highly familiar for the seventeenth century. Let us remind ourselves how Charles Webster summed up the findings of his *Great Instauration:*[47]

Each group . . . tended to develop an attitude towards nature consistent with its social, political and religious position . . . strongly contrasting styles of science were being evolved in response to differing intellectual standpoints . . . The borderlines between the various groups were never defined rigidly; certain individuals gradually reoriented themselves . . . nevertheless, at any one point in time it is possible to discern a mosaic of competing groups wedded to different value systems. The various groups identify themselves both by the type of phenomenon chosen for investigation and by their method of approach . . .

Adding medicine to science, and incorporating practical innovations as well as theoretical investigations, this can serve as an apt description of the picture I have tried to paint of some key developments in early Hanoverian London.

[47] Webster *Great Instauration*, pp. 497–8.

V

Conflict, Consensus and Charity: Politics and the Provincial Voluntary Hospitals in the Eighteenth Century*

THE voluntary hospitals were amongst the most original and enduring monuments of Georgian England. Financed on the seemingly flimsy basis of voluntary benefactions and annual subscriptions,[1] they nevertheless flourished in the eighteenth century and subsequently became the leading medical institutions of the industrial age. By entitling even the small subscriber to recommend patients, they recruited substantial support amongst the large class of shopkeepers and traders; by weighting this power in proportion to the size of the contribution, they nevertheless preserved the pre-eminence of local magnates. By making subscription open to men and women of all confessions, they worked for the hegemony and unity of property against the threat of religious divisions; by enlisting subscribers as governors, they rewarded the act of giving with a share of power. Managed by honorary committees elected annually from the subscribers themselves, they enabled the shopkeeper to join the grandee in a common enterprise; by restricting committee-membership to male subscribers, they kept within bounds the participation of 'the sex'. Through the annual publication of the financial accounts, the subscribers' names, and the numbers of patients 'cured' and 'relieved', they ensured probity of management, gave publicity to the subscribers great and small, and assured those subscribers that their money had been well spent. With their strong local roots, they promoted a sense of civic identity; by bringing together local medical men as honorary consultants, they helped to forge a professional medical community; by constructing a new context for medicine, they led to innovations in medical practice and teaching. And by making charity dependent upon the channel of personal recommendation, they exacted

* This study has been supported by the Wellcome Trust, and has used the facilities of the Birmingham Central Library, the Brotherton Library (University of Leeds), Cambridge University Library, the Thackray Medical Museum at Leeds, and the library of the Wellcome Institute for the History of Medicine. While any errors are my own responsibility, I wish to thank many individuals for their help. Mark Jenner and Bill Speck gave me initial guidance and also commented on the first draft. For responses to that draft I am grateful also to Amanda Berry, Ann Borsay, Geoffrey Cantor, John Christie, Patrick Curry, Roger French, Ann Hargreaves, Ben Marsden, Frank O'Gorman, John Pickstone, Roy Porter, John Woodward and David Wykes. Special thanks go to Timothy Ashplant, John Cannon, Paul Langford and Katherine Webb, and also to a reader for the *English Historical Review*, for detailed observations and information which have led to many revisions of the text; and particularly to Mike Woodhouse, who has helped very generously with advice, comments and information.

1. Addenbrooke's at Cambridge (1766) and the Radcliffe at Oxford (1770) each benefited from personal legacies made some decades earlier, and duly took their names from the respective benefactors; both of them, however, owed their actual foundation to collective local action and functioned as county hospitals.

146

a political tribute from the sick poor who sought the benefit of their facilities. To each individual patient the hospitals made available a massive though brief donation of help in a time of need. To the poor collectively they offered a profound and highly visible subordination, translating the practice and rhetoric of personal dependence into an institutional setting.[1]

Although the voluntary-hospital form was invented in London, where the Westminster Infirmary was founded in 1719, the wider hospital movement which dates from the 1730s was just as strong in the provinces as in the capital. Like 'Sylvanus Urban', the pseudonymous editor of the *Gentleman's Magazine*, the provincial infirmaries elegantly united country and town – the two synergistic sources of polite Georgian culture. Most such infirmaries were county hospitals; all of them were situated in substantial towns, and had some sense of responsibility towards the town. Sometimes this dual identity was enshrined in the infirmary's very name, from the *Winchester County* Hospital (1736) to the *Kent and Canterbury* Hospital (1793). Elsewhere the connection took other forms. The Infirmary at Newcastle upon Tyne (1751) served the counties of Northumberland and Durham and the town itself, whose corporation made available a permanent site at a nominal rent. At Lincoln the County Infirmary (1769) conferred *ex officio* membership of its governing board on the mayor and aldermen of the town.[2]

Just as each individual infirmary linked county and town, so collectively the provincial voluntary hospitals displayed both national and local features. On the one hand, they were linked in a national movement. Four of the first five provincial infirmaries were inspired by two individuals: Alured Clarke, successively prebendary at Winchester and cathedral dean at Exeter, who set up the county hospitals at Winchester and at Exeter (1741), and Lady Elizabeth Hastings, who helped to initiate both the York County Infirmary (1740) and the Bath General Hospital (1742).[3] Their leading role was continued by such activists as Martin Benson and Isaac Maddox, bishops of Gloucester and Worcester, and Thomas Secker, Archbishop of Canterbury.[4] Several subse-

1. For overviews of hospital procedures, see Anne Borsay, ' "Persons of Honour and Reputation": The Voluntary Hospital in an Age of Corruption', *Medical History*, xxxv (1991), 281–94, and Adrian Wilson, 'The Politics of Medical Improvement in Early Hanoverian London', in *The Medical Enlightenment of the Eighteenth Century*, ed. Andrew Cunningham and Roger K. French (Cambridge, 1990), pp. 4–39, at pp. 24–34.

2. S. Middlebrook, *Newcastle upon Tyne: Its Growth and Achievement* (Newcastle upon Tyne, 1950), p. 122; G. H. Hume, *The History of the Newcastle Infirmary* (Newcastle upon Tyne, 1908), p. 7; Francis Hill, *Georgian Lincoln* (Cambridge, 1966), p. 71.

3. Roy Porter, 'The Gift Relation: Philanthropy and Provincial Hospitals in Eighteenth-Century England', in *The Hospital in History*, ed. Lindsay Granshaw and Roy Porter (London 1989), pp. 149–78; Ann Borsay, 'Cash and Conscience: Financing the General Hospital at Bath, c. 1738–1750', *Social History of Medicine*, iv (1991), 207–29, at 207; Beatrice Scott, 'Lady Elizabeth Hastings', *Yorkshire Archaeological Journal*, lv (1983), 95–118, at 110.

4. For Benson (1689–1752, Bishop of Gloucester from 1735), see Hume, *History of the Newcastle Infirmary*, p. 125; D[ictionary of] N[ational] B[iography], s.v.; and Donna T. Andrew, 'On Reading

quent infirmaries were modelled on individual predecessors: thus the Winchester Hospital was the model for the Salop Infirmary (1747), the rules of the Bristol Infirmary (1737) were copied by the Worcester Infirmary (1746), and those of Northampton (1743) were imitated at Newcastle.[1] And many later infirmaries asserted a wider emulation: thus at Liverpool it was stated in 1748 that 'the advantages of Infirmary Hospitals are now ... evident from their own good effects', and the town's own Infirmary opened in the following year.[2]

On the other hand, each infirmary necessarily had strong local roots, making for variety: thus different hospitals had distinct management practices, medical activities, and local relationships.[3] And the most striking aspect of this diversity concerns the very origins of these institutions – for as Table 1 reveals, the chronology and geography of hospital foundation show no easily explicable pattern. Indeed, the eighteenth-century movement was not exactly national in scope, for not all towns or counties were persuaded of the 'evident advantages' of infirmaries. Thus in the early 1740s attempts were made to create county infirmaries in Berkshire, Lincolnshire and Norfolk, but without success.[4] Each of these plans attracted some backing: the Norfolk proposal was published in the *Norwich Gazette* in 1744, and reiterated in 1750;[5] that for Berkshire reached the pages of the *Gentleman's Magazine* in 1743 and 1744;[6] and the Lincoln proposal came from 'several lords and gentlemen of the county', was supported by the high sheriff and grand jury, and issued in a twenty-seven-page printed plan.[7] Yet all three attempts lapsed – in contrast with contemporary initiatives in three

Charity Sermons: Eighteenth-Century Anglican Solicitation and Exhortation', *Journal of Ecclesiastical History*, xliii (1992), 581–91, at 583 (the 1736 sermon mentioned there seems to have been for Christ's Hospital); Isaac Maddox, *The Duty and Advantages of Public Infirmaries* (London, 1743); id., *The Duty and Advantages of Public Infirmaries ... Further Considered* (London, 1744); id., *The Necessity of Persisting in Well-Doing* (Worcester, 1748). For Secker, see John R. Guy, 'Archbishop Secker as a Physician', *The Church and Healing*, ed. W. J. Sheils (Ecclesiastical History Soc., Oxford, 1982), pp. 127–35, at pp. 132, 135; Porter, 'The Gift Relation', p. 163; cf. *infra*, p. 604, n. 4.

  1. Porter, 'The Gift Relation', p. 151; Joan Lane, *Worcester Infirmary in the Eighteenth Century* (Worcester Historical Soc., Occas. Pubs., vol. vi, 1992), p. 1; W. E. Hume, 'The Origin and Early History of the Infirmary of Newcastle upon Tyne', *Archaeologia Aeliana*, 4th ser. xxii (1954), 72–99, at 78.

  2. George McLoughlin, *A Short History of the Liverpool Infirmary, 1749–1824* (Chichester, 1978), p. 16.

  3. Porter, 'The Gift Relation', p. 151.

  4. And also an unsuccessful proposal for a dispensary at Coventry: see *infra*, p. 605, n. 5.

  5. P. Eade, *The Norfolk and Norwich Hospital 1770 to 1900* (Norwich, 1900), p. 17; Kathleen Wilson, 'Urban Culture and Political Activism in Hanoverian England: The Example of Voluntary Hospitals', in *The Transformation of Political Culture: England and Germany in the Late Eighteenth Century*, ed. E. Hellmuth (Oxford, 1990), pp. 165–84, at p. 170, n. 11. In 1751 it was thought in Newcastle that the Norwich initiative had succeeded: see Frederick J. W. Miller, 'The Infirmary on the Forth, 1753–1906', *Archaeologia Aeliana*, 5th ser. ix (1986), 143–65, at 143.

  6. *Gentleman's Magazine*, xiii (1743), 640 and ibid., xiv (1744), 47. I am grateful to Mike Woodhouse for these references.

  7. Hill, *Georgian Lincoln*, pp. 70–1; D. Mary Short, *A Bibliography of Printed Items Relating to the City of Lincoln* (Lincoln Record Soc., vol. lxxix, 1990), p. 315.

Table 1.   Provincial Voluntary Hospitals Founded before 1800, with Dates of Foundation and Associated Constituencies

County	Hospital name	Date	Borough
Hants*	Winchester CH	1736	Winchester
Somerset	Bristol I	1737	Bristol*
Yorks*	York CH	1740	York*
Devon*	Devon & Exeter H	1741	Exeter*
Somerset	Bath GH	1742	Bath
Northants*	Northampton CI	1743	Northampton*
Worcs*	Worcester I	1746	Worcester*
Salop*	Salop I	1747	Shrewsbury
Lancs	Liverpool I	1749	Liverpool*
Northumb'd, Durham	Newcastle I	1751	Newcastle*
Lancs	Manchester PI	1752	–
Cheshire*	Chester I	1755	Chester*
Gloucs*	Gloucester I	1755	Gloucester*
Cambs*	Addenbrooke's H	1766	Cambridge
Staffs*	Stafford CH	1766	Stafford
Wilts*	Salisbury CH	1766	Salisbury
Yorks	Leeds GI	1767	–
Lincs*	Lincoln CH	1769	Lincoln*
Oxon*	Radcliffe I	1770	Oxford*
Leics	Leicester I	1771	Leicester*
Norfolk*	Norfolk & Norwich H	1771	Norwich *
Herefs*	Hereford GI	1776	Hereford*
Warwickshire	Birmingham GH	1779	–
Notts*	Nottingham GH	1782	Nottingham*
Yorks	Hull I	1782	Kingston-upon-Hull*
Somerset*	Somerset CI	1792	Taunton
Kent*	Kent & Canterbury H	1793	Canterbury*
Yorks	Sheffield I	1797	–

Notes:
1. Asterisks in the county and borough columns identify the 'hospital constituencies' discussed in the text.
2. Key to names of hospitals:

   H   Hospital
   I   Infirmary
   C   County
   G   General
   P   Public

149

other counties[1] – and they were not revived until a generation later in Lincolnshire and Norfolk, and almost a century later in Berkshire.[2] The fate of such early initiatives did not depend in any simple way upon a town's demographic size or local importance. Of the regional capitals, Bristol, York and Exeter all acquired hospitals by 1741, and Newcastle followed suit in 1751, but Salisbury not until 1766 and Norwich only in 1771 (despite the attempt of 1744). The counties, too, behaved in very different ways: for instance, in the West Country, Devon entered the movement early (1741), as we have seen; Somerset joined it very late (1792); and Dorset and Cornwall had still not joined it by 1800, even though a Cornish Infirmary was projected without success in 1799.[3] In short, the hospital 'movement' was patchy and its complexities remain unexplained. Many counties and substantial towns still lacked an infirmary in 1800; and it is far from clear why (say) Northampton, Leicester and Nottingham founded hospitals in the eighteenth century, whereas (for example) Derby, Bury St Edmunds and Great Yarmouth did not.

Equally unresolved is the question as to the political and religious identity of the hospitals. The prevailing view sees them as associated with elite or class consensus – as a focus through which Tory and Whig, Anglican and Dissenter could unite in the pursuit of common objectives.[4] This account looks forward implicitly, and sometimes explicitly, to the nineteenth century, when the mechanism of voluntary subscription – of which the hospitals were early exemplars – served as an instrument to unite the middle class and indeed, it has been argued, to forge the very identity of that class.[5] While this interpretation matches much of the hospitals' own eighteenth-century rhetoric, at least until the 1770s,[6] it is still unclear how well it describes their real origins, activities and bases of support. Only seldom has this view been backed up by systematic study of the records, and even then with ambiguous results.[7] In those few hospitals whose conjunctures of founding or leading governors have been investigated, distinct political or religious

1. In the 1740s county infirmaries were established at Northampton (1743), Worcester (1746) and Shrewsbury (1747).
2. The Lincoln County Infirmary was established in 1769, the Norfolk and Norwich Hospital in 1771, and the Royal Berkshire Infirmary in 1839.
3. Porter, 'The Gift relation', p. 160. Somerset had acquired the Bath General Hospital in 1742, but this was not designed for local patients. However, it apparently treated a disproportionately large number from Somerset: see Borsay, 'Cash and Conscience', 218, n. 68.
4. Porter, 'The Gift Relation'; Borsay, 'Cash and Conscience', 219; Donna Andrew, *Philanthropy and Police: London Charity in the Eighteenth Century* (Princeton, 1989).
5. R. J. Morris, 'Voluntary Societies and British Urban Elites, 1780–1850: An Analysis', *Historical Journal*, xxvi (1983), 95–118, at 97–8; id., *Class, Sect and Party: The Making of the British Middle Class, Leeds, 1820–1850* (Manchester, 1990); Wilson, 'Urban Culture and Political Activism'.
6. It seems that the appeal in charity sermons to 'the pacific and unifying effects of joint charitable activity', common at mid-century, disappeared 'after the 1770s': Andrew, 'On Reading Charity Sermons', 583, 585.
7. P. Langford, *Public Life and the Propertied Englishman, 1689–1798* (Oxford, 1991), pp. 128–30; see further *infra*, p. 605, n. 2.

institutional identities have repeatedly emerged, both in London (just as in the endowed hospitals there) and in the provinces.[1] Thus the very first voluntary hospital, the Westminster Infirmary, began as a Tory project in the wake of the calamitous political defeats of 1714–15; the London Hospital, created in 1740, was 'patronized by the great Whig families, and was dominated by Whig officers and Whig subscribers'; and a preliminary investigation suggests that the Middlesex Hospital, established in 1745, was equally Whig.[2] Similarly, the Bristol Infirmary was 'largely governed by Quakers'; the governors of the Bath General Hospital were predominantly Tories; while at Leicester the Tory corporation 'gave not a penny towards the founding of the infirmary, which was managed by a cabal of prominent Whigs'.[3] These findings suggest that a case can be made for linking the hospitals back to the 'first age of party', rather than forwards to the age of class.

One reason for this uncertainty as to the political and religious meaning of the hospitals is that political historians have taken little interest in these institutions. The main activists behind the national hospital movement – Lady Elizabeth Hastings, Alured Clarke, Isaac Maddox, Thomas Secker – are seldom discussed, even though each of these individuals had particular allegiances in politics and religion.[4] Though political historians are increasingly widening their focus from parliamentary and electoral processes to other activities, such as petitions, addresses, sermons and charities, the infirmaries have for the most part remained beyond their horizon.[5] This is all the more regrettable since many of the hospitals were established in towns notable for

1. See Craig Rose, 'Politics and the London Royal Hospitals, 1683–92', in *The Hospital in History*, pp. 123–48.

2. Wilson, 'The Politics of Medical Improvement'; Langford, *Public Life and the Propertied Englishman*, p. 129; Adrian Wilson, *The Making of Man-Midwifery: Childbirth in England, 1660–1770* (London, 1995), ch. 11.

3. M. Fissell, *Patients, Power and the Poor in Eighteenth-Century Bristol* (Cambridge, 1991), p. 90; Borsay, 'Cash and Conscience', 219; Porter, 'The Gift Relation', p. 154.

4. Hastings was associated with Henry Hoare, Mary Astell and the SPCK, suggesting a Tory allegiance. Clarke and Maddox were comprehensionists, working for an eventual union between the Established Church and the Dissenters; Secker was apparently sympathetic to this view. For Hastings, see Borsay, 'Cash and Conscience', 207, and Scott, 'Lady Elizabeth Hastings', *passim*. For Clarke and his circle, see Barbara Carpenter Turner, *A History of the Royal Hampshire County Hospital* (Chichester, 1986), p. 4, and *DNB, s.v.* 'Charlotte Clayton, lady Sundon'. For Maddox, see W. H. McMenemy, *A History of the Worcester Royal Infirmary* (London, 1947), and Philip Doddridge, 'Compassion to the Sick Recommended and Urged' (1743), in *Works*, ed. Edward Williams and Edward Parsons (10 vols., Leeds, 1802–5), iii. 93–116, at 107. For Secker, see Geoffrey Nuttall, 'Doddridge's Life and Times', in *Philip Doddridge 1702–51: His Contribution to English Religion*, ed. Nuttall (London, 1951), pp. 11–31, at pp. 25–6.

5. John Money, *Experience and Identity: Birmingham and the West Midlands, 1760–1800* (Manchester, 1977); James E. Bradley, *Religion, Revolution, and English Radicalism: Nonconformity in Eighteenth-Century Politics and Society* (Cambridge, 1990); Linda Colley, *Britons: Forging the Nation, 1707–1837* (New Haven/London, 1992). This historiographic boundary is strikingly apparent in Bradley's excellent study, which mentions charities only in passing and only for Bristol (p. 209), without discussing the Infirmary there. Yet at Newcastle, which is the focus of another of Bradley's case-studies, Kathleen Wilson has found that 'several radical leaders served their political apprenticeships in the ... Infirmary, or took a leading role in founding similar charities': 'Urban culture and Political Activism', p. 182.

151

their continuous political traditions.[1] The one political historian who has directly researched any of the hospitals, Paul Langford, has produced a contradictory set of findings. On the one hand, 'Propertied combination was meant to unite rather than divide'; 'the clearest test case is perhaps that of the infirmaries'; and in support of this thesis, the Northampton Infirmary of 1743 showed 'no hint of party bias'. Yet on the other hand, 'even the voluntary bodies found it difficult to steer completely clear of party politics', as was shown by party troubles affecting the infirmaries at Shrewsbury, York and Liverpool.[2] The historiographic exception confirms the rule: it remains unclear just how the infirmaries fitted on to the eighteenth-century political map. Here we have one reflection amongst many of the persistent gulf between 'social' and 'political' history.[3] The present essay attempts to bridge this divide by relating the foundation of the hospitals to electoral contests. For strategic reasons this exercise will be conducted at the national level, though as we shall see the subject demands intensive local research.

To the extent that the hospitals have been connected with eighteenth-century politics at all, the link between the two spheres has been seen as eirenic. Specifically, Roy Porter has observed that infirmaries were designed to transcend party and religious divisions; and Langford has taken this further, arguing that these institutions actually helped to create a unified propertied interest.[4] That is, hospitals were intended to reduce party conflict, and they succeeded in mitigating its effects. While such claims were a commonplace of sermons in support of the hospitals, at least one eighteenth-century observer suggested that the association ran in the opposite direction. In 1744 one 'W.H.', attempting to revive a plan put forward three years earlier for a dispensary at Coventry, wrote in the *Northampton Mercury*:[5]

> The following plan was drawn up at Coventry in August 1741 during the epidemic fever that then raged there. ... [The plan] being communicated to a few of the leading inhabitants, they hinted many difficulties which, from the rancour of party, at that time too predominant, would inevitably retard, if not wholly defeat the attempt. Their diffidence of its success suppressed its publication; yet this very plan enlarg'd, partly gave rise, in the year 1743, to ... the County Infirmary at Northampton: And as I am persuaded (from the

1. Five of the twelve boroughs listed by O'Gorman as having the most active and continuous traditions of party politics were hospital towns (Bristol, Gloucester, Leicester, Nottingham, York). Eight of the twenty-two boroughs in O'Gorman's next most politically-active grade of boroughs were hospital towns (Chester, Exeter, Lincoln, Liverpool, Newcastle upon Tyne, Norwich, Oxford, Worcester). Together these account for almost half (13:28) of all the provincial hospitals, for more than half (13:24) of the hospitals in borough towns, and for over a third (13:34) of the most politically-active boroughs. See Frank O'Gorman, *Voters, Patrons, and Parties: The Unreformed Electoral System of Hanoverian England, 1734–1832* (Oxford, 1989), pp. 350–6.
2. Langford, *Public Life and the Propertied Englishman*, pp. 128–30.
3. See my 'A Critical Portrait of Social History', in *Rethinking Social History: English Society, 1570–1920, and its Interpretation*, ed. Wilson (Manchester, 1993), pp. 9–58.
4. Porter, 'The Gift Relation'; Langford, *Public Life and the Propertied Englishman*, pp. 128–30.
5. *Northampton Mercury*, 10 Mar. 1743–4. I thank Mike Woodhouse for this reference.

152

present general harmony, owing, perhaps, to our frequent amicable meetings at the late summer-evening entertainments, contriv'd by the ingenious Mr Spires[1]) we may now put the ... plan into immediate execution ... I have ... at last obtained the benevolent author's permission to print the aforesaid plan ...

The 'rancour of party' in 1741 was hardly surprising in an election year, particularly in a borough as often contested as Coventry. (As it happened, 'W.H.' proved too sanguine, for his attempt to revive the Coventry dispensary scheme was unsuccessful.) The point to notice is the suggestion that the successful launching of a hospital (or in this case, a dispensary) required a *pre-existing* political harmony – precisely the inverse of the usual claim.

Thus eighteenth-century testimony can be used to suggest that the putative eirenic associations of hospitals ran in either direction, or in both. But such testimony was by no means disinterested. On the contrary, it was a standard trope of political rhetoric to present a particular interest as the general interest, a party move – particularly in the realm of charity – as an anti-party initiative.[2] Thus contemporary claims that hospital foundation either reflected or promoted a spirit of party co-operation, a burying of political hatchets, ought to be treated with at least a measure of suspicion. Further, it has to be admitted that the eirenic picture as a whole still rests on a mere handful of such rhetorical claims: a general case has been made from only a few examples, and it remains to be seen whether these can be generalized. (We know that Joseph Priestley supported the Leeds General Infirmary in 1768, but did he back the Birmingham General Hospital in the 1780s?)[3] In short, if we are to assess the accuracy of the prevailing picture, it will be necessary both to move beyond such rhetorical testimony, and to use a more systematic method than the mere assembling of examples.

One possible way of approaching this task is to use the incidence of contests at general elections as an index of political conflict, and to set this against the presence or absence of infirmaries in the relevant county and borough constituencies.[4] Admittedly, the frequency of electoral contests will supply at best only an oblique measure of political tension, since, as O'Gorman has stressed, 'the absence of contested elections does not allow us to conclude that party conflict was absent'. In some constituencies contests were avoided simply because support for the two parties was known to be equally balanced; further, there were many

1. This doubtless refers to the concerts of vocal and instrumental music at Spires's Spring Garden. See Peter Borsay, *The English Urban Renaissance: Culture and Society in the Provincial Town, 1660–1800* (Oxford, 1989), pp. 333, 351.

2. Wilson, 'The Politics of Medical Improvement', pp. 7–8.

3. Porter, 'The Gift Relation', pp. 163–4; I find no mention of Priestley in this connection in Money, *Experience and Identity*. Priestley moved to Birmingham in 1780: William Hutton, *An History of Birmingham* (2nd edn., Birmingham 1783), p. 117.

4. The authorities cited below also list contested by-elections; but I have excluded these, since it is not clear whether the absence of a by-electoral contest (which was the usual state of affairs) indicates no contest (as with general elections) or simply no by-election. Thus the incidence of by-electoral contests is not formally comparable with the incidence of general-election contests.

'aborted contests' - elections where a poll was avoided when informal canvassing established in advance what the result would be.[1] Nor were electoral contests, when they did occur, necessarily affairs of party: on the contrary, from the 1740s to the 1760s (a period in which over half the hospitals were founded) such contests were more commonly stimulated by dynastic rivalry in the counties and by such issues as oligarchic control in the boroughs.

Despite these ambiguities, it will still be worth comparing the pattern of hospital foundation with the incidence of electoral contests. For it is only if we *fail* to find the 'expected' association between hospitals and (apparent) political quietude that these considerations will come into play. If it turns out that hospitals *were* associated with a relatively low incidence of electoral contests, this will also suggest that, despite the qualifications just mentioned, the frequency of contests reflected, to some extent at least, the intensity of political conflict in the various constituencies.[2] And only by attempting the exercise can we discover whether this was the case. Let us therefore proceed to compare the frequency of contests in constituencies with and without a hospital, and to ask how this related to the moment of hospital foundation.[3] If local political calm was the precondition for hospital foundation, then we would expect that 'hospital constituencies' experienced a relatively low rate of contests *before* the moment of hospital foundation. Conversely, if hospitals promoted political harmony, we would expect this to emerge *after* the respective hospitals were founded. In view of the hospitals' associations with both town and county, we need to pursue this investigation both in the counties and in the boroughs. In each case the definition of comparable 'hospital' and 'non-hospital' constituencies is not quite straightforward.[4]

Relevant county constituencies: I have used England, less Monmouthshire, as the sphere of comparison. Nineteen of the thirty-nine counties (identified by asterisks in Table 1) belonged to the 'hospital' category, i.e. they acquired before 1800 a hospital named as a county infirmary or at least situated in the county town. Fifteen counties belonged to the

1. O'Gorman, *Voters, Patrons, and Parties*, pp. 342 (and cf. p. 341), 111–12.

2. In addition, Paul Langford notes (personal communication) that the frequency of contests might not capture the putative effects of hospitals, for a new, extra-party arena might conceivably have been created without necessarily reducing partisan activity in its traditional domains of parliamentary elections and corporation politics. The same applies to this as to the issues raised in the text: it will make a 'negative' finding difficult to interpret, but will not affect a 'positive' finding.

3. Just two hospitals were founded in election years. The Devon and Exeter Hospital (23 July 1741) *post-dated* the election of that year (19 May): see Romney Sedgwick, *The House of Commons, 1715–1754* (2 vols., London, 1970), i. 46, and John Caldwell, 'Notes on the history of Dean Clarke's Hospital, 1741–1948', *Reports and Transactions of the Devonshire Association for the Advancement of Science, Literature and Art*, civ (1972), 175–92, at 175–6. Although the Salop Infirmary opened in 1747, its inaugural meeting *pre-dated* this election by some years (Mike Woodhouse, personal communication).

4. Constituency characteristics were taken from the Appendix tables given in Sedgwick, *The House of Commons, 1715–1754*; Sir Lewis Namier and John Brooke, *The House of Commons, 1754–1790* (2 vols., London, 1964); and R. G. Thorne, *The House of Commons, 1790–1820* (2 vols., London, 1986).

154

'non-hospital' category, in that they did not acquire a county infirmary before 1800. Five counties had to be excluded from the comparison. Middlesex, where a hospital was founded in 1745, has been excluded because both its electorate and its hospital were effectively part of London, and it is thus not comparable with other counties.[1] Northumberland and Durham were jointly served by a single hospital, the Newcastle Infirmary; as a result this hospital could not be associated with a specific county constituency, nor could these counties be assigned to the 'non-hospital' category.[2] Finally, Lancashire and Warwickshire were special cases of a different kind. Lancashire was served by the Manchester Infirmary, founded in 1752 (though not by the Liverpool Infirmary, established three years earlier, which was restricted to the town and drew the great bulk of its support from urban subscribers).[3] Yet the basis of the Manchester Infirmary was not so much the county as the region, that is 'eastern Lancashire and Cheshire' – at least until the Chester Infirmary was created in 1755.[4] Similarly in Warwickshire, the Birmingham General Hospital (1779) was designed to serve 'the populous county about it' as well as Birmingham itself; but this may have referred to the town's practical hinterland, which cut across county boundaries, embracing parts of Worcestershire and Staffordshire, but excluding much of Warwickshire itself.[5] (The parallel between these two hospitals was no accident: both towns were rapidly growing centres of manufacture, situated near the geographical edges of their respective counties.) It may well be that after closer examination, either or both of the hospitals at Manchester and Birmingham should be regarded as county hospitals; but in the first instance, their counties cannot clearly be allocated to either the 'hospital' or the 'non-hospital' category.

Relevant borough constituencies: Of the twenty-eight voluntary hospitals founded before 1800, twenty-four were situated in towns which enjoyed a borough franchise.[6] But that franchise took several different

---

Contests were identified from John Cannon, *Parliamentary Reform, 1640–1832* (Cambridge, 1973), App. 3 (pp. 276–89).

1. Since Middlesex was removed from the 'hospital' counties because of its association with London, it might be argued that Essex, Hertfordshire and Surrey should be excluded from the 'non-hospital' counties for the same reason (I thank John Cannon for drawing my attention to this point). The analyses reported below were therefore repeated with these three counties excluded; this lowered the rate of contests in the 'non-hospital' counties (see Fig. 2), but otherwise did not affect the findings.

2. Hume, 'The Origin and Early History of the Infirmary of Newcastle upon Tyne', 78; Wilson, 'Urban Culture and Political Activism', pp. 173, 176.

3. McLoughlin, *A Short History of the Liverpool Infirmary, passim*; Wilson, 'Urban Culture and Political Activism', p. 174.

4. J. V. Pickstone, *Medicine and Industrial Society: A History of Hospital Development in Manchester and its Region, 1752–1946* (Manchester, 1985), p. 13 (quoted); cf. William Brockbank, *Portrait of a Hospital, 1752–1948* (London, 1952), pp. 11–12, and id., 'The Manchester Publick Infirmary, Lunatic Hospital and Dispensary', *Manchester University Medical School Gazette*, xxvi (1947), 131–5, and xxvii (1948), 31–5, at 134.

5. Money, *Experience and Identity*, p. 9.

6. The four exceptions were Manchester, Leeds, Birmingham and Sheffield.

forms – freeman, burgage, corporation, scot and lot, householder – and was associated with electorates of very different sizes, which behaved electorally in different ways. Thus if we are to compare 'hospital boroughs' with 'non-hospital boroughs' we must restrict attention to some comparable type or types of constituency. In fact, seventeen of the twenty-four 'hospital boroughs' had large electorates (1,000 voters or more), either for all of the period in view (fifteen cases) or at least from before the respective hospitals were founded (the remaining two cases).[1] Of these seventeen, sixteen were freeman boroughs and the remaining one, Northampton, had a householder franchise. Thus the simplest way of making a valid comparison between 'hospital' and 'non-hospital' boroughs is to restrict attention to boroughs with a freeman or householder franchise, whose electorates were or became 'large' during the eighteenth century. This means that we have eleven 'non-hospital boroughs'[2] for comparison with seventeen 'hospital boroughs' (the latter are identified by asterisks in Table 1).[3]

Figures 1 and 2, treating the boroughs and the counties respectively, display the frequencies of electoral contests in 'non-hospital' constituencies and in 'hospital' constituencies, both before and after these acquired their hospitals. Here the period from 1716 to 1806 has been divided into five phases, each spanning three general elections. (Some such aggregation is required because the small numbers of county contests make for random fluctuations in the apparent rate of contests if a single-election focus is used. The five-phase division used here is arbitrary, but is largely justified on political grounds.) The first result of this exercise is to suggest that the frequency of contests may indeed have reflected not only such contingent influences as dynastic rivalry, but also the underlying state of political relations in the various constituencies. For both in the boroughs and in the counties, 'hospital constituencies' experienced fewer electoral contests than did 'non-hospital constituencies' – just as we were led to expect. But the form of this association, and its clarity, differed between the boroughs and the counties. In the boroughs (Figure 1) the pattern was clear-cut: before obtaining their hospitals, 'hospital boroughs' experienced the same rate of contests as did 'non-hospital boroughs', whereas after hospital foundation they had proportionately fewer contests. Thus, in line with

1. The electorates at Lincoln (county infirmary 1769) and at Kingston upon Hull (town infirmary 1782) expanded from 'medium' to 'large' at mid-century. On electoral sizes I have followed the various volumes of *The House of Commons*.

2. All these eleven were freeman boroughs. The electorates in six of these boroughs were 'medium' until 1747, but 'large' from 1754: Bedford, Carlisle, Maidstone, Dover, Evesham and Beverley. The remaining five were 'large' throughout the period: Durham, Colchester, Lancaster, Bridgnorth and Coventry. Strictly speaking, Preston (a householder borough) should have been included, since its electorate eventually expanded from 'medium' to 'large'; but this occurred so late (c. 1790) that it was thought best to exclude Preston throughout.

3. The hospital boroughs excluded were Winchester, Cambridge, Shrewsbury and Stafford, with freeman franchises and 'small' electorates; Bath and Salisbury, with corporation franchises and 'small' electorates; and Taunton, with a householder franchise and a 'medium'-sized electorate.

156

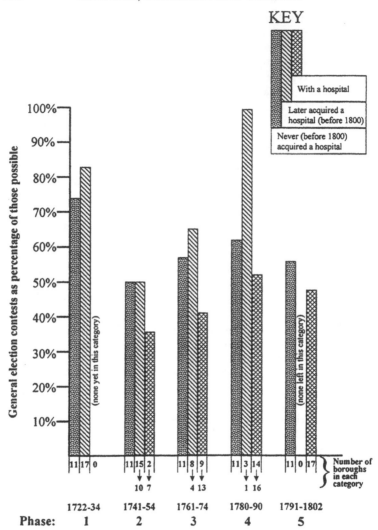

Fig. 1.   Borough contests: distinguishing boroughs which never acquired a hospital from those which later acquired one.

Langford's argument, it appears that hospitals tended to promote a degree of political peace in the boroughs; but contrary to what 'W.H.' suggested in 1744, it did not require a pre-existing harmony in the borough for a hospital to be founded. Yet the claim of 'W.H.' was at least partly borne out by the counties. For we see from Figure 2 that even before the moment of hospital foundation the 'hospital counties' tended to experience a lower incidence of contests than did 'non-hospital counties'. Admittedly, this tendency was reversed in the (pooled) elections of 1741, 1747 and 1754 – when contests were infrequent in counties of all types – and was slight in the 1780s. But in the (pooled) elections of 1761–74 the disparity between the two groups of counties was sufficiently strong to suggest that a real effect was at work.[1] In addition, it appears that the frequency of contests fell after the moment of hospital foundation, once again in agreement with Langford's argument.

In the boroughs, then, it seems that hospitals promoted political peace rather than reflecting it; whereas in the counties there obtained to some extent a reciprocal relationship between political peace and the founding of infirmaries. Yet the pattern in the counties is not entirely clear, perhaps because the various hospitals were founded across a wide time span – from the 1730s to the 1790s – during which the incidence of electoral contests fluctuated considerably. In order to clarify this issue we may approach the matter from a different angle. In each 'hospital constituency' we can compare the incidence of electoral contests before and after the moment of hospital foundation. A suitably broad 'window' for this purpose will be ten general elections: four preceding and six succeeding the year in which the given hospital was founded. We can then pool the results from all the hospitals into a composite 'window' having ten 'cells', representing the numbers of contests in 'hospital constituencies' at distances of ($-4, -3, -2, -1, +1, +2, +3, +4, +5$ and $+6$) general elections from the moment of hospital foundation. A 'control' pattern can be derived from the frequency of contests in the 'non-hospital constituencies'. For each cell in the 'window', the 'control pattern' will show the number of contests which *would have* occurred in the pooled 'hospital constituencies', *if* these had shown the same incidence of contests as the 'non-hospital constituencies'. This will allow for any possible distortion arising from the changing incidence of contests throughout the period. Further, the 'control pattern' will enable us to compare the incidence of political contests in the two classes of constituency, independently of the dates at which hospitals were founded.

The results are shown in Figure 3 for the boroughs, and Figure 4 for the counties. The pattern in the boroughs confirms that here the hospitals promoted harmony rather than reflecting it. Before the creation of a hospital, the incidence of contests in 'hospital boroughs' was effectively identical with the rate in 'non-hospital boroughs' (in fact, for the first three elections in the 'window' it was slightly higher, though not significantly so). After the creation of a hospital, the frequency of contests was reduced by almost one-third: in the next three elections pooled, where

1. At these three (pooled) elections, the 'hospital counties' which had not yet obtained a hospital experienced only 2:23 possible contests, whereas 'non-hospital counties' experienced 28:49 possible contests. The probability that this disparity could occur by chance is less than 1 in 100 (0.0096) by Fisher's exact-probability test, for which see Sidney Siegel, *Nonparametric Statistics for the Behavioural Sciences* (New York, 1956), pp. 96–104. A more conservative assessment can be obtained by deriving the chance probability that such a disparity could occur in *any* of the five relevant comparisons; even this attains conventional 'statistical significance', i.e. a probability of under 1 in 20.

158

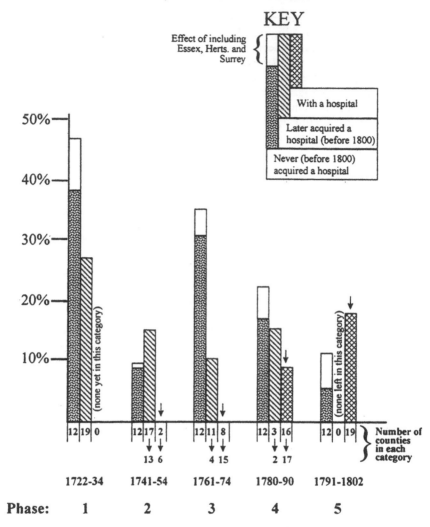

Fig. 2.   *County contests: distinguishing counties which never acquired a hospital from those which later acquired one.*

the 'control pattern' would suggest about twenty-eight contests in all, we find only twenty. However, the effect was temporary, for in subsequent elections the frequency of contests rose again, becoming the same as the 'control pattern'. Thus the hospitals' apparent soothing effect on borough constituencies lasted for just three general elections, i.e. for no more than twenty years.

In the counties (Figure 4) the results are more complex. On the one hand it is confirmed that hospitals both reflected and promoted county political harmony. In the combined four general elections *preceding* the moment of hospital foundation, contests in the 'hospital counties' were about half as frequent as in the 'non-hospital counties'; in the combined three general elections *after* hospital foundation, this proportion fell to about a quarter. Overall it seems that the two underlying phenomena – political harmony promoting hospital foundation, and the converse – were roughly equal in strength.[1] The effect of the hospitals on the county constituencies was slightly greater than their impact on the boroughs, reducing the frequency of contests by one-half as against one-third. However, it was similar in duration, apparently lasting for about three elections, since in subsequent elections the rate of contests in the 'hospital counties' seems to have been returning towards the level (in relation to the 'control pattern') that had obtained before the hospitals were founded.[2] On the other hand, we also find an unexpected anomaly: the election *immediately preceding* the moment of hospital foundation saw a peculiarly large number of contests, which uniquely attained the level of the 'control pattern'. That is, six county infirmaries – almost a third of such hospitals – were founded in the wake of general-election contests in the respective counties. As Table 2 shows, the six cases in point were spread across the entire period in view, from the 1730s to the 1790s – which explains why our earlier analysis (Figure 2) did not detect this phenomenon. This apparent association between contested elections and hospital foundation might be a coincidence, but the odds are against it: it is much more likely that some systematic effect was at work.[3]

The exercise of linking the foundation of hospitals with electoral contests has uncovered three findings. First, the eirenic effect of the hospitals, posited by Langford, was indeed felt in the arena of electoral politics. Though this impact was rather brief, disappearing after three general elections, it was strong while it lasted – reducing the incidence of electoral contests by one-third or more – and was seen in both the

1. In the combined four elections preceding hospital foundation, contests in the hospital counties were 0.47 times as frequent as the 'control' estimate. Supposing, for the sake of argument, that the effect of the hospitals was as great again, we would expect the corresponding ratio in the subsequent three elections to be .47 × .47, i.e. 0.22. This would mean that in the hospital counties there were 3.6 contests in these three elections pooled, or 4 rounded; and there were in fact 4 such contests.

2. Pooling the final three cells in the window, we would expect 8 contests (rounded) if the incidence of contests (in relation to the 'control pattern') returned to the level that had obtained before hospital-foundation, and only 4 contests if this continued to follow the pattern that had obtained in the first three elections after hospital-foundation. In fact there were 7 contests.

3. Had we expected to find such a concentration of contests in the preceding election, the probability of its occurring by chance would have been about 1 in 66, easily attaining conventional statistical significance. Given that we did not anticipate this phenomenon, we ought perhaps to assess the probability that such a concentration of contests could occur by chance in *any* of the elections in the 'window': this turns out to be about 1 in 7 (.1416). The latter, more conservative estimate does not attain statistical significance, but the odds are still against a chance explanation of the pattern. See further *infra*, p. 616, n. 1. This calculation has used binomial probability, for which see Murray R. Spiegel, *Probability and Statistics* (New York, 1975), p. 108.

160

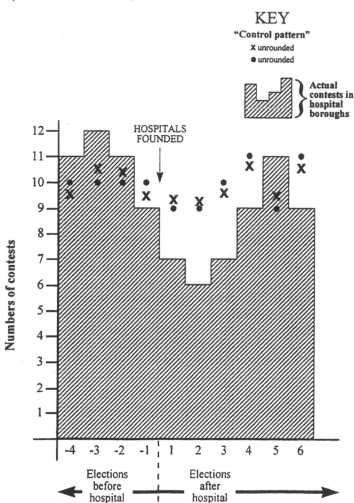

Fig. 3.   *Seventeen 'hospital boroughs': numbers of contests before and after hospital-foundation, compared with 'control pattern'.*

boroughs and the counties. Second, in the counties, though not in the boroughs, there was also an equally strong influence working in the opposite direction: that is, it was counties which already had a relatively low incidence of contests which tended to obtain hospitals. But third, and cutting across this, several hospitals were founded after contested county elections. We must now assess the meaning of this unexpected pattern.

In fact, it was not simply a contested county election which tended to precede the foundation of a hospital.[1] Rather, it was a run of two (or more) *uncontested* elections followed by a single *contested* election: this was the pattern in all the six cases listed in Table 2.[2] It is precisely for this reason that the last election before the moment of hospital foundation stands out in Figure 4. When the matter is viewed from this angle, a chance explanation becomes the more improbable.[3] In some of these six cases (though not in all[4]) a contested election, coming after a sequence of at least two uncontested elections, probably helped in some way to stimulate the creation of a county infirmary within the next two to six years. This result is strengthened by the cases of Lancashire and Warwickshire. It will be recalled that these two counties were excluded from consideration because the hospitals at Manchester and Birmingham served a hinterland which cut across county boundaries, though they were nevertheless associated with Lancashire and Warwickshire respectively. It is thus striking to find that both these hospitals were founded after contested elections in the respective counties, and that in each case the preceding two (and more) elections had been uncontested. In Lancashire there was no electoral contest between 1727 and 1741; the general election of 1747 was contested, and the Manchester Infirmary was founded in 1752.[5] Warwickshire saw no contests between 1708 and 1768; the contest of 1774 (occasioned by the retirement of the long-standing MP, Sir Charles Mordaunt) was followed by the creation of the Birmingham General Hospital in 1779. Thus the pattern of two uncontested elections, then a contested election, then the creation of an infirmary now extends to eight counties – over a third of all the counties which acquired infirmaries before 1800.

1. Between 1734 and 1796 there were 242 elections in counties without a hospital, i.e., 'non-hospital counties' plus 'hospital counties' which had not yet obtained their hospital. Amongst these, 13 out of 190 uncontested elections (one in 14.6) and 6 out of 52 contested elections (one in 8.7) were followed by hospital foundation. If electoral contests had no effect, about four hospitals (4.1), rather than six, would have been founded after contested elections. The disparity is slight in statistical terms, being associated with a probability of about 0.45 by the chi-square test (Siegel, *Nonparametric Statistics*, pp. 104–11).

2. The two cases of contests in the second cell of the 'window' arose from the counties of Staffordshire and Oxfordshire, not from the counties experiencing a contest in the fourth cell (the latter are listed in Table 2).

3. Between 1722 and 1790 there were 242 three-election sequences in counties without a hospital (i.e. 'non-hospital counties' plus 'hospital counties' which had not yet obtained their hospital). Some 33 of these sequences took the form (no contest, no contest, contest); six of these were followed by hospital-foundation, i.e. one in 5.5. Of the remaining 209 sequences, 13 were followed by hospital foundation, i.e. one in 16.1. This difference is statistically significant by the chi-square test.

4. The frequency of hospital foundation after all other electoral sequences combined (i.e. one in 16.1: see previous note), applied to the 33 instances of the sequence (no contest, no contest, contest), would produce just two hospitals. This would suggest that the sequence played a part in triggering the foundation of four of these six hospitals.

5. The Liverpool Infirmary was mooted in 1748 and founded in 1749, also fitting the pattern. Even though this hospital did not serve the county (see *supra*, p. 608, n. 3), its foundation may also have been triggered by the 1747 contest.

162

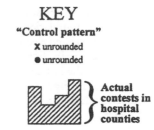

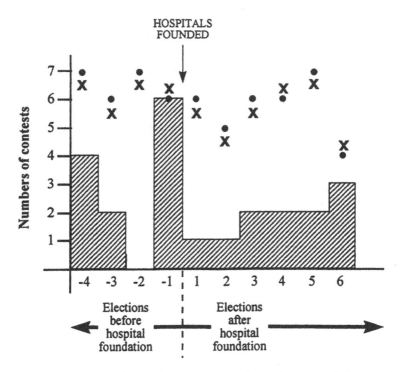

Fig. 4. Nineteen 'hospital counties': numbers of contests before and after hospital-foundation, compared with control pattern'.

It is most unlikely that this pattern was a coincidence;[1] but a statistical association of this kind does not demonstrate a concrete connection. In order to discover whether hospital foundation was actually stimulated by an electoral contest coming after two uncontested elections, as this finding suggests, detailed local research will be required. Certainly in the

1. If Warwickshire and Lancashire are added, then the chance-probabilities given *supra*, p. 613, n. 3, become 1 in 554 (.0018) instead of 1 in 66, and 1 in 55 (.0179) instead of 1 in 7. Even the more conservative of the two now attains conventional statistical significance.

Table 2.   County hospitals founded after a contested election

County	Date of contested election	Date of foundation of county infirmary
Hampshire	1734	1736
Yorkshire	1734	1740
Worcestershire	1741	1746
Norfolk	1768	1771
Herefordshire	1774	1776
Kent	1790	1793

case of the Birmingham General Hospital there are good grounds for suspecting that its successful re-launching in the 1770s, reversing an ignominious failure of the 1760s, was indeed assisted by the Warwickshire electoral contest of 1774.[1] This suggests that it will be worth investigating whether such was the case in any of the other seven hospitals founded in the wake of such contests. Here we have a starting-point from which to address the explanatory puzzle posed by the foundation of provincial infirmaries. How might county elections have played such a role? By way of conclusion, I shall sketch two alternative hypotheses.

What we may call the 'eirenic hypothesis' might run as follows. As is well known, members of the county elite deeply disliked electoral contests in the eighteenth century: not just because contests were personally expensive for the candidates and their backers, but more particularly because they were held to disturb 'the peace of the county'.[2] And contests may have appeared especially troubling against a background of previous harmony. Thus an electoral contest occurring after a sequence of no contests could have led to a special concern to restore the pre-existing political quiescence. Perhaps this stimulated men such as Alured Clarke to propose an infirmary, with the deliberate aim of smoothing over party differences; perhaps it simply strengthened their hand, disposing the local gentry and aristocracy to back them. In either case, this conjuncture tended to favour the creation of an infirmary: for instance the Winchester County Hospital, the very first county infirmary, was founded at Clarke's behest just two years after the election of 1734, which had seen Hampshire's first contest for over twenty years.[3] If this was indeed the motive behind the founding of some infirmaries, it had the desired effect, though only for about a generation

1. Adrian Wilson, 'The Political Origins of the Birmingham General Hospital' (paper in preparation). See also Money, *Experience and Identity*, pp. 9–11, and Conrad Gill, *History of Birmingham* (3 vols., Birmingham, 1952–74), i. 130–1.

2. O'Gorman, *Voters, Patrons, and Parties*, pp. 60, 112–13; Langford, *Public Life and the Propertied Englishman*, pp. 122–4; Money, *Experience and Identity*, p. 213, quoting Sir Roger Newdigate (here notice also Samuel Aris using the phrase 'the peace of the town', in 1790; cf. *infra*, p. 618, n. 4).

3. Clarke, who had been a prebendary at Winchester since 1723, made his first known moves towards the Winchester hospital in the summer of 1736: Carpenter Turner, *History of the Royal*

164

(the next three general elections). As a bonus, the hospitals also had a similar soothing effect on the local borough electorates.

An alternative explanation, which may be termed the 'agonistic hypothesis', can be derived from the case of Warwickshire. In that county, at least, the 'eirenic hypothesis' is poorly supported by the available evidence. For at the 1780 election, held a year after the re-founding of the Birmingham General Hospital, what prevented a contest was not peace in the county but, on the contrary, the self-assertiveness of the Birmingham freeholders, who had shown their electoral muscle in support of Sir Charles Holte in 1774 and now 'applied to Sir Robert Lawley' to stand on their behalf. (Holte had decided to retire as MP; Lawley was being invited to serve as his replacement.)[1] The move achieved instant success, for it persuaded the 'county' candidate William Holbech not to stand, with the effect that Lawley was returned unopposed (along with Holbech's fellow 'county' candidate, Sir George Shuckburgh). This was a classic 'aborted contest' (one of several at the 1780 election), that is, a trial of strength conducted in advance.[2] Here, then, the 'peace of the county' was secured at the price of a major political concession, attesting not to the absence of conflict but rather to the equal balance of contending forces. What part did the founding of the Birmingham General Hospital play in this process? Certainly the Hospital provided a link between the town's leaders and Sir Robert Lawley;[3] perhaps it also helped to unite the Birmingham freeholders into a formed 'interest'.[4] This would give a political edge to the strong civic meaning which Money has rightly stressed for the hospital.[5] The 'agonistic hypothesis' would be that it was forces of this kind which were at work in the foundation of infirmaries.[6] Hospitals would thus be expressions of particular interests, in ways which may well have varied from place to place. It might then emerge that county consensus was the public mask of local conflict.

Whichever of these interpretations one favours (and in different counties, both may perhaps be true), our findings suggest that politics and charity were reciprocally related, and thus that the eighteenth-century infirmary falls within the purview of the political historian. With twenty-eight provincial infirmaries founded before 1800, there is a vast wealth of material here to explore. In up to seven further counties

Hampshire County Hospital, p. 3. (Hampshire's previous contest had been in 1713: Cannon, Parliamentary Reform, p. 278.)

1. Namier and Brooke, The House of Commons, 1754–1790, i. 399–400.
2. O'Gorman, Voters, Patrons, and Parties, pp. 111–12.
3. Money, Experience and Identity, p. 10 (and cf. pp. 176–7); Birmingham Central Library, MS 1423/2 (Birmingham General Hospital Committee of Trustees Minute Book, 1766–1784), 19 June 1777.
4. Hence the fact that Samuel Aris could write of 'the peace of the town' in 1790 (cf. supra, p. 617, n. 2). By the latter date Birmingham had become a sphere of interest and contest in its own right.
5. Money, Experience and Identity, ch. 1.
6. This has been suggested for Norwich by Wilson, 'Urban Culture and Political Activism', pp. 181–2.

(Hampshire, Yorkshire, Lancashire, Worcestershire, Norfolk, Here-fordshire, Kent), hospital foundation may have been stimulated by an electoral contest, as it very probably was in Warwickshire; but this possibility needs to be tested by local research. And in the rest of the kingdom we do not yet know why hospital schemes came to be con-ceived, nor how they were brought to fruition. Why was the idea put forward before 1800, so far as we know, in only about half the counties of England? Why did hospital initiatives succeed in some counties, such as Hampshire, but fail in others, such as Berkshire? Our starting-point must be the successful attempts, and these left ample documentary traces. In most cases, the initial lists of hospital subscribers have sur-vived; it will often be possible to link these with poll-books, and thus to reconstruct the political and social profile of hospital founders.[1] Equally important was the precise local political conjuncture, together with the network of institutions both old (such as cathedral chapters and town corporations) and new (assembly rooms, debating societies).[2] Here we have an inviting field for research, covering a wide canvas. Perhaps this theme can serve as a focus through which to connect the politics of boroughs and counties. Certainly it bids fair to act as a bridge between local and national issues – and between historians of society and his-torians of the State.

Originally published in *The English Historical Review* 111 (1996). Reproduced by permission of Oxford University Press.

1. The subscribers were listed in the printed annual reports, produced by all provincial infirmaries; I am in the process of compiling a list of surviving reports. In many cases local newspapers also printed lists of subscribers, particularly at the moment of foundation. Printed poll-books (though not manuscript ones) are listed in John Sims (ed.), *A Handlist of British Parliamentary Poll Books* (University of Leicester History Department/University of California Riverside Occas. Pub. no. 4, 1984).
2. The cathedral chapter played an important part at Winchester: see Carpenter Turner, *History of the Royal Hampshire County Hospital*, p. 4. On new cultural initiatives, see Borsay, *The English Urban Renaissance*.

VI

The Birmingham General Hospital and its public, 1765–79

This chapter seeks to relate Habermas's concept of *bürgerliche Öffentlichkeit*, the 'bourgeois public sphere', to the voluntary hospitals of eighteenth-century England, and particularly to the origins of such hospitals. As a test case I shall use the Birmingham General Hospital, which is of particular interest because it was in effect founded twice: first and unsuccessfully in the 1760s, then again a decade later, when the Hospital was relaunched, this time with success. I shall conclude by asking what light this troubled history sheds upon Habermas's conception.

The premise of this study is a point emphasized in Steve Sturdy's introduction to the present volume: that the concept of the *bürgerliche Öffentlichkeit* needs to be refined so as to take on board the founding of institutions, over and above those (such as coffee houses and newspapers) which by definition belonged to that sphere as sites for what Habermas called 'rational-critical debate'. It is a truism, but one that bears repeating, that institutions did not arise, in this or any other setting, by 'spontaneous generation';[1] rather, their genesis needs to be seen in each case as a concrete initiative arising from a specific socio-political context. Thus the creation of any new institution within the 'public sphere' must reflect the very nature of that 'sphere'; and this point acquires special force in the setting of eighteenth-century Britain. For it was there, according to Habermas, that the *bürgerliche Öffentlichkeit* first came into being;[2] we also find there a remarkable array of new institutions; and many of these initiatives arose precisely within the 'public sphere'. In this context, therefore, the birth of new institutions ought to shed light on the birth, or at least the development, of the 'public sphere' itself.

The dominant component of the eighteenth-century British polity was England; and in this period England was especially rich in such novel institutions – assembly rooms, banks, debating societies, dispensaries, infirmaries, libraries, literary and philosophical societies, music festivals, newspapers, theatres and more. Although London of course played its part in this process,[3] the most striking feature of these developments was that they took place in dozens of provincial towns, from Lancaster to Norwich and from Exeter to Newcastle. Without doubt this 'urban renaissance', as Peter Borsay has dubbed it,[4] was closely bound up with what Habermas depicted as the development of the

'bourgeois public sphere'.[5] Consequently, the 'urban renaissance' presents a trea-
sure-trove of initiatives through which to explore the emergence of the *bürgerliche
Öffentlichkeit* in England.

With respect to medicine, the key such institutions were the voluntary hospitals and dispensaries – and especially the hospitals, for these preceded the
dispensaries,[6] outnumbered them until the nineteenth century[7] and had a much
more conspicuous public profile. Thus the topic of medicine and the 'public
sphere' directs our attention to the foundation of these hospitals; and here we
have an *embarras de richesse*, for by 1800 there were twenty-eight provincial infirmaries,[8] along with another dozen or so voluntary hospitals in London.[9] This
raises the question as to how to make manageable such a plethora of examples;[10] the strategy that I have chosen is to restrict attention to a single infirmary,
treating this not in the mode of institutional biography (for that genre tends to
treat the genesis of the given institution as a matter for celebration rather than
explanation),[11] but rather within the framework of a local study that attempts to
reconstruct the specific conjuncture in which that hospital was founded.[12]

The particular infirmary whose origins I shall be examining is the
Birmingham General Hospital, which was first launched in 1765 but did not
open until 1779. One reason for this choice is that the history of eighteenth-
century Birmingham is unusually accessible, thanks to the existence of John
Money's pioneering *Experience and Identity*.[13] The other consideration, mentioned
already, is that the Birmingham General Hospital was founded not once but
twice, which makes it easier to problematize such acts of foundation as I am
seeking to do. It should be remarked that this hospital was not alone in failing
initially, for the same had already happened in four other cases,[14] while at least
three of those infirmaries that got off the ground at the first attempt had faced
local opposition.[15] Thus, although no such individual infirmary can be taken as
'representative', the difficulties which the Birmingham General Hospital experienced were by no means unusual. And we shall see that the reasons for those
difficulties, though highly specific in their local expression, were anchored in
issues that obtained throughout the counties of England.

Before proceeding to this case study, let us recall the salient characteristics of
the voluntary hospitals in general.[16] They originated in the eighteenth century:
the first of them, the Westminster Infirmary, was established in 1719, and as
we have seen, some forty such hospitals had been created by the end of the
eighteenth century. The reason that they are called 'voluntary' is that they were
financed by voluntary subscriptions (regular annual gifts) and benefactions (one-
off donations). They were thus wholly dependent on the goodwill of their
subscribers; and indeed in a very real sense they revolved around those
subscribers.[17] For the subscribers not only funded the hospitals but also managed
them (typically through an elected committee), and were therefore also called
governors; it was these subscribers/governors who appointed the medical staff
(commonly a salaried apothecary and rotas of honorary surgeons and physicians); and the subscribers had a considerable say as to the patients who were
admitted, for although prospective patients were vetted by the medical staff,

patients normally required a letter of personal recommendation from a subscriber in order to be considered for admission. These arrangements had specific medical consequences, for admissions were typically restricted to curable illnesses, which assured the subscribers that their gifts had produced tangible results. So too the voluntary hospitals embodied a distinctive set of social arrangements: a line of inequality was drawn between the donors and the recipients of charity; above that line, that is, among the subscribers, there were further social gradations, both by size of donation and by traditional rank; and yet, as we shall see, there was theoretical equality with respect to the management of the given hospital itself.

In the long term the voluntary hospitals acquired massive importance, in both their medical and charitable aspects. On the charitable front their contribution, though outweighed in the nineteenth century both by the burgeoning dispensaries and by the new Poor Law hospitals, was nevertheless considerable, not least because large-scale industrial firms came to be enrolled as subscribers. In medical terms, the voluntary hospitals became pre-eminent both as centres of medical innovation and as sites of medical education,[18] and they maintained their elite position until they were finally nationalised in 1948, as part of the creation of the NHS.

In their original, eighteenth-century setting, these hospitals belonged firmly within the 'bourgeois public sphere' as Habermas depicts it; we have seen this on general grounds, and the point is strengthened by several of their specific features. First, one of their defining characteristics was *public accountability*, associated with extensive use of the print medium. Further, when the subscribers met each year to receive the accounts and to elect a new committee, the humble tradesman who subscribed merely half a guinea had an equal voice with a lord, a bishop, a merchant or a captain of industry whose annual subscription could be several times that sum; this *formal equality* among the subscribers corresponds well with the picture that Habermas paints of the notional equality that prevailed within the bourgeois public sphere.[19] Again, the hospitals' ideology was in line with the Habermasian conception: for they studiously invoked the *public interest* as what they furthered.[20] In short, just as the 'English urban renaissance' in general corresponds well to Habermas's account of the eighteenth-century 'bourgeois public sphere', so this is particularly true of the voluntary hospitals.

Thus to recapitulate, the character of the 'bourgeois public sphere' should be illuminated by investigating the origins of any such hospital: in the present case, the Birmingham General Hospital, which stumbled into life between 1765 and 1779. I shall next outline the setting of the Hospital's foundation, which comprised not only Birmingham but also its county, Warwickshire, along with the singular institution that notionally linked the two, namely the Bean Club; I shall survey Birmingham, Warwickshire and the Bean Club from around 1750 to the late 1770s. The third section will examine the founding, abandoning and refounding of the Hospital itself, and the chapter will conclude by relating the findings to Habermas's concept of the *bürgerliche Öffentlichkeit*.

88

Birmingham, Warwickshire and the Bean Club, c.1750–80

In the late eighteenth century Birmingham, though not enfranchised in its own right, was to become effectively the political hub of Warwickshire, displacing the two enfranchised boroughs of Warwick and Coventry. There are several signs that this process was under way as early as the 1740s; of these I shall pick out just two, from the beginning and end of the decade.[21] First, in 1741 Thomas Aris founded the *Birmingham Gazette*, and although he had a rival in the form of *Jopson's Coventry Mercury*, which began publication in the same year, *Aris's* swiftly outstripped *Jopson's*, becoming not only the major newspaper of the Midlands but also the principal voice in Warwickshire affairs. Second, in May 1749 the Bean Club, a convivial association of 'high-flying' – that is, extreme – Tory gentlemen, led by a small but potent group of aristocrats, was refounded in Birmingham.[22] While the Club quickly acquired a national dimension, it was primarily oriented to Warwickshire, as is signalled by its close connection with the county's Parliamentary representation. Not only were both Knights of the Shire – Warwickshire's MPs – drawn from the Club's membership throughout the next several decades; in addition, the selection of those representatives was controlled by the same men who supplied the Club's leadership, that is to say, Barons Craven and Leigh and, from the mid-1750s, the Earl of Denbigh. Conversely the equally aristocratic family of Finch, holders of the Earldom of Aylsford, whose Toryism was of a far more moderate kind, were excluded throughout the 1750s and 1760s both from the Bean Club and from determining the representation of the county.[23] The Bean Club, then, was the key social forum for the clique of high Tories who effectively ran Warwickshire, and the fact that the Club initially based itself at Birmingham was a mark of the town's significance.

The reason for Birmingham's rising importance was of course the remarkable growth of its prosperity and population, which had been under way for several decades and was now gaining increasing momentum.[24] From its seventeenth-century base in iron-smelting, Birmingham capitalism was expanding in many directions: into gun-making, which had been under way since before 1700; to the working of metals in general, notably brass but eventually also silver and gold; into the production of metal buckles, buttons, trays and trinkets ('toys'), and thence into their decoration by such techniques as japanning; into the metal-dependent trade of printing, whence John Baskerville's famous typography; eventually, thanks to Matthew Boulton and James Watt, into the manufacture of steam-engines; and, meanwhile, as a result of the local demand for capital and for credit, into banking, notably through the firm of Taylor and Lloyd, the progenitor of Lloyds bank. Birmingham's numerous and thriving manufacturers large and small were a varied lot, comprising natives and immigrants, Anglicans and Dissenters, well-born men and self-made ones. This diversity can be illustrated schematically, at the upper reaches of prosperity, by the individual figures of Matthew Boulton and William Hutton. Boulton was a Birmingham-born Churchman who inherited his father's business in 1757 and expanded it mightily, building the vast 'manufactory' at Soho, near Handsworth, which became one of the wonders of the kingdom;[25] Hutton was an immigrant Presbyterian who began in 1750 as a book-pedlar with borrowed capital, yet by 1756 had opened his own paper warehouse, exploiting an opportunity arising from the town's expanding printing industry.[26]

The siting of the Bean Club in Birmingham reveals that Warwickshire Tories were showing an interest in the town at mid-century; the same was true of the Whig aristocracy, particularly the recently ennobled Archers of Umberslade;[27] and like any substantial English town at this period, Birmingham offered each party a natural constituency. On the one hand, the town had a high-Tory pedigree, perhaps indeed a Jacobite one,[28] whence its choice for the refounding of the Bean Club. On the other hand, although the great majority of the people of Birmingham as of other places belonged to the Church of England, and a few to its new Methodist offshoot,[29] there were several Dissenting churches:[30] a small congregation of Baptists,[31] a larger Quaker group and three Presbyterian meetings.[32] There was thus the potential for considerable conflict in Birmingham – as would become only too clear, and tragically so, in the anti-Priestley riots of 1791[33] – but at this stage in the town's history, that is to say, in the middle of the eighteenth century, four circumstances conspired to hold such tensions at bay. In the first place, Birmingham's burgeoning economy made for calm, by providing employment for the poor and niches for the enterprising of all persuasions. Second, its manorial government had evolved in such a way as to give both Dissenters and Anglicans a say in the running of the town,[34] and while the Birmingham Tories may not have been happy with this arrangement, they managed to tolerate it. Third, although Thomas Aris was a Tory and belonged to the Bean Club, his *Birmingham Gazette* cultivated a discreet rhetoric that avoided offending any section of his readership. Last but not least, Birmingham's potential electoral muscle had never been exercised, for it so happened that there had been no contest for Warwickshire's two Knights of the Shire since 1705. The Tory aristocrats and gentlemen of the county, who controlled its representation, had carefully avoided any by-electoral contest when sitting members died, and the handful of Whigs amongst the Warwickshire aristocracy had calculated that it would be fruitless to disturb what was called 'the peace of the county' by provoking such a contest at a general election. The absence of county electoral contests, combined with the fact that Birmingham was not enfranchised, meant that political differences never came into focus there in the way that they did, notoriously, in Coventry.

Although Birmingham prospered throughout the 1750s, the same cannot be said for relations between the town's Tories and the Bean Club, nor indeed for the Club itself.[35] Even in the early 1750s, the Club's link with Birmingham was weakening; by 1755 there were 387 members, yet only forty-two of these were from Birmingham; and, in that year, there emerged signs of tension between the Birmingham members and the country gentlemen. Just why this gap opened up between the Tories of Birmingham and of Warwickshire is not clear, but what can be said is that this presaged a wider decline in the Club's vitality. As early as 1753, the meetings were cut back from weekly to monthly; from 1756 onwards,

90

fewer than half of these meetings were actually held, and the recruitment of new members plummeted; at the end of 1759 the monthly meetings were abandoned, leaving the annual anniversary meeting and dinner as the only occasions in the Club's calendar.

The decline of the Bean Club's momentum in the latter half of the 1750s reflected the fact that the Tory interest throughout the kingdom was disintegrating, under the impact of national political events: the breaking-up of the 'Old Corps' of Whigs; the emergence of Pitt; the impact of the fall of Minorca in 1756; and last but not least, the reform of the militia, which offered the Tory gentry opportunities for local office that had no precedent since the accession of George I in 1714.[36] Ironically, the collapse of proscription threw the Tories into disarray, by depriving them of their oppositional *raison d'être*. Thereupon, individual Tories went in a remarkable variety of different political directions,[37] and this process continued, and acquired new twists, after the accession of George III in 1760. It is thus intelligible that the Bean Club continued to be troubled into the 1760s. Its link with Birmingham remained feeble: symptomatic of this was the fact that after Thomas Aris died in July 1761, leaving the *Birmingham Gazette* to his son Samuel, no attempt was made to elect Samuel Aris as a member, even though he had inherited not only the newspaper but also his father's Anglicanism, his Toryism and his masterly editorial discretion. The Bean Club's failure to recruit so important a Birmingham Tory as the new editor of *Aris's Birmingham Gazette* suggests that its leaders had lost their political touch. And so they had, for throughout the 1760s the Club stumbled through a series of little catastrophes, repeatedly seeking to revive itself and yet falling back again, sometimes within a matter of months.

In sharp contrast with the Bean Club, Birmingham in the 1760s not only continued to expand rapidly but also embarked on a new self-assertiveness. The first sign of this was the publication in 1763 of James Sketchley's *Birmingham Directory*, one of the first provincial directories of the kingdom;[38] this was followed in 1765 by the project for the Birmingham General Hospital, to be considered in the next section; and as this was under way there came the successful launching of the Birmingham Canal Navigation, which was opened in 1768 to much rejoicing, and understandably so, for it almost halved the price of coal in the town.[39] But the climax of these developments came in March 1769, when Birmingham at long last came to play a role in Warwickshire politics. For a by-election held in that month returned Thomas Skipwith, a disaffected member of the Bean Club, as one of the two Knights of the Shire, and Skipwith owed his selection to the freeholders, to whom he had appealed directly by advertising his candidacy in the newspapers, in particular *Aris's Birmingham Gazette*.[40] This tactic, which was wholly novel in Warwickshire, had at a stroke unleashed the hitherto-dormant power of the Birmingham freeholders; Skipwith's selection as Member of Parliament, which was ritually completed at a county meeting held at Warwick on 29 March, was a triumph as much for the freeholders as it was for Skipwith himself.

Even though Skipwith himself was a gentleman and a Bean Club member, the effect of his campaign was to wrest the representation of Warwickshire from aristocratic and gentry control for the first time in living memory. This posed an unprecedented political threat to the high-Tory interest in the county, which had hitherto controlled the selection of the Knights of the Shire. And in response to that threat the Bean Club shook off its torpor and reinvented itself, beginning at the first available opportunity, that is, at the anniversary meeting of August 1769. The Club now adopted a new organizational form, by appointing two annual 'stewards', and, significantly, one of the two stewards chosen was none other than Thomas Skipwith, suggesting that a concerted effort was being made to heal wounds and close ranks in the wake of the by-election.[41] Initially this was no easy matter, because the next few months saw much pressure from Birmingham for a county petition in support of John Wilkes, and equally determined resistance from the county aristocracy, a passage of events which widened the rift between town and county.[42] But in the following year, when the Wilkes issue was dying down in the region, the attempt to re-establish the Club began to bear fruit, for ten new members were elected – and significantly, six of them hailed from Birmingham, including Samuel Aris himself, editor of the *Gazette*.[43] This was the beginning of a sustained and successful recruitment effort, which was targeted in particular to Birmingham. Between 1770 and 1773 the Club acquired fifty-one new members, that is to say, more than had been elected in the whole of the 1760s; over two-thirds of these (thirty-six of them) came from Birmingham, and these new Birmingham members included four merchants, two brass-makers, two mercers, two buckle-makers, two button-makers and a 'toyman', showing that there was now a policy of bringing Birmingham manufacturers into the Club.

These moves succeeded, for the quarterly meetings were revived in 1771, and subsequently, as John Money has shown, the Bean Club played a major role in the affairs of Birmingham and managed to create a more or less stable link between the town and the local landed interest,[44] principally of Warwickshire. Yet the Bean Club's links with both town and county were highly selective, for the Club continued to be deeply partisan in both politics and religion. Even though some of its individual members (such as Thomas Skipwith) had now forged new, Whig allegiances,[45] the Club as a whole remained specifically Tory: for strikingly, the Warwickshire Whig aristocratic families of Greville, Conway and Archer did not contribute a single member. Correspondingly, the Club continued to be exclusively Anglican; not a single Dissenter was ever elected to its ranks. And what is equally significant, the Club's Birmingham recruitment was still narrower than this, for there were some remarkable absentees even among Birmingham Churchmen: namely Matthew Boulton and the gun-maker Samuel Garbett, the town's two most eminent entrepreneurs. On the face of it, both Boulton and Garbett were supremely qualified for membership of the Bean Club, not just as leading capitalists but also in political terms: for Boulton was thoroughly conservative in outlook,[46] and his business partner John Fothergill had joined the Club in 1761, while Garbett had a longstanding link with Lord Denbigh. Yet neither Boulton nor Garbett was ever admitted – an omission that seriously weakened the Club's pretensions to leadership in Birmingham. The reason for their exclusion can readily be surmised: despite

92

their Anglicanism and their conservative views, Boulton and Garbett were unfit, for each of them was also closely associated with Dissenters.[47]

It can be seen that Birmingham during the 1760s and 1770s brought into play a complex array of political interests, involving differences of locality, class, party, religion and family. Such were the circumstances of the founding of the Birmingham General Hospital, which took place in two stages: from 1765 to 1768, and from 1776 to 1779.[48]

The making of the Birmingham General Hospital

When a Birmingham hospital was proposed in the autumn of 1765, the circumstances were apparently favourable in three ways. First, the town was going from strength to strength as we have seen. Second, charitable help to the poor was particularly needed at this time, since local grain prices had been rising almost continuously for over a year and a half.[49] Third, in the summer of this year the Bean Club had experienced one of its little revivals of the 1760s;[50] and this was propitious for the intended Hospital because Dr John Ash, the leading spirit behind the Hospital proposal, was also a longstanding and well-respected member of the Club, which gave the Hospital's activists good reasons to hope for landed support. Sure enough, the Hospital was initially backed by a broad coalition of local interests, with the effect that funds came in quickly. In short, the Hospital had every prospect of success. Yet as we are about to see, the initiative failed disastrously, so much so that it took ten years to revive it.

It seems to have been the launch of a county infirmary in Staffordshire in 1765 that stirred some of Birmingham's leaders to initiate the hospital proposal. On 30 September 1765, through a letter published in *Aris's*, the town's Overseers of the Poor mooted the idea of a Birmingham hospital, in emulation of their Staffordshire neighbours.[51] No doubt part of their motive was to find a way of catering for the medical needs of Birmingham's numerous immigrant poor, many of whom would have been entitled to relief only in their home parishes, not in Birmingham itself.[52] Hence the specific proposal that was put forward in *Aris's* five weeks later, on 4 November 1765:

> A General Hospital for the relief of the sick and lame, situated near the town of Birmingham, is presumed would be greatly beneficial to the populous country about it, as well as [to] that place.[53]

The proposed Hospital was called 'General' to demonstrate that its benefits would be available to all, not just to natives of Birmingham or for that matter of Warwickshire, and the reference to 'the populous country about it' alluded to the fact that Birmingham's hinterland extended to Staffordshire, Worcestershire and to some extent Shropshire. The advertisement went on to call a public meeting on 21 November 'of the nobility and gentry of the neighbouring country, and of the principal inhabitants of this town', in order to 'consider of proper steps to render effectual so useful an undertaking'.

To all appearances this initial meeting was auspicious. It was attended – as the next issue of *Aris's* reported – by 'a considerable number of gentlemen both of the country and the town';[54] a subscription to fund the proposed Hospital was opened on the spot; donations totalling over £1,100 were 'sent in' on the day from some sixty-eight wealthy benefactors;[55] and in addition, over £200 per annum was pledged in subscriptions. Equally encouraging, though of course not mentioned in *Aris's*, was the fact that this support came not just from both 'country' and 'town' but also from a broad politico-religious spectrum within the Birmingham elite. Donations from the town were headed by the firm of Boulton and Fothergill (50 guineas), and came also, typically in sums of 10 or 20 guineas, from longstanding members of the Bean Club;[56] from moderate Churchmen such as Samuel Garbett and the attorney Joseph Carles; from the Quakers Samuel Galton and Sampson Lloyd; and from such Presbyterians or Unitarians as John Taylor (Lloyd's partner in the then-incipient bank) and William Russell. As for the 'country', this was represented by the Earls of Aylesford and Dartmouth, along with both of their wives; by baronets such as Sir Roger Newdigate (30 guineas);[57] by gentlemen such as Richard Geast;[58] and last but not least, by the two Knights of the Shire for Warwickshire – William Bromley and Sir Charles Mordaunt – who each gave 30 guineas, this however after most of the other benefactions (sixty-four of the sixty-eight) had been received.

The participation of both Warwickshire MPs draws attention to a curious and significant feature of the Hospital's landed support: despite the care of its activists to represent it as a regional initiative, not a county-specific one, almost all of its 'country' benefactors hailed from Warwickshire. Indeed the only significant landed contribution from outside the county came from the Earl and Countess of Dartmouth (50 guineas between them),[59] who were seated in Staffordshire, and there were several contingent reasons for Dartmouth's particular involvement.[60] Why was it that, apart from Dartmouth and one or two gentlemen, the Hospital failed to draw in landed backing from outside Warwickshire? Part of the reason was that Worcestershire and Shropshire already had county infirmaries, both established in the late 1740s, and Staffordshire was now following suit as we have seen, so that the available support in these counties was already committed elsewhere. Yet a deeper consideration was probably at work: namely that gentlemen and aristocrats throughout the region were oriented primarily towards their own counties. This localism may have involved an element of etiquette, in which case Dartmouth was breaching that etiquette. But it also made political sense: for although Birmingham had a considerable immigrant population, very few of these immigrants would have had freeholds in Worcestershire, Staffordshire or Shropshire, with the effect that there were not many votes to be gained in Birmingham for elections in any of those counties. Conversely, county loyalties lay behind the fact that the two Warwickshire MPs added their contributions once the Hospital had already amassed substantial support: for it was part of the recognized duty of Knights of the Shire to lend their backing impartially to any initiative arising within their respective counties, provided that the given project was not actively opposed there by some contending interest.

94

Thus the Birmingham General Hospital was immediately propelled towards becoming – contrary to its name and to the original intention – the *de facto* county infirmary of Warwickshire. In order for this to succeed, it would be necessary to maintain the double coalition that was manifested in the initial group of benefactors: between the Birmingham elite and the Warwickshire gentry, and between Churchmen and Dissenters within the town.

In the next few weeks and months the project seemingly continued to thrive. By 9 December the benefactions had reached over £1,900, and the promised subscriptions had come to £600 a year.[61] Further, by 16 December about a hundred small tradesmen from Birmingham had been enrolled as subscribers, mostly pledging an annual guinea or two apiece,[62] and this expansion of the Hospital's base of support was no doubt helped by the fact that its proceedings were being reported in *Aris's*. Thus encouraged, the subscribers met on Christmas Eve, agreed to build a hospital, and appointed a thirty-one-member committee to superintend this. And the composition of this committee reflected the broad base of the Hospital's support: its members came equally from the landed classes and from Birmingham (sixteen and fifteen men respectively), while those from Birmingham comprised nine Churchmen and six Dissenters.[63] Less than three months later (March 1766) the committee purchased a seven-acre site just north of the town, a plan was promptly commissioned, and work started on the building in the summer of 1766.[64]

Yet it swiftly turned out that the funds were insufficient, partly because the builders over-ran their original estimate. As a result the building had to be boarded up in November 1766, just when the structure had almost been completed.[65] Thereafter the project limped ahead for another year and a half,[66] beset by a squeeze between rising costs and insufficient income, which was met by a series of temporary expedients:[67] notably the bankers, Taylor and Lloyd – who were also amongst the Hospital's trustees, as we have seen – supplied a loan against future subscriptions. Eventually, in May 1768, the hospital was said to be ready 'for the immediate reception of patients';[68] but in fact this was whistling in the wind, for no such 'reception of patients' took place. The enterprise had now run into serious difficulties, for over £2,000 was owing to the bank, and the promised subscriptions were not coming in. Some help came in September from a three-day music festival, which raised almost £800, but this still left the Hospital massively indebted. And what was equally significant, the meeting of trustees scheduled for the first day of the festival (7 September) went unrecorded in the minute-book.[69] Perhaps the meeting was simply inquorate; more probably, the trustees were now unable to agree among themselves as to how to proceed; but whatever the reason, this signalled a collapse in morale, for at this point, that is, in September 1768, the operation was effectively suspended,[70] and the building was closed again, this time with no prospect of completing it. An initiative that had begun so brightly had become an ignomin-ious failure: the hospital now existed solely as a debt that lay on the books, accumulating interest, and a boarded-up building that stood as a mute reproach to all concerned.

What had gone wrong? The hospital's governors probably made a tactical mistake in building a full-scale infirmary at the outset, rather than starting in small premises and then gradually expanding,[71] and the upward drift of the costs suggests that they were unlucky, or perhaps unwise, in their choice of builders. Above all, however, what let them down was that the hoped-for backing from the Warwickshire landed interest did not materialize, for the initial lead of a dozen or so gentlemen did not produce any wider financial support from the landed interest. Furthermore, the sixteen landed gentlemen on the building committee seem to have played no active part in its proceedings: from an early stage the Birmingham members were left to manage the Hospital on their own, and, indeed, as we shall shortly see, the gentlemen may even have withdrawn from the project altogether within as little as three months.

The first sign of the problem was implicit in the list of initial supporters, specifically at aristocratic level. For that list included only two lords, the Earls of Aylesford and Dartmouth – both probably recruited by Matthew Boulton[72] – and since Lord Dartmouth was seated in Staffordshire, Aylesford was the sole Warwickshire noble who backed the Hospital. Furthermore, Aylesford was in Warwickshire terms a political eccentric, for his moderate Toryism set him apart from the high-Tory peers who had long controlled the representation of the county (Craven, Leigh and Denbigh), yet cannot have endeared him to the local Whig lords (the Earls of Warwick and Hertford, and their junior partner Baron Archer). This, then, was not only a very narrow aristocratic base but was also an unpromising nucleus for drawing in further support – either from the aristocracy itself, both Whig and Tory, or from the gentry, who of course were overwhelmingly Tory. And the absence of support from Craven, Leigh and Denbigh reveals that Dr John Ash had been unable to make effective use of his Bean Club connections to draw in the landed interest.

Sure enough, the weakness of landed backing became apparent as early as March 1766 – that is, when the site for the Hospital was acquired – and this in two ways. For one thing, the set of twelve trustees who were now appointed to hold the land on the Hospital's behalf consisted wholly of Birmingham men: not a single gentleman lent his name, even in a token capacity. Hence the suspicion that by this time the sixteen gentlemen on the committee had withdrawn. For another, when announcing the purchase of the site the committee entered a plea that '*the nobility and gentry who are inclined to promote this universal charity, and have not yet signified their intentions, are earnestly requested to send their benefactions*'.[73] The wording of this appeal makes it clear that the landed interest was failing to support the Hospital – this within three months of constituting the committee, and well before the problem with the building costs emerged. The same pattern recurred after that problem had been announced: for in the following year, 1767, an appeal for a second tranche of benefactions brought in £180 or so from some sixteen Birmingham men, but not a single contribution from the aristocracy or the gentry.[74] And further proof of the Hospital's inability to recruit landed support came in May 1768 – that is, when the Hospital was allegedly ready 'for the immediate reception of patients', though in fact it was in desperate straits. At

96

this time the committee sent two separate and carefully worded personal appeals to seven aristocrats and two gentlemen.[75] The fact that the governors could only come up with the names of two gentlemen to approach shows that Ash could not deliver so much as the hope of support from members of the Bean Club, while the list of seven peers was highly deficient, omitting as it did the most eminent Warwickshire lords of both political sides (the Tory Baron Craven, the Whig Earl of Hertford). And equally telling was the response, or rather the lack of it: for both letters fell on deaf ears.[76]

Now the Hospital's failure was not solely due to the collapse of landed support, for by this time its Birmingham backing had also subsided alarmingly. This is particularly revealed by the contrasting fortunes of the Birmingham Canal Navigation – a 'cut' from Birmingham to Wolverhampton, aimed principally at bringing in cheap coal from the Staffordshire collieries. The Navigation was set up in January 1767, that is, just after the Hospital was first boarded up (November 1766); within the ensuing seven months (January to August 1767), it drew in capital of £50,000,[77] most of it from inhabitants of Birmingham, including the very men who were promoting and running the Hospital project. At this time the Hospital could have cleared its debts with a modest £2,000 or so; yet as has been mentioned already, an appeal made in June brought in a mere sixteen benefactions, which between them amounted to a paltry £180. And since twelve of these donors belonged to the Hospital committee, while another had been among those who contributed in 1765,[78] it can be seen that this appeal brought only three more Birmingham men[79] to support the Hospital – whereas the Canal had over a hundred shareholders. In part, the dramatic divergence between the fates of the two initiatives reflected the very different attractions of profit on the one hand and charity on the other, but it is unlikely that this was the sole reason at work, since the Canal's success was by no means guaranteed in advance. In all probability, the decline in support for the Hospital in Birmingham was itself a result of the failure to secure any significant backing from the landed interest. For the project had from the outset sought to draw in the aristocracy and gentry; the failure to achieve this, which by this time (1767) was only too apparent, must have eaten into the morale of the Birmingham activists themselves, whence the fact that only about half of them contributed to their own appeal in June; the thinness of landed patronage implicitly stigmatized the project in the eyes of Birmingham at large, which was why hardly anyone else contributed at this time.

The final attempt to garner support for the Hospital in the 1760s, namely the music festival of 7–9 September 1768, though seemingly a success, actually set the seal on the Hospital's failure to draw in landed backing. An advertisement in *Aris's* reported that the festival attracted a 'concourse of nobility and gentry from this and the neighbouring counties', which 'gave the whole a most splendid appearance, and at the same time showed their desire to concur with the inhabitants of this place in support of a charity so beneficial and extensive'.[80] Yet there is every reason to suspect that this account greatly exaggerated the degree of 'support' from the 'nobility and gentry'. For one thing, the seven committee members who had organized the festival were all Birmingham men: that is, not a single gentleman had been involved, just as none of them had been named as land trustees two years before. For another, as we have already seen, the festival raised less than £800, which fell far short of the Hospital's debt. Further, the occasion cannot have induced any of the local 'nobility and gentry' to drum up any further support from their friends, since the Hospital's proceedings thereupon closed. And strikingly, the only 'nobility' who were actually *named* as being present were the same two Countesses who had backed the Hospital in the first place, namely Dartmouth and Aylesford.[81] The fact that the Hospital's aristocratic patronage was still limited to the families of Dartmouth and Aylesford – both of them, in different ways, outsiders in Warwickshire affairs – confirmed how narrow was its 'support' from the 'nobility', and doubtless from the gentry as well.

To sum up, the reason that the Birmingham General Hospital failed in 1765–8 was that its hoped-for coalition between town and country interests was weak from the outset and soon collapsed. As for its other, complementary dimension of coalition – that is to say, *within* the town, between Birmingham Churchmen and Dissenters – this seems to have held together throughout these troubled three years, albeit with one qualification: the Dissenters on the committee were more active, or perhaps more persistent, in their support for the Hospital than were the Churchmen.[82] It seems, therefore, that the Churchmen among the Hospital's Birmingham activists were especially discouraged by the withdrawal of the landed gentry – which is intelligible, since the gentry were of course their co-religionists.[83] By the time the festival took place, it will be recalled, the Hospital's land trustees were unable to decide how to proceed; and it is possible (though this is speculation) that they were divided on confessional lines.[84]

Now the Hospital's failure to recruit landed support mirrored a difficulty that had long been experienced by the Bean Club. As we saw earlier, the Club's links with Birmingham had faded within a few years of its refoundation in 1749 and remained feeble throughout the 1760s; conversely, the Birmingham initiative for the Hospital now proved unable to forge links with the landed gentlemen who belonged to the Club. But if these were two sides of the same problem, that problem acquired an additional twist in the case of the Hospital, thanks to the prominence of Dissenters among its leaders; and against this background, it is instructive to recall the subsequent development of the Bean Club and to compare this with what happened to the Hospital project. We have seen that in the wake of the 1769 by-election, the Bean Club was revived on a new basis, involving the election of annual stewards; the intended recouping of Thomas Skipwith, the new Knight of the Shire; the successful revival of quarterly meetings in 1771; and the recruitment of Birmingham members on an unprecedented scale.[85] Here at last was an institutional link between Birmingham and the landed interest of Warwickshire, which in theory could have made it possible to revive the Hospital project. But no such revival took place at this time, and the reason is not far to seek: the Bean Club had always been specifically Anglican and Tory, and it remained within these limits, whereas the Hospital rested on an alliance between Churchmen and Dissenters.[86]

It is thus perhaps significant that the first sign of renewed interest in the Hospital was the work of a Dissenter. In 1774 – that is, some six years after the Hospital's closure in 1768 – a young and pious Birmingham Baptist named Mark Wilkes (apparently no relation of his famous namesake) attempted to bring the project back to public attention by publishing an imaginary *Dialogue between the Hospital and the New Play House*.[87] It has been claimed that this piece sold 'an immense number of copies', and that it effectively shamed 'the public' into reviving the Hospital;[88] yet this is doubtful, for it was another two years before any attempt was made to reactivate the Hospital. Nevertheless, such an attempt was indeed made – whether prompted by Wilkes's dialogue or by some other stimulus is unclear – in September 1776, and this was the beginning of a process of revival that eventually attained success. A reconstituted committee solicited funds, organized another music festival, negotiated over the Hospital's debts and completed and furnished the building. Yet even now this was a protracted struggle, which took three years to reach completion, for it was not until September 1779 that the Hospital was finally opened for the admission of patients. [89]

There is not space here to trace these developments, but what we must notice is the social composition of the reconstituted Hospital committee. This time, the initial leadership came solely from Birmingham, for *every one of the sixteen landed or titled men who had served on the ill-fated committee of 1765 had now dropped out*, and no others were found to replace them. In contrast, over half of the Birmingham men who had been involved in 1765 (eleven out of twenty-one) were still active in 1776–9,[90] and twenty-three new activists had now been recruited, *all of them from Birmingham*. Thus, although the size of the core group was much as it had been before – thirty-four men, as compared with thirty-one in 1765 – its composition was radically different. Further, the strong contribution of Dissenters was maintained and indeed increased: four Dissenters from the 1765 committee were still involved,[91] while of the new activists, at least nine and probably ten were Dissenters.[92] Thus in all, Dissenters now comprised some thirteen or fourteen of the Hospital's thirty-four activists. In confessional terms, this was precisely in keeping with the retreat of the landed gentry, all of whom of course belonged to the Established Church. It is no surprise to find, therefore, that the Hospital once again had only limited success in attracting landed backing: its successful revival rested almost exclusively on benefactions and subscriptions from Birmingham itself. In effect Birmingham's leaders had learnt the lesson of self-reliance.

Nevertheless the Hospital did now manage at long last to acquire a Warwickshire aristocratic patron. And the man they found to back them was one whose politics were precisely in line with the strong presence of Dissenters on the new committee: namely the sixth Baron Craven, who was now of Whig allegiance. Curiously enough, Craven had begun his political life as a Tory, [93] as was to be expected in view of his family's tradition; but after succeeding to the barony in 1769, he had gradually migrated in a Whig direction,[94] a move that achieved its consummation in 1780, when he became the co-patron (along with Lord Archer) of the Dissenting corporation of Coventry.[95] Thus when Craven became the first President of the Birmingham General Hospital in 1779, this was precisely in line with the position that he had reached by the late 1770s; the fit between Craven's politics and the Hospital's confessional basis illustrates the fact that party and religion remained intertwined.[96]

Conclusion

What lessons concerning Habermas's concept of *bürgerliche Öffentlichkeit* – the 'bourgeois public sphere' or 'bourgeois publicness' – might emerge from this case-study? I want to draw out three points.

First, the question arises as to the *limits* of 'bourgeois publicness' in any given historical setting. What raises this issue is the fact that the Birmingham General Hospital's institutional closure in 1768 was accompanied by another kind of closure: the Hospital immediately *disappeared from the public arena*, and it remained so to speak out of sight for several years – and this despite the physical presence of the boarded-up building. This conspiracy of silence was remarkably widespread, taking in at least three distinct sets of interests: the country gentlemen who stopped subscribing; the Hospital's creditors; and, last but not least, Samuel Aris, the editor of the *Gazette*, who seems to have dropped all mention of the Hospital as soon as the problems began to emerge. While Habermas's stress on 'publicness' helps to bring this issue into prominence, this episode of silence conversely reveals that 'publicness' was not automatic but contingent in any given setting.

Second, the case of Birmingham in the 1760s and 1770s suggests that the public sphere was an arena not just of 'rational-critical debate' – the aspect that Habermas stressed – but also of difference and of contest. Habermas tended to minimize this agonistic character of the public sphere, because he sought to portray that 'sphere' as a single shared interest, over against the state; but while this may indeed have been the case over the long term and in an emergent manner, it is probably at odds with what happened in any specific setting. Rather, the 'bourgeois public sphere' – certainly in eighteenth-century Britain, and arguably in the French and German settings as well – was differentiated, and this in complex ways: not just by gender and class (as Habermas recognized, up to a point),[97] but also as between town and country, and by confessional differences. As John Money has shown, both the Bean Club and the General Hospital came to play prominent roles in Birmingham's public life,[98] yet these rested on very different constituencies: the one was constituted by an alliance between urban and landed elites, united by the bond of religion; the other rested on an alliance between Churchmen and Dissenters, united by their shared interest in furthering the emerging civic interest of Birmingham itself; and although a few men (notably Ash and, after 1779, Craven) belonged to both groups, the two remained largely distinct. Furthermore it may be suspected that the 'bourgeois public sphere' in general was actually *constituted* by the clash of different interests, in which case an adequate understanding of that 'sphere' will require us to recapture the dynamics of struggle within it.[99]

100

Third, the persistent importance of confessional divisions in Birmingham during the 1760s and 1770s raises the question as to the role of religion in Habermas's story, and here we encounter a curious paradox. On the one hand, religion was depicted as part and parcel of *repräsentative Öffentlichkeit*[100] – the earlier form of 'publicness' that, according to Habermas's analysis, preceded the development of *bürgerliche Öffentlichkeit* – and indeed as emblematic of it;[101] and what was more, the Reformation was assigned the leading role in the transition from *repräsentative Öffentlichkeit* to *bürgerliche Öffentlichkeit*.[102] On the other hand, when Habermas came to describe the subsequent development of the *bürgerliche Öffentlichkeit* itself, religious themes were systematically written out of his account: for instance when considering Britain, Habermas referred to the Exclusion Crisis of 1679 only in order to dismiss from consideration the very issue that had prompted that crisis, namely the Catholicism of James, Duke of York.[103] I shall not attempt to explain the contradiction between these two utterly different roles that Habermas assigned to religion – first as the prime mover in the genesis of *bürgerliche Öffentlichkeit* (though a highly abstract and stylized prime mover),[104] then as a complete irrelevance in the development of that form of *Öffentlichkeit*. Nor is this the place to suggest how Habermas's concept of the *bürgerliche Öffentlichkeit* might be modulated so as to accommodate religion, though I suspect that this could be done. What is clear is that some such modulation of the concept is required, both because the coherence of Habermas's entire conception is at stake and because religion was a vital aspect of eighteenth-century Britain, the very polity that Habermas took as his 'model case'.

The burden of my argument has been that Habermas's conception of the *bürgerliche Öffentlichkeit* stands in need of enlargement and enrichment: not only to embrace the founding of new institutions (this, it will be recalled, was my initial premise), but also to take account of differences and contests within the *bürgerliche Öffentlichkeit*, and especially to deal with religious issues. The theme of religion in particular will surely require considerable modification of Habermas's picture. But the converse may also apply: that is, a *rapprochement* between religion and the concept of the *bürgerliche Öffentlichkeit* may perhaps shed new light upon early-modern religion itself. And, in that case, historians of the early-modern period may still have much to learn from Habermas's *Strukturwandel der Öffentlichkeit*, forty years after that work was published.

Acknowledgements

For help with this chapter I wish to thank Jon Hodge, Sarah Kattau, Josephine Lloyd, John Money, Mike Woodhouse, David Wykes and the staffs of the Birmingham Central Reference Library (BCRL), the Warwickshire County Record Office (WCRO) and the Brotherton Library, University of Leeds. Special thanks go to Steve Sturdy both for his helpful comments and for his editorial patience.

Notes

1 Cf. A. Wilson, 'The politics of medical improvement in early Hanoverian London', in A. Cunningham and R.K. French (eds), *The Medical Enlightenment of the Eighteenth Century*, Cambridge: Cambridge University Press, 1990, pp. 4–39, at p. 7.

2 J. Habermas, *The Structural Transformation of the Public Sphere: An Inquiry into a Category of Bourgeois Society* (German original 1962), trans. T. Burger with the assistance of F. Lawrence, Cambridge: Polity Press, 1989, p. 57.

3 See for instance M.D. George, *London Life in the Eighteenth Century* (orig. pub. 1925), Harmondsworth: Penguin, 1966, and D. Andrew, *Philanthropy and Police: London Charity in the Eighteenth Century*, Princeton: Princeton University Press, 1989.

4 P. Borsay, *The English Urban Renaissance: Culture and Society in the Provincial Town 1660–1800*, Oxford: Clarendon Press, 1989.

5 Cf. Habermas, *Structural Transformation*, pp. 20–22, 27, 31–2, 38–9, 58–62.

6 Voluntary hospitals began in 1719 in London, and in 1737 in the provinces; dispensaries began in the 1770s.

7 In the provinces only some nine or ten dispensaries were founded before 1800, as against twenty-eight hospitals. On dispensaries see I. Loudon, 'The origins and growth of the dispensary movement in England', *Bulletin of the History of Medicine*, 1981, vol. 55, pp. 322–42, and R. Kilpatrick, '"Living in the light": dispensaries, philanthropy and medical reform in late eighteenth-century London', in Cunningham and French (eds), *Medical Enlightenment*, pp. 254–80.

8 These are listed in J. Woodward, *To Do the Sick no Harm: A Study of the British Voluntary Hospital System to 1875*, London, Routledge, 1974.

9 For overviews see Andrew, *Philanthropy and Police*, and S. Lawrence, *Charitable Knowledge: Hospital Pupils and Practitioners in Eighteenth-Century London*, Cambridge: Cambridge University Press, 1996.

10 The usual approach is to construct a composite picture by using selected examples from different localities; see R. Porter, 'The gift relation: philanthropy and provincial hospitals in eighteenth-century England', in L. Granshaw and R. Porter (eds), *The Hospital in History*, London: Routledge, 1989, pp. 149–78; K. Wilson, 'Urban culture and political activism in Hanoverian England: the example of voluntary hospitals', in E. Hellmuth (ed.), *The Transformation of Political Culture: England and Germany in the Late Eighteenth Century*, Oxford: Oxford University Press, 1990, pp. 165–84; P. Langford, *Public Life and the Propertied Englishman 1689–1798*, Oxford: Clarendon Press, 1991, pp. 493–500. For an attempt at a comprehensive survey, which yielded only crude and broad-brush results, see A. Wilson, 'Conflict, consensus and charity: politics and the provincial voluntary hospitals in the eighteenth century', *The English Historical Review*, 1996, vol. 111, pp. 599–619.

11 An example of such a study is W. Brockbank, *Portrait of a Hospital 1752–1948*, London: Heinemann, 1952.

12 H. Marland, *Medicine and Society in Wakefield and Huddersfield 1780–1870*, Cambridge: Cambridge University Press, 1987; M.E. Fissell, *Patients, Power and the Poor in Eighteenth-Century Bristol*, Cambridge: Cambridge University Press, 1991; J. Lane, *Worcester Infirmary in the Eighteenth Century*, Worcester Historical Society Occasional Publications No. 6, Worcester, 1992; A. Borsay, *Medicine and Charity in Georgian Bath: A Social History of the General Infirmary, c.1739–1830*, Aldershot: Ashgate, 1999.

13 J. Money, *Experience and Identity: Birmingham and the West Midlands, 1760–1800*, Manchester: Manchester University Press, 1977.

14 The Bath General Hospital got going in 1742 but only after four previous initiatives that went back to 1711; the county hospitals of Lincolnshire, Norfolk and Berkshire all failed in the early 1740s and were not revived until a generation or more later (Borsay, 'Cash and conscience', p. 208; Wilson, 'Conflict, consensus and charity', pp. 601–2).

102

15 This is attested at Winchester, Exeter and Leicester. See respectively A. Clarke, *A Sermon Preached in the Cathedral Church of Winchester, before the Governors of the County-Hospital…at the Opening of the Said Hospital*, London, 1737, pp. 20–2, and the attached 'A Collection of Papers', pp. 8–11; J. Caldwell, 'Notes on the history of Dean Clarke's Hospital 1741–1948', *Reports and Transactions of the Devonshire Association for the Advancement of Science, Literature and Art*, 1972, vol. 104, pp. 175–92, at pp. 176–7; and Porter, 'The gift relation', p. 154, quoted in Wilson, 'Conflict, consensus and charity', p. 604.

16 For more detailed accounts see Porter, 'The gift relation'; Borsay, 'Cash and conscience'; and Wilson, 'Conflict, consensus and charity'.

17 See the diagram in Wilson, 'The politics of medical improvement', p. 12.

18 Though in London, the three endowed hospitals of St Bartholomew's, St Thomas's and Guy's were even more important: see Lawrence, *Charitable Knowledge*.

19 Habermas, *Structural Transformation*, p. 36.

20 So too Habermas's account fits with the geographical and cultural associations of the voluntary hospitals: not only were they always located in towns, but more particularly they were commonly associated with forms of polite culture that were moving away from court patronage and towards a market orientation. Emblematic of this was the benefit performance of Handel's Messiah in 1749 for the London Foundling Hospital: see R.K. McClure, *Coram's Children: The London Foundling Hospital in the Eighteenth Century*, New Haven: Yale University Press, 1981.

21 For another such sign see note 27 below.

22 The original records of the Bean Club have not been found; I have used the transcripts in W.K.R. Bedford, *Notes from the Minute Book of the Bean Club, 1754–1836*, 1889, BCRL 131399, and J.B. Stone, 'Annals of the Bean Club, Birmingham', MS of *c*.1900, BCRL 345313.

23 Here my account differs from the standard view, which is that the Warwickshire representation in the 1750s and 1760s was managed by Baron Craven and the Earls of Warwick, Aylesford and Hertford: L. Namier and J. Brooke, *The House of Commons 1754–1790*, 2 vols, London: HMSO, 1964, vol. 1, p. 399, and Money, *Experience and Identity*, p. 171. The issue is discussed in A. Wilson, 'The peace of the county: Warwickshire, Birmingham and the Bean Club, 1746–1774' (forthcoming).

24 W. Hutton, *An History of Birmingham*, Birmingham, 1780 and 1783; reprinted with an introduction by C.R. Elrington, Wakefield: EP Publishing, 1976; C. Gill, *History of Birmingham*, vol. 1: *Manor and Borough to 1865*, London: Oxford University Press, 1952; Money, *Experience and Identity*.

25 See for instance S. Smiles, *Lives of Boulton and Watt*, 2nd edn, London: John Murray, 1866; H.W. Dickinson, *Matthew Boulton*, Cambridge: Cambridge University Press, 1937; R.E. Schofield, *The Lunar Society of Birmingham: A Social History of Provincial Science and Industry in Eighteenth Century England*, Oxford: Clarendon Press, 1963.

26 See Elrington's introduction to Hutton, *History of Birmingham*.

27 In 1746 – that is, the year before his ennoblement as first Baron Archer – Thomas Archer purchased the lordship of the manor of Birmingham at a cost of £1,700 (Hutton, *History of Birmingham*, p. 181); in 1752 his younger brother Henry Archer helped to set up a Birmingham Court of Conscience for the recovery of small debts.

28 E. Cruickshanks, *Political Untouchables: The Tories and the '45*, London: Duckworth, 1979, p. 107.

29 Hutton, *History of Birmingham*, pp. 124–5.

30 Ibid., pp. 116–21.

31 BCRL, BC/1 and BC/2.

32 The Old Meeting dated from the 1690s, the New Meeting from 1730, and the Carr's Lane Meeting split off from the Old Meeting in 1748: Hutton, *History of Birmingham*, pp. 116–18.

33 Money, *Experience and Identity*, pp. 222–4.

34 See J.T. Bunce, *History of the Corporation of Birmingham, with a Sketch of the Earlier Government of the Town*, vol. 1, Birmingham: Cornish Brothers, 1878, and Hutton, *History of Birmingham*, pp. 196–202.
35 What follows is discussed more fully, with supporting references, in Wilson, 'The peace of the county'.
36 J.R. Western, *The English Militia in the Eighteenth Century: The Story of a Political Issue 1600–1802*, London: Routledge, 1965, *passim*; L. Colley, *In Defiance of Oligarchy: The Tory Party 1714–60*, Cambridge: Cambridge University Press, 1982, p. 285.
37 M. Peters, 'The *Monitor* on the constitution, 1755–1765: new light on the origins of English radicalism', *The English Historical Review*, 1971, vol. 86; Colley, *In Defiance of Oligarchy*, pp. 288, 360 n. 67.
38 This directory is not extant; for its existence see J. Hill, *The Bookmakers and Booksellers of Old Birmingham*, Birmingham: privately printed, 1907, p. 65.
39 Hutton, *History of Birmingham*, p. 266.
40 For accounts of this by-election see Money, *Experience and Identity*, pp. 171–2, and Wilson, 'The peace of the county'.
41 Equally significant, the other steward was William Craven, the new Lord Craven (the sixth Baron), who immediately before his accession to the peerage had been in contention with Skipwith at the by-election. (Craven had been forced to withdraw because by a remarkable twist of fate, his uncle and namesake, the 5th Baron Craven, died on 17 March, whereupon the barony passed to him, making him ineligible to serve in the Commons. On the sixth Baron Craven see further below, at note 95.)
42 Money, *Experience and Identity*, pp. 172–3; and cf. pp. 106–7, 169.
43 All these members were elected on 11 September 1770.
44 Money, *Experience and Identity*, pp. 100–1 and *passim*.
45 For Skipwith see ibid., pp. 208–10 and F. O'Gorman, *The Rise of Party in England: The Rockingham Whigs 1760–82*, London: Allen & Unwin, 1975, pp. 320, 430–1, 596 n.19. Skipwith's so-to-speak leftwards political move was echoed in the early 1770s by Sir Charles Holte; and later in the decade Lord Craven, the sixth Baron Craven, went even further in the same direction (see below, at note 95).
46 Money, *Experience and Identity*, *passim*.
47 Garbett's partner Dr John Roebuck was in the late 1740s a trustee of the Presbyterian New Meeting, and in the 1760s Garbett was on very friendly terms with the Unitarian John Taylor and the Quaker Sampson Lloyd, partners in the firm of Taylor and Lloyd: Hill, *Bookmakers and Booksellers of Old Birmingham*, p. 89, and R.S. Sayers, *Lloyds Bank in the History of English Banking*, Oxford: Clarendon Press, 1957, pp. 6–7. For Boulton see Schofield, *The Lunar Society*, and Dickinson, *Matthew Boulton*.
48 For accounts of the Hospital's origin and development see J. A. Langford, *A Century of Birmingham Life*, vol. 1, Birmingham, 1968, pp. 153–74; Gill, *History of Birmingham*, vol. 1, pp. 130–1; and Money, *Experience and Identity*, pp. 9–11.
49 Money, *Experience and Identity*, p. 166.
50 Between May and August 1765 three meetings were held (as many as in the previous three years) and ten new members were elected (as many as in the previous four years).
51 *Aris's*, 30 September 1765.
52 For titles to settlement and relief see R. Burn, *The History of the Poor Laws, with Observations*, London, 1764, pp. 106–7; G.W. Oxley, *Poor Relief in England and Wales 1601–1834*, London: David & Charles, 1974, pp. 19–21; and K.D.M. Snell, *Annals of the Labouring Poor: Social Change and Agrarian England 1660–1900*, Cambridge: Cambridge University Press, 1985, *passim*, particularly pp. 71, 77.
53 Langford, *Birmingham Life*, p. 154, punctuation modified.
54 *Aris's*, 25 November 1765.
55 Birmingham General Hospital Quarterly Board of Governors Minute Book 1765–1842, entry for 21 November 1765, BCRL, MS. 1423/1. Some of these

104

benefactors had probably been present at the meeting, while others sent their gifts through the hands of friends.

56 Samuel Birch (elected 1751) and Richard Hicks (elected 1753).

57 On Newdigate see Money, *Experience and Identity*, p. 2.

58 One of the refounding members of the Bean Club in 1749; of Blythe Hall, a few miles north-east of Birmingham. Another Richard Geast, presumably his son, was to join the Club in 1775; his address was given as Birmingham.

59 This was the third Earl, William Legge (1731–1801), grandson of the second Earl, with whom he has sometimes been confused. The third Earl succeeded on 15 December 1750, but did not take his seat in the House of Lords until 31 May 1754; see A. Collins, *The Peerage of England*, 3rd edn, 5 vols in 6, London, 1756, vol. 3, p. 344.

60 Dartmouth's seat of Sandwell-Hall was only four miles from Birmingham; he was both a neighbour and a confidant of Matthew Boulton (see Money, *Experience and Identity*, p. 58), whose firm was, we have seen, one of the strongest supporters of the Hospital; Dartmouth may have been cultivating a Birmingham connection at this time, for when the Birmingham Canal Navigation was launched two years later, he was to be a major shareholder.

61 *Aris's*, 9 December 1765.

62 Ibid., 16 December 1765.

63 The Dissenters were Samuel Galton, John Kettle, Sampson Lloyd, Dr William Small, John Taylor and John Taylor Junior.

64 Langford, *Birmingham Life*, pp. 155–7.

65 Birmingham General Hospital Quarterly Board of Governors Minute Book 1765–1842, p. 19 (Friday 7 November 1766), BCRL, MS. 1423/1.

66 Birmingham General Hospital Committee of Trustees Minute Book 1766–84, entries for 1766–8, *passim*, BCRL, MS. 1423/2.

67 For instance, the secretary agreed to have his salary held back for a year, and as will emerge below, further benefactions were solicited.

68 BCRL, MS. 1423/2, 3 May 1768.

69 BCRL, MSS 1423/1 and 1423/2.

70 Save only that three further meetings were held: on 13 September, mainly to take out insurance on the building; on 22 November, which meeting was adjourned, supposedly for three months; and on 2 May 1769, when the secretary was requested to bring in exact accounts of the moneys owing: BCRL, MS. 1423/1.

71 As for instance at Manchester (see Brockbank, *Portrait of a Hospital*).

72 See Money, *Experience and Identity*, pp. 58 (Dartmouth; cf. note 60 above), 175 (correspondence with Aylesford's Countess).

73 Langford, *Birmingham Life*, pp. 156–7.

74 The appeal was made on 1 June 1767; its outcome was reported in *Aris's*, listing the individual donations (this probably in an attempt to shame others into contributing), on 25 January 1768. See Langford, *Birmingham Life*, pp. 157–8.

75 BCRL, MS. 1423/1, entry for 3 May 1768.

76 No reply to either letter was recorded in the minutes, and none of the recipients thereafter became a benefactor. A fitting emblem of the indifference of the county aristocracy is supplied by Lord Denbigh. Denbigh was a prime candidate to approach, for in his youth he had made a point of cultivating a Birmingham interest, and he was associated with two of the Hospital's leading activists (Samuel Garbett and Henry Carver); yet so little did he care about the Hospital's plight that he did not even trouble to record its communication in his letter-book: WCRO, CR 2017/C243.

77 C. Hadfield, *The Canals of the West Midlands*, Newton Abbot: David & Charles, 1969, pp. 63–4.

78 Mr Francis Goodall (5 guineas).

79 William Bentley (10 guineas), Edward Hector and James Farmer (5 guineas each).

80 *Aris's*, 12 September 1768, quoted in Langford, *Birmingham Life*, p. 159.
81 Cf. above, at note 72. After the Thursday morning performance of music from Handel and Boyce, held in St Phillip's Church, these Countesses (it was reported) 'very obligingly stood to receive at the church door for the benefit of the charity'.
82 Thus the appeal made in 1767 drew in contributions from five of the six Dissenters, but from only about half of the others (including contributions from relatives, such as Francis Garbett Esq., whom I take to have been related to Samuel Garbett); the Dissenters were disproportionately prominent on the little sub-committee that organized the music festival of 1768, contributing as they did three of its seven members (Dr William Small, John Taylor Esq., and Mr John Taylor Junior; others on the sub-committee were Dr John Ash, Henry Carver Junior, Mr Brooke Smith and Isaac Spooner Esq.).
83 Nevertheless, at least two of the three new donors in 1767 (note 79 above) were Churchmen: Edward Hector, a Bean Club member since 1751, and William Bentley, who was to be elected to the Club in 1774.
84 Above, at note 69. The Churchmen could well have been suspicious of the double role played by John Taylor and Sampson Lloyd, that is, as members of the committee and as the Hospital's bankers. Conversely the Dissenters may have resented the fact that members of the Established Church had delivered far less support to the Hospital than they themselves had produced.
85 Above, at note 43.
86 An emblem of the contrasting approaches underlying the Hospital and the Club is the case of Matthew Boulton. As a manufacturer, Boulton was in fierce rivalry with John Taylor, and there was no love lost between them in commercial matters (Taylor to Boulton, 16 July 1772, BCRL, Matthew Boulton papers, 256/42); yet Boulton served alongside Taylor on the Hospital committee, and he was to remain staunch in his support for the Hospital. But precisely because he associated freely with Dissenters like Taylor, he was excluded from the Bean Club, as we have seen (above, at note 47).
87 The full title was *Poetical Dream, Being a Dialogue between the Hospital and the New Play House*. See Langford, *Birmingham Life*, pp. 160–1.
88 J.W. Showell in *Aris's*, 1856, quoted in Langford, *Birmingham Life*, p. 162.
89 See the extracts in Langford, *Birmingham Life*, pp. 162–7.
90 Dr John Ash, William John Banner, Matthew Boulton, Henry Carver, Samuel Galton, John Kettle, Sampson Lloyd, Francis Parrott, Joseph Smith, John Taylor and John Turner.
91 Samuel Galton, John Kettle, Sampson Lloyd and John Taylor.
92 Known Dissenters were Samuel Galton Junior, Samuel Harvey, William Hunt, Michael Lakin, Charles Lloyd, Sampson Lloyd Junior, John Richards, John Rickards and William Russell, while a possible case was Samuel Freeth. What is particularly striking is that several of these new men – five or six of them – came from the Presbyterian Old Meeting, which had not contributed a single member to the original committee: Harvey, Hunt, Lakin, Richards, Rickards and possibly Freeth (perhaps the husband of Martha Freeth of the Old Meeting). Members of the Old Meeting have been identified from the MS. Register of their resolutions, 1771–91, in BCRL.
93 In the 1769 by-election he had initially offered himself against Skipwith, and his candidacy had been backed by Lord Denbigh: see note 41 above.
94 Perhaps under the influence of his wife: Money, *Experience and Identity*, p. 78 n.76.
95 Craven had attained a more liberal stance by 1774 (signalled by his backing Lord Guernsey as prospective candidate for the Warwickshire election), and he opposed the American war in 1775. See Money, *Experience and Identity*, pp. 69, 78 n. 67, 78 n. 76, 175–6, 216 n. 58.
96 At the same time, the question needs to be asked as to why Craven, only very lately a Whig, was chosen in this role, rather than the Earl of Hertford, the Earl of

106

Warwick or Baron Archer, all of whose Whig allegiances were of much longer standing. This is connected with a larger puzzle that I have not yet resolved: why was it that no effective links had developed between these Whig aristocrats and the Dissenters among the Birmingham elite? This is all the more of a conundrum in view of the Archers' earlier interest in Birmingham (note 27 above). There was at least one such link, between John Taylor and Lord Warwick, which is attested in 1769 and had no doubt developed earlier, but this merely intensifies the question as to why the Hospital made so little of connections like this. For the Taylor–Lord Warwick connection, see S.H.A. Hervey (ed.), *Journals of the Hon. William Hervey, in North America and Europe, from 1755 to 1814; with Order Books at Montreal, 1760–1763. With Memoir and Notes*, Suffolk Green Books, No. 14, Bury St Edmunds: Paul and Mathew, 1906, p. 217.

97 See for instance Habermas, *Structural Transformation*, pp. 33, 55–6.

98 Money, *Experience and Identity*, pp. 9–11, 100–1 and *passim*.

99 It is important to register that what we might call the 'internal' relations of the public sphere were themselves contingent upon 'external' relations with the state, at least in the setting that has been considered here. What defined an aristocrat was his family's membership of the House of Lords; what made a man a gentleman, in the full sense of the word, was his appointment to the county Commission of the Peace, an appointment that was made by the Crown; and what gave force to religious divisions was that the Church of England and this alone was *Established*, that is, formally united with the state. Thus the conflicts within the 'public sphere' lead us not away from the state but back towards it: cf. my 'A critical portrait of social history', in A. Wilson (ed.) *Rethinking Social History: English Society 1570–1920 and its Interpretation*, Manchester: Manchester University Press, 1993, pp. 9–58, at pp. 13–20.

100 In the English translation, *repräsentative Öffentlichkeit* has been variously rendered as 'representative publicness' (Habermas, *Structural Transformation*, pp. 10, 11), as 'the publicity of representation' (p. 9), and as 'the publicity that characterized representation' (p. 8); in view of the difficulties of translation, it seems safest to stick to Habermas's German words. Speaking approximately, *repräsentative Öffentlichkeit* was a ceremonial display of the status of those who held power (pp. 7, 8). More precisely, *repräsentative Öffentlichkeit* was a display of the *virtues* held to be associated with that power: qualities such as 'excellence, highness, majesty, fame, dignity, and honour' (p. 7, apparently quoting Carl Schmitt; cf. the next note). This was quite different in kind from 'representation' as we tend to think of it, that is, 'representation in the sense in which the members of a national assembly represent a nation, or a lawyer represents his clients' (p. 7). Rather, what was represented was the ensemble of noble virtues; the way that this ensemble of virtues was represented was through the being of the ruler. Habermas suggested that *repräsentative Öffentlichkeit* took a succession of different forms – first courtly-knightly, then Renaissance-humanist and finally monarchic-aristocratic (pp. 9–11).

101 Habermas, *Structural Transformation*, pp. 8–9. This phase of Habermas's argument leaned heavily on the writings of Carl Schmitt, published in the 1920s and 1930s.

102 Ibid., pp. 11–12.

103 Ibid., p. 63. Again, when Habermas turned to France its Catholicism was not even noticed; the 1685 revocation of the Edict of Nantes was registered merely in a footnote and even there only obliquely (p. 263, n.23 to p. 67); the religious concerns of the early *philosophes* were mentioned only to dismiss these as non-political (p. 68). And with respect to Germany Habermas excluded all mention of religion, not only from his initial discussion of its political development (pp. 71–3), but also from his subsequent account of the thought of both Hegel and Marx (pp. 117–29).

104 Habermas described the Reformation as bringing about, or as equivalent to (it was not clear which), 'the so-called freedom of religion' (ibid., p. 11).

VII

ON THE HISTORY OF DISEASE-CONCEPTS:
THE CASE OF PLEURISY

It is, I believe, uncontentious to suggest that concepts of disease — both in general and with respect to particular ailments — have changed and developed historically in the long history of the Western medical tradition. And it is obvious, too, that diseases (taking that term in its widest sense, to embrace illnesses at large) were and are precisely the distinctive concern of medicine. On principle, therefore, we might expect that *the history of disease-concepts* plays a central part in the historiography of medicine, just as the histories of celestial, physical and vital concepts do in the historiographies of the respective natural sciences; yet paradoxically, this is far indeed from being the case. That strand of medical history which focuses on medicine's cognitive content has devoted far more attention to anatomical and physiological knowledge than to pathology; the history of medical practice is often written without reference to the disease-categories by which past practitioners apprehended the illnesses of their patients; and as we shall see, histories of actual diseases have tended to treat their objects as timeless entities, thereby blocking off the very possibility of considering disease-concepts historically.

This paper proposes that the history of disease-concepts deserves far more attention than it has traditionally been accorded, not least because this theme is relevant to the full range of medical history's existing concerns, from anatomy to medical practice. I shall proceed in three stages. Part 1 sketches the historiographic state of play with regard to disease-concepts. Part 2, which makes up the bulk of the paper, seeks to illustrate the possibility of treating such concepts historically by means of an example, namely the disease of *pleuritis* or *pleurisy*; I shall trace the shifting meanings of this term first amongst the ancients and then, on a very selective basis, in the early-modern period. Finally Part 3 will meditate briefly on the results of this case-study, returning to the general historiographic theme and suggesting some points of wider application.

1. HISTORIOGRAPHY

There is already a substantial tradition of scholarship which treats concepts-of-disease as historical products, and which has traced their histories in a series of particular cases. That tradition could be said to begin in the 1930s and '40s, with three pioneering studies: Ludwik Fleck's *Genesis and development of a scientific fact*, which stressed that "syphilis" was a historically-changing concept;[1] Owsei Temkin's *The Falling Sickness*, a history of concepts of epilepsy from ancient

190

to modern times;[2] and Georges Canguilhem's *The normal and the pathological*, a critical dissection of the mid-nineteenth-century shift in the definition of the pathological, which was written as a doctoral thesis in the 1940s and was published in 1966.[3] The tradition was renewed in the 1970s and '80s, most explicitly by the school of "social-constructivists"[4] but also by various other medical historians working from a range of different perspectives;[5] in the 1990s it is still alive and well, as various recent studies attest.[6] And this now substantial body of work has consistently demonstrated the historicity of disease-concepts — not just for putatively "soft" diseases such as epilepsy, chlorosis[7] and hysteria,[8] but also for diseases which all observers regard as having a physical, bodily basis. This can be illustrated with reference to four examples: syphilis (arguably the classic case, since Fleck historicized it as long ago as 1935); asthma (which has often been assigned a "psychosomatic" component, but which has always been seen as thoroughly "somatic" as well); coronary thrombosis; and Bright's disease.

(1) The historicity of "syphilis" was the fundamental premise of Fleck's *Genesis and development of a scientific fact*: the book opened with a little history of "how the modern concept of syphilis originated",[9] and Fleck went on to argue that every relevant development in knowledge entailed a change in the very definition of what we know as "syphilis". This impact of knowledge upon disease-concepts was particularly marked in the cases of the two great discoveries of the early twentieth century — the micro-organism *Spirochaeta pallida* (first detected in 1905) and the Wassermann reaction (first reported in 1906, gradually refined into a serological test).[10] Of the Wassermann reaction, which was the central concern of his study, Fleck wrote that it "*redefined* syphilis",[11] and indeed he argued that the very success of that reaction as a diagnostic test required such redefinition of the disease.[12] And with respect to the discovery of the spirochaete, he remarked:[13]

> The statement, "Schaudinn discerned *Spirochaeta pallida* as the causative agent of syphilis" is equivocal as it stands, because "syphilis as such" does not exist. There was only the then-current concept available on the basis of which Schaudinn's contribution occurred, an event that only developed this concept further. Torn from this context, "syphilis" has no specific meaning....

The reason that Fleck thus historicized "syphilis" was that he was seeking to problematize scientific knowledge and its making, using the Wassermann reaction as his case-study. I shall shortly have occasion to look more closely at Fleck's conception of knowledge; for the moment, what commands attention is the fact that he depicted the "modern concept of syphilis" precisely *as* a concept, that is, as a human product.

(2) Asthma, John Gabbay showed in a paper of 1982,[14] began in the ancient world as a symptom; it changed its nature in the Renaissance, becoming a disease in its own right, and one located in the abdomen; subsequently, in the eighteenth century, it moved its abode to the thorax; it was repeatedly reinterpreted throughout the

nineteenth century; and it went on being transmuted until the mid-1970s. In short, the entire course of asthma's long history was a story of change, to the very eve of the time that Gabbay was writing.

(3) Coronary thrombosis has a history of a very different kind, since this disease was only discovered, or invented, in the 1920s; but from Christopher Lawrence's study it emerges that coronary thrombosis was and is just as much a constructed and contingent "entity" as asthma.[15] For instance, coronary thrombosis was stabilized only with great difficulty, if indeed it was stabilized at all;[16] its relation to ECG findings (its supposed clinical test) was consistently problematical;[17] and Lawrence went on to suggest that it was disappearing as a clinical category in the 1990s. It seems, then, that coronary thrombosis is perhaps a disease-concept with an end as well as a beginning; and just this pattern is revealed by my final example.

(4) What was called "Bright's disease" — that is, a particular kind of dropsy which Richard Bright distinguished in 1827 — has been elegantly interrogated by Steven Peitzman.[18] We thus learn that "Bright's" was not one but three diseases; that its signs and symptoms were always variable, as were its putative causes (cold according to Bright himself, microbes according to a later generation, immunological changes still later); and that in the twentieth century "Bright's disease" went into terminal decline. By about 1950 "Bright's" had given up the ghost, ironically yielding place to the older category "nephritis", which was succeeded by "renal failure", which in turn gave way, in the age of dialysis, to "end-state renal disease";[19] and each of these new names designated a different clinico-pathological concept, for all that these various concepts overlapped.

The collective import of these and other such studies has been that concepts-of-disease, like all concepts, are human and social products which have changed and developed historically, and which thus form the proper business of the historian. Yet this insight has been held in check by another approach, in which diseases *throughout history* have been identified with their *modern* names-and-concepts. Under this very different rubric, *responses to* diseases, both on the part of individual patients-and-doctors and on a larger scale in the form of such political measures as quarantine, are permitted to vary historically; but this historiographic permission is withheld from *diseases themselves*, since those diseases are all taken to coincide with their respective modern concepts. And the effect of this approach is to construct a conceptual space in which the historicity of all disease-concepts, whether past or present, has been obliterated. Past concepts of disease have simply been written out of existence; and the historicity of modern disease-concepts (or what are taken to be modern ones) is effaced, because those concepts have been assigned a transhistorical validity.

These two approaches have now been running side-by-side for some decades; yet the tension between them has attracted remarkably little comment.[20] Since one chief purpose of the present paper is to bring that tension to light, it will be worth

274

comparing the different ways in which these two traditions have approached a single disease. The most convenient example to choose is the disease which came to be known as "syphilis" — for this was precisely the disease-concept which Fleck historicized in his *Genesis and development of a scientific fact*, and it is also the theme of a highly-regarded history-of-disease study, namely Claude Quétel's *Le mal de Naples* (1986), translated in 1990 as *History of syphilis*.

Quétel's *Le mal de Naples* is (as its Introduction puts it) a study of "syphilis as a cultural phenomenon".[21] Seen strictly within its own terms of reference this is an admirable work, which beautifully captures many of the cultural responses evoked over the centuries by what was variously called the "*mal de Naples*", "great pox", "*morbus Gallicus*", "*morbus venereus*", "*lues venerea*", or "syphilis". But Quétel's terms of reference are precisely what is at issue here, for his inquiry rigorously excludes from consideration the various *concepts* associated with this motley welter of names. The reason for this exclusion is that one such concept, namely the modern concept, has been privileged as the factual mirror of Nature: *Le mal de Naples* is entirely premised upon retrospective diagnosis. Early-modern disease-descriptions are consistently read through the conceptual grid of the modern concept of "syphilis"; as Quétel depicts it, Schaudinn's *Spirochaeta pallida* was (or rather, is) simply "the syphilis microbe", and the Wassermann reaction yielded a diagnostic test for an implicitly unchanged "syphilis". And as a result, the little that emerges concerning disease-concepts presents a series of paradoxes which are in radical tension with the book's premises and are accordingly left entirely unresolved. For instance, the very name "syphilis" presents a riddle: coined by Fracastoro in the early sixteenth century, it lay dormant until the eighteenth century, when it somehow displaced "the great pox" and other terms which had been used for the previous two hundred years; yet this profound shift of terminology emerges only in asides.[22] Again, the "great pox" included, as one of its symptoms, a "gonorrhoea" (that is, a flux-of-seed),[23] which in the early nineteenth century came to be seen as a separate disease;[24] yet Quétel barely notices that this puts in question his own identification of the "great pox" with "syphilis".[25] In sum, disease-concepts lie beyond the conceptual horizon of *Le mal de Naples*; they enter Quétel's discourse only to be instantly dismissed from consideration.

Ironically enough, it turns out that this very approach to the history of diseases had already been described, criticized and explained in Fleck's *Genesis and development of a scientific fact*. In order to bring out this point, it will be necessary to outline Fleck's larger theses concerning the nature of scientific knowledge.

We saw earlier that Fleck sought to problematize both the content and the making of scientific knowledge. What we must now notice is that in the pursuit of this aim, Fleck consistently depicted the development of such knowledge as a social process. "Not only the principal ideas but also all the formative stages of the syphilis concept", he wrote, "are the result of collective, not individual, effort";[26] and he went on to portray scientific knowledge in general as embedded in a "thought style", associated with a specific "thought collective". Thus a "scientific fact" such as the Wassermann reaction was "a stylized signal of resistance in thinking ... by the thought collective".[27] Equally important, the subsequent *maintenance* of any such fact, that is, its historical stability, required "social reinforcement";[28] and Fleck proceeded to elaborate the social mechanisms by which historically-produced knowledge was maintained and stabilized.[29] Here Fleck's key concept was what he called "popular science" or "science for nonexperts": that is, a drastically-simplified version of scientific knowledge, whose aim is "the apodictic valuation" of "a certain point of view".[30] In "popular science", the uncertainty which is characteristic of scientific research has been replaced by certainty; the need for arduous proof is eliminated by creating a "vivid picture"; and *the historicity of concepts is necessarily eliminated*, for certain of those concepts are assigned the quality of eternal truths. This erasure of history, Fleck explained, has its own particular rhetorical mechanisms: in particular, the collective character of knowledge-making is obliterated and is replaced with a mythical, individualized picture,[31] involving a Manichean conflict between "the 'bad guys', who miss the truth, and the 'good guys', who find it".[32] But the key point is that the historical development of concepts is thereby erased. And in the particular case of *disease*-concepts, this means that the modern concept is extended backwards in time: the disease as presently conceived is seen as a permanent entity,[33] and it is assumed that it can be diagnosed retrospectively on the basis of earlier texts which in fact conceived that disease in radically different terms from those underlying the modern concept.[34] In sum, Fleck not only demonstrated the historicity of "syphilis"; he also showed that the contrary picture — the view which eternalizes the modern concept of "syphilis" — is intelligible as a necessary by-product, within "popular science", of the modern concept itself.

Le mal de Naples is obedient in every particular to the "popular-science" view of syphilis and its history, exactly as Fleck sketched it. As we have seen, the very foundation of Quétel's approach is the assumption that the "*mal de Naples*", the "great pox", and so on, are all to be identified with one another under the sign of the modern concept of "syphilis", and this entails that the actual meanings of these various disease-concepts are suppressed. Inevitably, therefore, Quétel's study scarcely considers the making of medical knowledge.[35] And to the extent that the development of medical knowledge is brought into view, it is depicted in strictly teleological terms (for instance, as a "step in the right direction"[36]) and is rigorously individualized[37] — precisely in line with the dictates of the "popular-science" conception of knowledge as delineated by Fleck.

The profound and pervasive contrast between the approaches of Fleck and of Quétel stems from a radical difference in conceptions of the cognitive, of the social, and of their interrelationship. Specifically, Fleck saw knowledge as socially-constituted, thereby placing the cognitive *within* the social, whereas Quétel has drawn a rigid boundary around the realm of the social and has placed knowledge *outside* that boundary. It should also be observed that Fleck went to some trouble to argue for his conception, whereas Quétel simply assumes his conception — and

276

symptomatically, Quétel nowhere mentions Fleck's work. The final irony is that this self-limitation radically restricts the scope of the responses-to-syphilis which Quétel allows himself to depict, thereby impoverishing the very argument which he was striving to develop, namely the vision of "syphilis as a cultural phenomenon". But what is significant in the present context is that Quétel's founding act of excluding the cognitive from the social has systematically obliterated the historicity of concepts-of-disease.

This contrast is by no means confined to the individual figures of Fleck and Quétel, or to the specific case of syphilis: on the contrary, it runs through the whole historiography of medicine. We might well describe it, using Fleck's own terms, as a difference in "thought styles" — specifically, "thought styles" concerning the nature of disease-concepts. By way of a convenient shorthand, I shall term these two thought styles 'the historicalist-conceptualist approach' and 'the naturalist-realist approach'. Their defining characteristics can be summarized as follows:

(a) The *historicalist-conceptualist* approach takes concepts of disease as objects of historical study: this is the tradition which I have illustrated by the studies of Fleck on syphilis, Gabbay on asthma, Lawrence on coronary thrombosis, and Peitzman on Bright's disease.

(b) The *naturalist-realist* approach excludes disease-concepts from historical investigation, because it takes modern disease-concepts as the mirror of natural reality: this is the countervailing tradition of which I have taken Quétel's study of syphilis as a specimen, and which is also illustrated by many other studies of responses-to-diseases and of historical epidemiology.

Now as I have already remarked in passing, the tension between these two approaches has scarcely been noticed.[38] And the reason for this, I suggest, is simply that *the naturalist-realist approach to diseases has played and continues to play a hegemonic role in the historiography of medicine.* That is to say, there has been no confrontation between the two approaches, because the naturalist-realist approach has been dominant. This makes intelligible the otherwise paradoxical fact that historians of medicine — in contrast to historians of science, from Thomas Kuhn onwards — have shown very little interest in Fleck's *Genesis and development of a scientific fact*.[39] The indifference of the historiography of medicine to Fleck's work, then, reflects a deeper problem: that the historicalist-conceptualist approach to the history of diseases has remained subordinate in medical history.

But perhaps the most telling index of the dominance of the naturalist-realist approach is that its assumptions pervade even some of the leading attempts to historicize medical knowledge in general, and apprehensions of disease in particular. I shall illustrate this by considering four classic works, spanning almost half a century; remarkably enough, we shall see in each of these cases that the historicity of disease-concepts has actually been written out.

(1) My first example is the very book which is usually cited as the paradigmatic example of the history of a disease-concept:[40] Owsei Temkin's *The Falling Sickness*, published in 1945. Now Temkin's approach to the history of epilepsy was admirably and rigorously historical, for he wrote in his preface that "we must above all find out what was meant by epilepsy", and "we must take the past seriously and try to understand it". But in the very act of defining this approach, Temkin placed severe boundaries upon its application — for he confined his vision of the historiography of disease-concepts to those diseases whose bodily riddles medicine had not (in his view) solved:[41]

> A history of epilepsy seems a premature, perhaps even a doubtful enterprise. There is no unanimity about the range of the concept of epilepsy, and the nature of the disease is yet obscure....
>
> All these doubts and questions suggest that a history of epilepsy cannot be written in the manner in which, for instance, a history of tuberculosis might be approached. In the latter case, we have definite and well-founded knowledge of the nature of the disease. *This knowledge we can apply as a critical standard to the past and can separate the true from the false.* At present such a procedure is not possible with regard to epilepsy, for we may easily decry as false what the future will prove to be true....
>
> This being the case, there seems but one way left. We must above all find out what was meant by epilepsy, what symptoms were attributed to it, how it was explained and how treated. That means we must take the past seriously and try to understand it.

That is to say, the attempt to "find out what was meant by epilepsy" and to "take the past seriously" was *only* appropriate *because* epilepsy was still not adequately understood. And conversely, Temkin assumed that when it came to such a disease as "tuberculosis", its history should be written strictly in naturalist-realist terms — defining "tuberculosis" along the lines which Koch had put forward in 1882,[42] and thereby obliterating the history of all the relevant concepts, including the concept of "tuberculosis" itself. This of course was precisely the anachronistic approach which Fleck had explained and criticized ten years earlier.

(2) A classic of a very different kind was Foucault's *Naissance de la clinique*, which was published in 1963 and was translated into English in 1973 as *Birth of the clinic*.[43] It may seem strange to suggest that *Birth of the clinic* blocked off the possibility of historicizing concepts-of-disease, for that work has widely been perceived precisely as having historicized medical knowledge, and specifically clinical knowledge,[44] and in one sense this was indeed the thrust of the book — as was only to be expected from a pupil of Canguilhem's. Yet in fact Foucault so constructed his theme as to erase the very possibility of writing the history of disease-concepts, and this in two ways. In the first place, the threshold which he depicted medicine as crossing with the "birth of the clinic" was a transition not within knowledge, but on the contrary from non-knowledge to knowledge.

278

Concepts-of-disease before *la clinique* were consigned to "the language of fantasy"; concepts-of-disease inaugurated by *la clinique* "made it possible ... for the patient's bed to become a field of scientific investigation"; the shift from the one to the other consisted simply in the fact that "language has turned into rational discourse".[45] Thus the historicity of disease-concepts consisted in one event and one event only, namely the transition itself — a transition which was neither more nor less than the move from darkness into light, from invisibility to visibility, from "fantasy" and "imaginary investments" to "scientific investigation" and "rational discourse".[46] And on neither side of this divide was there any further story to be told.[47]

Secondly, in line with the larger "archaeological" vision which he was then in the process of constructing, Foucault conceived this transition in language, this "mutation in discourse",[48] as strictly *syntactic* in nature: that is, as concerned not with the meanings of words but purely with their mutual arrangement. Having asked at the outset "From what moment, by what *semantic or syntactical* change, can one recognize that language has turned into rational discourse?",[49] he went on to argue — at the climax of his preface — that the semantic dimension was irrelevant and that the "mutation in discourse" could be identified at the level of syntactics alone:[50]

> But is it inevitable that we should know of no other function for speech (*parole*) than commentary? *Commentary* questions discourse as to what it says and intended to say ... in other words, in stating what has been said, one has to re-state what has never been said. In this activity ... is concealed a strange attitude towards language: to comment is to admit by definition an excess of the signified over the signifier; a necessary, unformulated remainder of thought....
>
> To speak about the thought of others, to try to say what they have said has, by tradition, been to analyse the signified. But.... Is it not possible to make a structural analysis of discourses that would evade the fate of commentary by supposing no remainder, nothing in excess of what has been said, but only the fact of its historical appearance? ... The meaning of a statement would be defined not by the treasure of intentions that it might contain ... but by the difference that articulates it upon the other real or possible statements....

Now in fact this formulation rested upon an "attitude towards language" no less "strange" than that of commentary itself: for in invoking "what has been said" as his object, Foucault simply reintroduced the very problem which he had been attempting to evade, namely the problem of meaning. The paradox of language, then, could not be resolved — for all of Foucault's efforts — by taking a stand on the side of syntax, of structure, of arrangements of words, and against meaning, intention, interpretation; on the contrary, Foucault's own claim that *la clinique* "turned" language into "rational discourse" rested precisely on a posited semantics, on the notion that language was "open[ed] up ... *to a whole new domain*", on the conception of "a new alliance *between words and things*".[51] Thus the purely structural analysis of language which Foucault claimed to envisage was in the strictest sense a contradictory enterprise.[52] Yet for all this, his conception carried powerful messages: that a line could be drawn between the meanings of words and the modalities of their arrangement, and that the former (semantics) was strictly subordinate to the latter (syntactics). And this formulation precluded any history of actual disease-concepts — for such a history would necessarily take the meanings of those concepts, that is, the semantic dimension of language, as its theme.

(3) In 1978 there appeared what was to become perhaps the best-known essay in the genre of "social constructivism": Karl Figlio's study of chlorosis in nineteenth-century Britain.[53] Subtitled "the social constitution of somatic illness in a capitalist society", Figlio's paper argued that the disease of chlorosis, or the "green sickness", was anchored in class relations. At first glance it seems that Figlio here historicized and relativized the concept of "chlorosis", and that he did so by presenting a narrative account of the rise and fall of that concept; yet these appearances are highly deceptive. In fact the paper offered no such narrative at all; it paid only the most cursory attention to the meaning of "chlorosis"; and it left wholly in suspense the question as to whether what changed historically was the *concept* of chlorosis or *the disease itself*. Indeed, as we shall see, the effect of Figlio's approach was to obscure the very distinction between what I am calling the historicalist-conceptualist approach and the naturalist-realist approach.

Chlorosis was classically a disease of young women. Figlio began by arguing that chlorosis was "a physical illness",[54] which was "limited to a definite life-span": it "emerged in the sixteenth century; it was first described clearly in the early eighteenth century and became common in the nineteenth century; it peaked around mid-century and was rare by the 1920s". In 1928, when it was being recognized that chlorosis had strangely disappeared, Henry Sigerist had argued that "the history of chlorosis is the history of young girls in society";[55] and Figlio's interpretation was an elaboration and refinement of Sigerist's view. Figlio summarized his own analysis as follows:[56]

> Capitalism developed increasingly by calling on youthful female labour. To the extent that the working-class girl was drawn into the labour process, the characteristics of the non-working girl were exaggerated, first by defining adolescence as a new child-like stage corresponding to the age of intensive labouring in the working class, and then by throwing into ever sharper relief the image of a-sexual, non-working, delicate femininity. Chlorosis reinforced this now polarized, dual nature of the youth become adolescent.

Despite these various narrative gestures — "a definite life-span", "developed", "first", "then", "now" — a narrative content was precisely what Figlio's essay *lacked*. The rise of chlorosis was not discussed at all. The period of its flourishing was depicted as entirely homogeneous, both with respect to the disease itself (examples were plucked indiscriminately from the 1780s, the 1830s, the 1860s, the 1880s and 1906)[57] and with respect to nineteenth-century British capitalism

280

(specific capitalist industries were scarcely identified, and there was no mention of, for instance, Chartism, empire, or compulsory education). But the most remarkable anti-narrative feature of the essay was that the decline of chlorosis — the very feature of its history that Sigerist had emphasized — was explicitly bracketed off from consideration at the very outset of the argument; and the form of this move was highly revealing. Here is how Figlio disposed of the issue (but with my emphases):[58]

> Explanations of its disappearance vary, but authors did reject the possibility that chlorosis vanished simply because it had received another name.... To go into these reasons in detail would get us into the risky business of retrospective diagnosis. But more important even than the explanations proposed to interpret its decline is the fact that the need met by attaching a medical label, with all the consequences that followed, was now *either* met in some way, *or* no longer existed.

Thus Figlio left it strictly indeterminate ("either ... or") whether concepts of disease had changed, or whether the physical disease of chlorosis had disappeared. The same ambiguity recurred in the body of the essay: sometimes Figlio hinted that capitalism had led to the very category "chlorosis",[59] sometimes he suggested that biological changes were involved,[60] and he never attempted to resolve the tension between these two interpretations. Indeed if anything, Figlio inclined towards the biological explanation — since in the passage just quoted, "the risky business of retrospective diagnosis" was invoked as the reason for not discussing the decline of chlorosis.

Although this ambiguity seems surprising, it is intelligible in the light of Figlio's purposes. All that mattered was that chlorosis could somehow be tied to "capitalist society": it was a matter of indifference whether this putative link was constructed by way of the concept or by way of the disease itself. And precisely for this reason, Figlio's essay had very little to say about the actual concept of chlorosis, or about its history. The ironies are considerable, for in fact chlorosis had undergone a dramatic mutation in the early nineteenth century (that is, at the beginning of the period with which Figlio was concerned), and this was linked to a larger and highly consequential shift of medical concepts. In the eighteenth century, chlorosis was a "cachexia", that is, a corruption of the blood;[61] in the early nineteenth century, it became an "anaemia"; and what brought about this transformation, or at least made it possible, was that the concept of "anaemia" itself — a concept which, unlike that of "chlorosis", is still with us — was invented at that time.[62] Thus attention to the concept of chlorosis rapidly opens a much wider horizon of historical inquiry. And conversely, the reason that Figlio failed to disclose such possibilities was precisely that he never brought chlorosis into focus *as a concept*.

(4) In 1992 Charles Rosenberg and Janet Golden published a collection of essays entitled *Framing disease*.[63] The volume was notable for including two papers which I have already cited as leading examples of the historicization of disease-concepts:

Lawrence's study of coronary thrombosis and Peitzman's essay on Bright's disease. Yet as Rosenberg's Introduction made clear, the book's very title was designed to marginalize, indeed to erase, the significance of those two essays and of the historicalist-conceptualist tradition as a whole. In a pivotal passage, Rosenberg spelt out the reasons for the collection's title, making it clear that diseases were to be seen as "framed" precisely in order that that they should *not* be seen as "constructed":[64]

> In the following pages I have, in fact, avoided the term social construction. I felt that it has tended to overemphasize functionalist ends and the degree of arbitrariness inherent in the negotiations that result in accepted disease pictures. The social-constructionist argument has focused, in addition, on a handful of culturally resonant diagnoses — hysteria, chlorosis, neurasthenia, and homosexuality, for example — in which a biopathological mechanism is either unproven or unprovable. It invokes, moreover, a particular style of cultural criticism and particular moment in time — the late 1960s through the mid-1980s — and a vision of knowledge and its purveyors as rationalizers and legitimators, ordinarily unwitting, of an oppressive social order. For all these reasons, I have chosen to use the less programmatically charged metaphor "frame" rather than "construct" to describe the fashioning of explanatory and classificatory schemes of particular diseases.

The effect of this passage was to identify the metaphor of "construction" with its particular instantiation as "social construction", that is, with the genre to which Figlio's study of chlorosis belonged — whence the allusion to that disease. And this move obliterated from view the essays of Lawrence and of Peitzman in the volume itself, not to mention Gabbay's study published ten years earlier and Fleck's *Genesis and development of a scientific fact* — all concerned with diseases which are generally regarded as involving "biopathological mechanisms", each of them demonstrating the contingent and constructed character of the disease-concept in question, none of them advancing "a vision of knowledge and its purveyors as rationalizers and legitimators ... of an oppressive social order". Rosenberg concluded:

> Biology, significantly, often shapes the varieties of choices available to societies in framing conceptual and institutional responses to diseases: tuberculosis and cholera, for example, offer different pictures to frame for society's would-be framers.

An accompanying footnote explained what such "different pictures to frame" meant: "The very different modes of transmission imply different relationships to relevant ecological and environmental factors."

Despite what Rosenberg was suggesting, the new metaphor "frame" was every bit as "programmatically charged" as the discarded metaphor "construct". For of course the purpose of this "framing" imagery was to do away with the notion of construction, and to depict diseases as natural entities — tuberculosis and cholera

200

282

being taken as examples. The historically-constructed categories "tuberculosis" and "cholera", complete with their "modes of transmission", that is, strictly following the post-Kochian definition of these diseases,[65] were assigned a timeless existence. Consequently, the scope of the historical was drastically restricted, in the standard manner of the naturalist-realist approach: "responses to" diseases were permitted to vary historically, but concepts of disease were not.[66] (And most of the studies in the book implicitly echoed this conception: that is, rather than exploring the historicity of disease-concepts in the manner of Lawrence or Peitzman, they treated diseases as real entities identical with their names,[67] and limited themselves to the various cultural "responses" which diseases, so construed, had evoked.) Yet ironically enough, the metaphor of pictures-and-framing undermined itself; for tuberculosis and cholera were depicted as "offer[ing] ... pictures" — and "pictures" are of course human-made. Thus Rosenberg's own rhetoric inadvertently conceded just what he was trying to deny:[68] that diseases are not simply "biological" entities in Nature but human constructs, as of course are the very concepts of the "biological" and the "biopathological".

To sum up, the naturalist-realist approach to the history of diseases has been remarkably tenacious: it comfortably survived the translation of Fleck's book into English, and it has even pervaded some of the major attempts to historicize medical knowledge. Consequently, the history of most disease-concepts still awaits investigation, as indeed does the history of the concept of "pathology" itself. And we have still to take the measure of Fleck's point, that the supposed timelessness of diseases, and the associated conception of medical knowledge, are themselves precisely human constructs.[69]

2. THE CASE OF PLEURISY

To adapt to the present context what Steven Shapin once wrote about the sociology of scientific knowledge,[70] one can either debate the possibility of the history of disease-concepts or one can go out and write such a history. In the previous section I sought to demonstrate the possibility; here I shall attempt to do it, albeit within certain limits. By means of a case-example I hope to show that investigating the history of disease-concepts yields rich rewards, and also that such an exercise does not require a technical medical competence, but simply calls for a modicum of exegetical care. The example I have chosen for this purpose is *pleurisy*, or to give it its original and ancient name, *pleuritis*.

"Pleurisy" — in inverted commas, that is, *concepts of* pleurisy — is a particularly eligible subject for such a study, for several reasons. In the first place "pleurisy", like "asthma", belonged and belongs to the entire history of the Western medical tradition. Its birth coincided with the birth of Western medicine itself, for it featured (as "pleuritis") in several of the Hippocratic texts; it was considered by all the subsequent leading medical authors of Antiquity; it reappeared in the medical writings of the Renaissance and the Enlightenment; in the epoch of *la clinique* it was discussed extensively by Laennec, who found for pleurisy its own distinctive auscultative sound; and people are diagnosed as suffering from "pleurisy" today. Thus pleurisy offers an example which should speak to historians of Western medicine working on any and every period. Secondly, it so happens that the first episodes in the history of "pleurisy" have already been charted by Wesley D. Smith, whose pioneering study of "pleurisy" (strictly speaking, "pleuritis") in the ancient texts considerably facilitates my own task.[71] Thirdly, "pleurisy" — *unlike* "asthma" — has always been seen (at least, in all the texts I have consulted) strictly as a bodily ailment, never as involving any "psychosomatic" component. Thus if, as I hope to show, "pleurisy" changed historically throughout the Western tradition, this mutability of the concept cannot be ascribed to any supposed "softness" on pleurisy's part: it always was as definite and bodily a disease as any ailment from which patients were seen as suffering. And yet a fourth reason for taking an interest in pleurisy concerns the particular modes of anatomical localization. Specifically, one school of thought held that pleurisy was located in the membrane lining the ribs: that is to say, not in an organ but rather in what would come to be designated, in the "age of Bichat",[72] as a tissue. Thus in one dimension of its history, pleurisy serves as an example — and as we shall see, a remarkably precocious one — of precisely that kind of localization which supposedly defined *la clinique*.

In line with the programmatic aims of the present paper as a whole, my discussion of "pleurisy" will be indicative rather than definitive. I shall not be telling a connected story, but merely depicting some salient episodes; thus what follows is to a history of "pleurisy" much as a series of snapshots is to a film. Further, the approach adopted here will be strictly "internalist" and textual. That is to say, I shall make no attempt to explain the various shifts of meaning which will emerge; rather, those shifts will be presented as offering a series of problems for further investigation. In short, the aim of this section is not to write the history of "pleurisy" — for as will become clear, that would require an entire book — but simply to demonstrate that "pleurisy" *had* a history of which an account *could* be written.

I shall begin with "pleuritis" in the ancient texts; here, thanks to Wesley Smith's help, it will be possible to give a more or less comprehensive overview. My discussion will then leap forwards to the Renaissance, from which point it will be necessary to be much more selective: I shall focus on just three authors — Vesalius, Baglivi and Morgagni — who between them will conduct us from the early stages of the medical Renaissance to the eve of *la clinique*. My emphasis throughout will be upon the *definition* of "pleuritis" or "pleurisy", even though several of the texts which I shall be considering were chiefly concerned with other matters: for instance, Vesalius's *Venesection letter* (the only work, amongst those to be discussed, which was devoted specifically to pleurisy) dealt with therapeutics. In different texts, therefore, we shall find the definition of "pleuritis" variously foregrounded and taken-for-granted; and it will emerge that this variety of focus is revealing in itself.

284

2.1. ANCIENT CONCEPTIONS OF PLEURITIS

We can schematically but conveniently distinguish three epochs within the ancient roots of Western medicine:

(i) the Hippocratics of the fifth century B.C., of whose works some have survived;
(ii) the Alexandrians of the third century B.C. and their "dogmatic" followers, whose writings have survived only in quoted "fragments"; and
(iii) the authors of the early Christian era, from whom (as from the Hippocratics) we have a number of extant works: principally Soranus (relayed through Caelius Aurelianus), Aretaeus, and above all Galen.

In his important and path-breaking essay on this subject, Wesley Smith has surveyed the accounts of "pleuritis" in (i) and in (iii), and has reconstructed the doctrines that were advocated in (ii).[73] What follows is much indebted to Smith's incisive study.

(i) In the Hippocratic writings, although there was no single picture of "pleuritis", the various different accounts had this in common, that they defined the disease — if they defined it at all — *symptomatically*. Many of the texts simply took the definition of "pleuritis" for granted, concentrating instead on prognostics,[74] on therapeutics,[75] or on speculative humoral pathology.[76] But pleuritis was described in *Affections*,[77] in *Diseases II*,[78] and in *Diseases III*,[79] and these three works gave closely-overlapping definitions of its characteristic symptoms. We may take as an example the description in *Diseases III*: [80]

> When pleuritis arises, a person suffers the following: he has pain [ὀδύνη] in his side [πλευρήν], fever and shivering; he respires rapidly, and he has orthopnoea [that is, he can breathe only when in an upright posture].[81] He coughs up somewhat bilious material the colour of pomegranate-peel, unless he has fissuring, then he coughs up blood too, from the fissures. In sanguinous pleuritis the sputum is charged with blood....

Of these various symptoms, the *pain in the side* was the critical element — which is just as we would expect from the etymology of the word "pleuritis". "Pleuron" meant "side" or "rib"; the suffix "-itis" seems to have meant an "affection", "affliction", "disease" or "trouble".[82] Thus "pleuritis" was a disease named after its chief symptom, namely pain-in-the-side — whence the fact that this symptom alone was named in those other Hippocratic texts which mentioned pleuritis without explicitly defining it,[83] while yet another work (*Regimen in acute diseases*) used the phrase "pain in the side" and the word "pleuritis" more or less interchangeably.[84] Yet while this was the common core of the various usages in the *Corpus Hippocraticum*, those usages varied in at least two ways. In the first place, one description, namely that in *Diseases II*, located the pain of pleuritis not in the side but instead "along the spine and in the chest" — as if the "pleur-" was here designating "ribs" rather than "side". However, as we shall see in a moment,[85] even *Diseases II* went on to revert to the normal usage, that pleuritis was pain in the side. We may take it, therefore, that pain in the side (rather than in the ribs) was the standard meaning.

A second and more significant source of variety within the Hippocratic texts was that "pleuritis" was seen sometimes as a single disease, and at other times as comprising, in effect, a family of different though related diseases. Indeed *Diseases III* itself, whose description of pleuritis I have quoted, deployed both of these usages in succession:[86] for that description was already in the process of distinguishing between "bilious" and "sanguinous" forms of pleuritis, and the text went on to speak of further "varieties" of pleuritis: first "dry pleuritises without expectoration"; then "pleuritis in the back"; and finally still further "pleuritises", in which "the sputum is clean, but the urine bloody" and "sharp pains extend along the spine to the chest and groin". Similarly *Diseases II*, having located the pain of pleuritis "along the spine and in the chest" as we have seen, immediately described "another pleuritis" involving "pain in the side and sometimes around the collar-bone", followed by yet "another pleuritis" in which the patient has "pain" in "his side" — thereby, we may notice in passing, transferring the pleuritic pain from the patient's "spine and chest" to its more typical location in the patient's side.[87] Although this pattern of usage seems inconsistent, it simply reflected the very origin of the term "pleuritis"; for different "pleuritises" were different constellations of symptoms which had in common pain in the side (or perhaps, taking *Diseases II* into account, in the ribs). Thus the term "pleuritis" was symptom-based: a "pleuritis", we might say, was what the patient reported to the doctor in the first place.[88]

(ii) A very different conception of pleuritis was advanced by the various so-called "dogmatic" medical writers who first appeared around 300 B.C., and chiefly in Alexandria: that is to say, the anatomists Herophilus and Erasistratus together with their teachers[89] and followers. For all of these authors — so we learn from the much later testimony of Soranus, as recounted still later by Caelius Aurelianus — defined pleuritis not symptomatically but *anatomically*.[90] Yet while the various "dogmatics" agreed over this radical shift of the mode of definition, they diverged as to its practical content; for amongst them (so Soranus/Caelius informs us) two very different opinions were advanced. Some, including Herophilus, saw pleuritis as affecting the *lung*; others, including Erasistratus, placed that affection not in the lung but instead in "the *membrana hypezocota* which girds the sides internally" — that is, in the "undergirding membrane" which lines the ribs. Those of the former opinion were presumably faced with the question as to how pleuritis was distinguished from that affliction of the lungs called *peripneumony*;[91] and at least one of these authors — namely Herophilus — offered an answer to that question: pleuritis, he suggested, arose when peripneumony was complicated by fever.[92] It seems that these two different anatomical interpretations of pleuritis, the one locating it in the lung, the other placing it in the *membrana hypezocota*, generated lively debate in the ancient world; for Soranus/Caelius gave an extended account of the arguments which had been advanced on each side. In addition, there was

286

probably also a third party in this debate, a party which Soranus/Caelius did not report — namely the "empirics", who argued that the location was irrelevant and that only therapeutics mattered.[93] We might well guess that the "empirics" defined pleuritis just as the Hippocratics had done, but unfortunately this information is lost to us. Nevertheless this much is plain: that the "dogmatics" all conceived pleuritis anatomically (while locating it variously in the lung and in the *membrana hypezocota*), in sharp contrast with the symptomatic conception of the earlier Hippocratics.

Further, there was at work here another shift; for in at least one respect the dogmatics gave pleuritis a new *symptomatic* content, over and above what was included in the Hippocratic writings. Specifically, the dogmatics observed that pleuritic patients characteristically have difficulty in lying on one particular side — not, curiously enough, on the side of the pain, but rather on the unaffected side.[94] Strikingly, the two contending anatomical schools of thought agreed on the presence of this symptom[95] — though they described and interpreted it in different ways, corresponding to their respective conceptions of the seat of the disease. Those who placed pleuritis in the lung (Herophilus and others) depicted the trouble-in-lying-on-the-unaffected-side as "difficulty in breathing";[96] but those who located pleuritis in the "undergirding membrane" (Erasistratus and others) portrayed the trouble-in-lying-on-the-unaffected-side as "pain".[97] And each school had its own distinctive anatomical account of the cause of that symptom — which was precisely why Soranus/Caelius, writing some centuries later, included it in his summary of the debate between them. Now what we must observe is that this symptom had *not* been mentioned in any of the accounts of pleuritis within the Hippocratic Corpus — despite their detailed descriptions of symptom-patterns, of prognostic signs, of different varieties of pleuritis. Moreover, there is no particular reason to assume that the much later testimony of Soranus/Caelius has exhausted the catalogue of such additional symptoms. It is therefore entirely possible that the "dogmatics" added to "pleuritis" yet further symptoms — perhaps, like the difficulty-in-lying-on-the-unaffected-side, common to both anatomical interpretations, perhaps specific to one interpretation or the other. This is of course entirely conjectural; yet we should not on that account rule it out as a possibility.

(iii) From the early Christian era we have discussions of pleuritis by at least three authors: in the first century by Soranus (relayed, as has been mentioned, through Caelius Aurelianus);[98] in the second century by Galen, in several of his works,[99] and by Aretaeus of Cappadocia in his treatise on acute diseases.[100] Although Soranus, Galen and Aretaeus were writing largely independently of one another, they were all heavily influenced by the writings of the preceding dogmatists; and while their orientations and emphases differed, they reveal a clear common core. For all three of them interpreted pleuritis anatomically, and specifically, they all followed what we may call the "Erasistratean" line, that is, that pleuritis was seated in the membrane lining the ribs. True, the anatomical orientation was much less prominent in Soranus/Caelius than in Aretaeus or Galen, for Soranus regarded the state of the whole body ("stringent" or "relaxed") as the key issue in the interpretation of diseases,[101] and he deployed this whole-body conception in his description of pleuritis just in his accounts of other acute diseases. Nevertheless Soranus also gave some weight to anatomical localization, to different degrees in different diseases;[102] and as it happened, he was particularly sympathetic to this approach in the case of pleuritis. As he summed up this point (from the Latin text of Caelius Aurelianus):[103]

> But when we see a case of *pleuritica*, let us view it not as a simple affection of the side but as an affection of the whole body accompanied by acute fever. For fevers involve the whole body. We shall be right, however, if we say that the *membrana hypezocota* is more particularly affected, for it is there that the pains are centred.

Thus even Soranus accepted a measure of anatomical localization for pleuritis — whence the fact that his account of the competing *definitions* of the disease did not mention Hippocrates,[104] whereas his subsequent discussion of competing *treatments* began with Hippocrates.[105] Further, the particular localization which Soranus endorsed was in the *membrana hypezocota*, not in the lung: thus the "Erasistratean" line had come to prevail over the "Herophilean" line. And in each of these respects Aretaeus and Galen, writing in the next century, were to take the same view as Soranus before them, simply going further than Soranus in their commitment to anatomical localization. In short, as Wesley Smith has well put it, there was by this time "a general understanding" as to the nature of pleuritis:[106] it was to be interpreted anatomically, and its particular seat was in the *membrana hypezocota*, the "undergirding membrane" which lined the ribs.

I shall consider the content and significance of this anatomical conception in a moment; first, however, we must pause to notice a further development on the symptomatic front. We have already seen, when considering stage (ii) of our three-epoch schema, that the anatomical approach inaugurated by Herophilus and Erasistratus brought with it a new symptom of "pleuritis", namely difficulty in lying on the unaffected side; and I suggested that other symptoms might well have been added to "pleuritis" at that time. Now that we have reached stage (iii) of our schema, another such symptom has indeed emerged; and as we shall see, it is possible that this, too, had been added at the time of Herophilus and Erasistratus.

The new symptom is the *quality* of the pain associated with "pleuritis". With one minor exception, which I shall note in a moment, the Hippocratic texts had all described pleuritis merely as pain-in-the-side, without distinguishing that pain in any way save by its location; but as Wesley Smith observes, the pain of pleuritis has now, in the writings of the early Christian era, become a pain of a particular kind.[107] Soranus/Caelius describes it as "pricking, throbbing, and burning";[108] Aretaeus mentions "acute" pain (specifically in the clavicles) and "acrid heat";

288

Galen describes the pleuritic pain as "nygmatodes", that is, "pricking",[109] or in Professor Smith's gloss, as "sharp or piercing as though from needle jabs". Now there are some further complexities here, for Soranus, Aretaeus and Galen described and interpreted this pain in slightly different ways.[110] Nevertheless they agreed in assigning to the pleuritic pain a particular quality, a certain sharpness or intensity; and this was almost wholly new as compared with the discussions of "pleuritis" in the Hippocratic texts. True, *Diseases III* had mentioned "sharp pains" [ὀδύναι τε ὀξέαι].[111] But even there, this sharpness of the pain was by no means seen as characteristic of "pleuritis", since these sharp pains were located not in the side but "along the spine to the chest and groin" — and this type of pain was associated only with one variety of "pleuritis", not with "pleuritis" in general. In short, even if the quality of the pleuritic pain as described by Soranus, Aretaeus and Galen was somehow derived from this little passage in *Diseases III*, it had radically changed its status since the days of the Hippocratics, for it had now been installed as a defining characteristic of pleuritis.

Thus the sharpness of the pain as a definitive symptom of "pleuritis" was added *after* the writing of the Hippocratic corpus. But just *when* was "pleuritis" endowed with this new quality? On this question, as with so many issues concerning ancient medicine, we have no clear evidence; and much depends on what we make of the precise description of the pleuritic pain. Galen's "nygmatodes" was apparently inherited from Archigenes, the leading Pneumatist who was active around 100 A.D.;[112] thus if Galen's term is taken as definitive, then this quality of the pleuritic pain may well have been a relatively late discovery.[113] But if we adopt a looser criterion, assimilating together the various descriptions of that pain supplied by Soranus, by Galen and by Aretaeus, there are grounds for assigning its discovery to the earlier dogmatics, and specifically to those who placed pleuritis in the *membrana hypezocota*.[114] It is therefore possible that the quality of the pleuritic pain dated from the era of Herophilus and Erasistratus, just as the difficulty-in-lying-on-the-unaffected-side did — though this is merely a hypothesis.

Although it is frustrating that this new symptom, the sharpness of the pleuritic pain, is so difficult to pin down historically, there is one sense in which this hardly matters. For whether we ascribe it to the earlier dogmatics or to the medical writers contemporary with the Roman empire — that is, to stage (ii) or to stage (iii) of our schema — the adding of that symptom confirms and extends what we already learnt from considering the difficulty-in-lying-on-the-unaffected-side: namely, that the shift from a symptomatic definition of pleuritis to an anatomical definition was accompanied by changes in the symptoms themselves. And as we shall see, this is intelligible enough, once we focus on what the anatomical conception of pleuritis entailed.

For a closer look at that anatomical conception in late Antiquity we may turn from Soranus to Aretaeus — for as we have seen, Aretaeus and Galen were more closely wedded to anatomical localization than was Soranus, and it happened that Aretaeus's treatise on acute diseases offered a more detailed and explicit account of pleuritis than did any of Galen's extant works. It is a fair presumption that the earlier Alexandrians, the originators of the anatomical approach — from whom we have no extant writings on the subject — had written along analogous lines to what we shall be seeing in Aretaeus. For our purposes, therefore, Aretaeus's interpretation of pleuritis can stand in lieu of that of those dogmatics (Erasistratus *et al.*) who had first placed this disease in the *membrana hypezocota*, though of course we have no such surrogate for the alternative (Herophilean) interpretation, that pleuritis was seated in the lung. Here are the opening sentences of Aretaeus's description of pleuritis:[115]

> Under the ribs, the spine and the internal part of the thorax as far as the clavicles, there is stretched a thin strong membrane, adhering to the bones, which is named *hypezokos*. When inflammation [*phlegmone*] occurs in it, and there is heat with cough and parti-coloured sputa, the affection is called pleuritis. But all these symptoms must harmonize and conspire together as all springing from one cause; for such of them as occur separately from different causes, even if they occur together, are not called pleuritis. It is accompanied by acute pain of the clavicles; acrid heat; lying down on the inflamed side easy ... but on the opposite side painful.... It is attended with dyspnoea, insomnolency, anorexia, florid redness of the cheeks, dry cough, difficult expectoration of phlegm, either bilious, or deeply tinged with blood, or yellowish; and these symptoms observe no order, but come and go irregularly....

This picture of pleuritis, when compared with the descriptions of pleuritis in the Hippocratic texts, reveals several interlinked changes which together amount to a profound transformation of medical categories. First and fundamentally, although pleuritis is still *identified* symptomatically (for of course only symptoms can be observed), it is now *defined* anatomically: specifically, as an inflammation in the membrane called the "*hypezokos*". That is to say, a word which had originally referred to *an experience of the patient* — pleuritis, pain in the side — is now being used to designate *a change in an anatomical structure*; and significantly, that structure is the starting-point of Aretaeus's entire description of pleuritis.

Second, the pain-in-the-side has strangely receded from view: Aretaeus assumes that pleuritis is an affection of the *side* (as becomes clear when he remarks that lying on the inflamed side is easier), and furthermore that it involves *pain*, yet he does not mention the pain-in-the-side itself. And the reason is that he has absorbed this, the experience of the patient, within the category "inflammation" [*phlegmone*]. Hence the fact that Aretaeus implicitly refers to that inflammation as a "symptom":[116] although this denomination is strictly illogical — for such inflammation of an interior structure is a medical inference rather than a presenting symptom — it is in fact entirely consonant with Aretaeus's redefinition of pleuritis. The patient's experience (pain) has been transformed into a process (inflammation), and has been remapped from a part of the experienced body (the side) onto an internal structure (the membrane called *hypezokos*); as we shall see in a moment, it has thereby changed its status, becoming the cause of the illness; and yet, for all this, it also retains traces of its original nature, namely the fact that it is a pain, and is thus a symptom.

Third, precisely because the pain-in-the-side has ceased to be definitive, "pleuritis" no longer embraces several different diseases, or a family of diseases; rather, it is a single condition. In this new conception it would be inconceivable to speak, as some of the Hippocratic texts had done, of "another pleuritis" (*Diseases II*), or of "some pleuritises" (*Diseases III*), each with different clusters of symptoms.

Fourth, as the corollary of this shift, the core symptomatic content has expanded: pleuritis is now characterized not by a single symptom (pain in the side) with which other and variable symptoms are loosely associated, but on the contrary by a precise constellation of symptoms. As we have seen already, this has involved the introduction of new and hitherto unsuspected symptoms: the piercing quality of the pain, the difficulty in lying on the unaffected side.

Finally, it is not the mere *concatenation* of these symptoms which establishes that unity which is "called pleuritis"; on the contrary, Aretaeus insists that this unity derives from the (supposed) *common causation* of those symptoms. And this completes the conceptual circle within which the new concept is inscribed; for of course the cause is neither more nor less than the defining anatomical event, namely the inflammation of the *hypezokos*.

In short, the entire conception of disease has been radically redefined. The installation of the new, anatomical element, and above all its privileging as the site of definition — these have necessitated a rearrangement of the old, symptomatic elements; or to use a different metaphor, what seem to be the same "moves" (the identification of certain symptoms) are in fact being played within a new and different "game".[117] Indeed, it is perhaps only now that the word "symptom" is appropriate, or that it gains the sense which we today confer upon it: that is, as something which reveals the disease, yet which is not that disease, and which thus in fact reveals the disease only obliquely.[118] It would seem that the new "game" involves a decisive shift of power from the patient to the doctor; for pain-in-the-side was an experience of the patient, whereas "inflammation of the *hypezokos*" is not something which the patient could conceivably experience or describe. Yet the patient's experience has by no means been swept aside; indeed, quite the contrary. For the anatomically-oriented writers have observed pleuritic symptoms which were precisely within the realm of the patient's experience, yet which the Hippocratics had ignored: the stabbing quality of the pain, the difficulty in lying on the unaffected side.

In view of this sharp disparity between Hippocratic "pleuritis" and the "pleuritis" of late Antiquity, we may well wonder what Galen had to say about "pleuritis"; for Galen adhered to the anatomical definition of that disease, yet he was concerned throughout his writings to portray his own medicine as *continuous* with the medicine of Hippocrates, repeatedly eliding the awkward problem that the Hippocratic texts were largely silent on matters anatomical.[119] Thus pleuritis was one of many themes which required Galen somehow to efface the differences between Hippocratic medicine and "dogmatic" (that is, anatomical) medicine. How did he tackle this task in the particular case of pleuritis? Within Galen's various commentaries upon Hippocrates, there were two particular points at which pleuritis was discussed: with respect to the *Aphorisms* and *Regimen in acute diseases*. In each case I give first the pertinent Hippocratic passage and then Galen's commentary upon it as translated by Wesley Smith.

(1) *Aphorisms:*[120]

> *Hippocrates:* Pleuritis that does not clear up in fourteen days results in empyema.[121]

> *Galen:* In pleuritis, acute fever with laboured breathing and cough and stabbing pain in the side are the essential signs by which we recognize the disease. Extension of the pain to the hypochondria or the collarbone are accessory, as is the greater ease of lying on the affected side rather than the other.

At first glance Galen here appears to be as "Hippocratic" as one could wish, for his description of pleuritis has no explicit anatomical content: it is confined to the realm of symptoms. Yet in fact his account is far removed from that of the Hippocratic texts, in two related respects. In the first place, the actual symptoms he describes are not Hippocratic but "dogmatic", for they include the very symptoms which the dogmatists had added to pleuritis, namely *stabbing* pain and the "greater ease of lying on the affected side". Secondly, Galen conceives these symptoms as "signs by which we recognize the disease", dividing these moreover into "essential signs" and "accessory" indications; and this conceptual grid, with its semiotic language, had no precedent in the Hippocratic writings.[122] No doubt it is the anatomical conception of pleuritis, positing as it does that the disease is an internal and invisible process rather than a reported experience of the patient, which has required and called into being this semiotic conception. And although the crucial anatomical element is wanting here, it will be supplied in another of Galen's commentaries, as we are about to see. What we should notice at this point is that by presenting this compact description of pleuritis within the context of his commentary on the *Aphorisms*, Galen has managed to identify the "pleuritis" of the later dogmatics, whose constellation of symptoms he is echoing, with Hippocratic "pleuritis".

(2) *Regimen in Acute Diseases:*[123]

> *Hippocrates:* ... Moreover, suppose the pain in the side continues and does not yield to the fomentations, while the sputum is not brought up, but becomes viscid without coction; should gruel be administered in these conditions without first relieving the pain, either by loosening the bowels or by venesection, whichever of these courses is indicated, a fatal termination will quickly follow.

292

> *Galen:* Let us recall that Hippocrates wrote the discussion of pleuritis as an example, and that this was shown to occur through the inflammation of the membrane lining the ribs. If one give barley broth [i.e., gruel] at the height of the inflammation, he will harm the patient greatly.

Here Galen has elegantly stitched together Hippocratic medicine and anatomical medicine. By the end of his first sentence he has established rhetorically that the "pleuritis" or "pain in the side" of Hippocrates was identical with the "pleuritis" of which Erasistratus and others wrote, that is, with "inflammation of the membrane lining the ribs". Then, in the next sentence, he rephrases the advice of Hippocrates in appropriate anatomical language: where Hippocrates had written that gruel should not be given to patients in whom "*the pain in the side* continues", adding a humoral gloss ("the sputum is not brought up, but becomes viscid without coction"), Galen reiterates the same warning but locates the time of danger — the danger of giving gruel —at "the height of *the inflammation*". And thus does Galen establish a putative Hippocratic lineage for the anatomical conception of pleuritis.

These little pieces of commentary by no means exhaust what Galen had to say about pleuritis; on the contrary, he adverted to it in several other works.[124] Although it is beyond my present scope to review all of Galen's discussions of the disease, we must take note of the way he considered it in his writings on the pulse — for in these treatises Galen added a further diagnostic sign of pleuritis, one which he did not mention in his commentaries on Hippocrates. Specifically, Galen taught that pleuritis is characterized by a "hard" pulse, its hardness arising not from strength (for it is not in fact a strong pulse, even though it seems to be) but rather from the fact that it is fast and frequent (*celer ... et creber*).[125] It is not clear whether Galen discovered this himself or whether he had derived it from earlier authors; the "hard" pulse as a diagnostic sign of pleuritis seems to have been unknown to the earlier dogmatists[126] — even to Herophilus, the effective discoverer of the pulse and inventor of its diagnostic use[127] — but it may have been Archigenes rather than Galen who made this innovation.[128] At all events, the "hard" pulse was now added as yet a further characteristic of pleuritis. Amongst the implications of this was that pleuritis was readily distinguished from peripneumony; for the latter disease was associated with a very different kind of pulse, namely one which was "large", "slow" and "soft" (*magnus, languidus, mollis*).[129] Characteristically, Galen had a rationale for the pleuritic pulse: the reason that it was "notably hard" was that in pleuritis, "it is a nervous part which is affected".[130] Characteristically, too, he berated those "vulgar physicians" who were ignorant of the diagnostic use of the pulse,[131] while conveniently omitting to mention the fact that this "ignorance" was shared by Hippocrates himself.

Galen's persistent elision of the differences between Hippocratic medicine and dogmatic medicine serves as a fitting ending to the strange tale of pleuritis in Antiquity. To reiterate, pleuritis began as a pain in the side, defined by that symptom; subsequently it acquired an anatomical seat, and this necessitated not just a different suite of symptoms but also, and more fundamentally, a different

211

conception of the very nature of diseases and of symptoms; those who agreed in giving pleuritis an anatomical location nevertheless differed for several centuries as to whether it was seated in the lungs or in the *hypezokos* membrane; eventually it was placed in the membrane, though the reasons for this consensus remain obscure. And finally, in Galen's hands, pleuritis changed yet again, in at least two ways. It now acquired a new sign, the hard pulse; and the very shift from a symptomatic conception to an anatomical one was obliterated, for an imaginary continuity was set up between Hippocratic pleuritis and the anatomical conception of pleuritis.

2.2. EARLY-MODERN CONCEPTIONS OF PLEURITIS

2.2.1. *Vesalius*

It happened that pleuritis played a critical role in the life and work of Vesalius — for it was the treatment of pleuritis which was at issue in the book which marked his first significant break with the authority of Galen, namely his *Venesection letter* of 1539. The controversy over bleeding in pleuritis had begun a generation earlier, in 1514, when Pierre Brissot launched a typically Renaissance attack upon "Arab" bleeding practices in the name of Hippocratic and Galenic purity.[132] Vesalius's intervention of 1539 arose from his discovery as to the anatomy of the "azygos vein" (that is, the "unpaired vein") and its branches: specifically, Vesalius had found that this single vein, which branched off from the vena cava on the *right* side, supplied the ribs of *both* sides (apart from the top three ribs). From this anatomical arrangement, and from the theory of phlebotomy as interpreted by Vesalius, there followed — so Vesalius argued — a new and decisive solution to the problem of where to bleed in pleuritis. For whether the pain was on the right side or on the left, and whether "derivative" or "reversionary" bleeding was desired, the pleuritic patient should always be bled from the *right* arm, since this was adjacent to the origin of all the costal veins.[133] At least, this was where bleeding should be carried out if the patient's pain was located in the lower nine ribs — and such was indeed usually the case in pleuritis, as Vesalius went on to argue, once again using anatomical reasoning.[134] Thus Vesalius's novel practice of dissecting for himself and of seeing (as he thought) with his own eyes had yielded its first decisive fruit: it had resolved an important therapeutic problem which had troubled physicians for a generation.

But what was "pleuritis" itself? That is, what was the condition whose treatment was at issue here? *A priori*, we should surely expect to find that Vesalius defined "pleuritis" anatomically: not only in view of his vehement convictions as to the importance of anatomy in general, but also and more particularly because the entire rationale of his argument in the *Venesection letter* itself was anatomical. Yet we are in for a surprise, for in fact Vesalius deployed a *symptomatic* definition of pleuritis, and moreover he was at pains to argue *against* the anatomical definition of that illness:[135]

212

294

> It does not worry me that perhaps someone more contentious might contend that where I have included under pleuritis, pain in the loins or ilium I am using the expression "pleuritis" incorrectly. To him I shall reply that the name of this disease belongs to the category of those which are derived from the position of the primary lesion such as nephritis, peripneumonia, ophthalmia and *coxendix*. The name pleuritis will signify to me an affection of the whole side and not of the membrane lining the ribs alone, as many who ignorantly call that membrane the pleura believe.

Here Vesalius at first appears to class pleuritis amongst diseases which are anatomically-defined — for what counts is "the *position* of the primary *lesion*", and the analogues he cites are all seemingly anatomical: nephritis was doubtless located in the kidney (*nephron*), peripneumonia in the lungs, ophthalmia in the eyes, *coxendix* in the coccyx or its vicinity. Yet it immediately becomes apparent that the meaning of "position" and of "lesion" here is in fact not anatomical at all. For whatever we make of "nephritis" *et al.*, Vesalius is locating pleuritis not in any particular organ or structure but on the contrary in the "side" of the patient, and in "the whole side" at that — that is, at a site defined in terms available to the patient, and localized only diffusely. And Vesalius goes on to contradict the alternative view, inherited as we have seen from the ancients, that pleuritis was an affection "of the membrane lining the ribs alone".[136] With respect to pleuritis, then, Vesalius has in effect gone back not, as we might expect, to Erasistratus or to Herophilus (who became his models for anatomy once he had broken with Galen),[137] but instead to Hippocrates,[138] that is, to a pre-anatomical conception; and accordingly his preferred terms for pleuritis were *dolor lateralis* (pain in the side)[139] and *morbus lateralis* (disease of the side).[140] Finally, as the finishing touch to his rigorously symptomatic definition of pleuritis, Vesalius specifically contests the use of the word "pleura" for the membrane-lining-the-ribs. That is, it would seem that Vesalius, precisely because he defined "pleuritis" as pain-in-the-side rather than an inflammation of the membrane in question, wanted to restore or reserve the term "pleura" as a name for the side of the body, rather than as a term for that membrane. (And he further asserted that "pleuron" as a term for a "primary position" did not mean "rib"; rather, he suggested that the Greeks had called the ribs *pleurai* merely "because they form the side",[141] which meant that "the side" was the true and original meaning of the Greek πλευρον.)

Now this terminological issue has taught us something more: that by the time of Vesalius, the membrane lining the ribs has acquired a new name. In the ancient world, that membrane had been called the "*hypezocota*" (or in Latin, the *membrana costas succingens*); but at some point since that time — we do not know when — it has come to be called, by some, the "*pleura*". Further, Vesalius indicates that those who have thus re-named that membrane are just those who interpret the disease "pleuritis" as an affection of that same membrane. As we have seen, the act of locating pleuritis within the "*membrana hypezocota*" was the work of a vast ancient tradition, from Erasistratus in the third century B.C. to Aretaeus and Galen four or five hundred years later; but the renaming of that membrane as the *"pleura"* has apparently happened since Galen's time. (I have not established who it was that proposed or adopted this new term; in view of Vesalius's hostility to it, we may presume that the "ignorant" re-namers of the membrane are men who do not know their Galen and do not dissect for themselves, but this leaves many possible candidates.[142]) Of course all acts of anatomical naming, throughout anatomy's complex and troubled history, are highly significant: to a large extent anatomical discovery amounted to anatomical nomenclature, for anatomy was inherently concerned with a domain of experience which went beyond the bounds of ordinary language.[143] But there is something very special about this particular re-naming: in this instance, the name of the *part* has apparently been influenced by the name of the associated *illness*. For the term which had originally referred to the patient's side or rib, namely *"pleura"* (Greek πλευρον) has so to speak migrated inwards, into the *"hypezocota"* — and this is the very path which had previously been traced by "pleuritis" itself. That is to say, the name *"pleura"* for that membrane is a piece of anatomical nomenclature which has followed in the footsteps of pathology.

True to the argument of the *Venesection letter*, Vesalius's *Fabrica* of 1543 gave the membrane its ancient name, that is, in its Latin form, the *membrana costas succingens*.[144] However, this was one battle which Vesalius lost; for by 1605, when Caspar Bauhin's *Theatrum anatomicum* was published, the term "pleura" had become the standard name for the membrane.[145] Just how and why this occurred I have not established; at least two alternative hypotheses suggest themselves. First, it is possible that the anatomical conception of pleuritis somehow came to prevail in the course of the late sixteenth century, and that this shift carried with it the name of the membrane: in other words, that Vesalius was defeated on both fronts. But second, there was in the late sixteenth century another and different development, which might also have led to the term *pleura*'s being preferred as a designation for that membrane. Specifically, by Bauhin's time that membrane had acquired another layer, a layer which invested the lungs (just as the peritoneum had long been seen as investing the abdominal organs);[146] and it is conceivable that this doubling of the membrane made the term *"succingens"* (undergirding) seem inappropriate. Whatever the reason, the anatomical aspects of the matter seem to have become consensual by the seventeenth century; for the double character of the membrane, and its naming as "the pleura", have been routinely accepted ever since. But what of pleuritis? As we shall see, consensus was to prove much more elusive in pathology than in anatomy.

2.2.2. *Baglivi*

Vesalius surprised us by defining pleuritis symptomatically when we expected him to define it anatomically; a century and a half later Giorgio Baglivi, in his *De praxi medica* (*On the practice of medicine*) of 1699, will spring upon us a complementary surprise. As it happened, pleuritis — in the English translation of 1723, "pleurisy" — was the very first disease which Baglivi used to illustrate what he called the "aphoristical way" of describing diseases.[147] Thus in order to appreciate what Baglivi had to say about pleurisy, we need to take note of this "aphoristical way" and of its place in Baglivi's larger argument. *De praxi medica* was just as much a Renaissance project as Vesalius's earlier anatomical investigations had been,[148] for Baglivi's central argument was that although the moderns had now excelled the ancients in medical *theory*, chiefly thanks to "experimental philosophy" and to the use of "geometrico-mechanical principles",[149] the ancients — which meant Galen as well as Hippocrates — were far superior to the moderns in all aspects of medical *practice*.[150] And in line with this orientation, Baglivi presented his "aphoristical way" as a revival of the literary practices of Hippocrates.

Baglivi described the "aphoristical way" as consisting of "short sentences, tied up to no rules of method or scholastic subtlety, but clearly and openly delivered"[151] — this in contrast with what he called the "methodical way", which "consists in tying it [physic] up to methods, and in digesting and adorning it with abstracted and useless notions".[152] The point of the "aphoristical way" was that it was a "loose" form of description, which precisely because of its unsystematic character left "void spaces ... for the insertion of the new and ever multiplicable voices of Nature".[153] Baglivi associated the "aphoristical way" not only with Hippocrates but also with Bacon;[154] and he presented it as the appropriate mode of recording for what he called the *Medicina Prima* — a concept which was surely meant to echo Bacon's *"Philosophia Prima"*.[155] The *Medicina Prima*, Baglivi explained, was "a pure history of diseases, obtained by sole observation at the sick man's bedside, and related by the patients themselves".[156] Baglivi argued strenuously that this *Medicina Prima* — the very foundation of medicine — was "not to be met with in books", because "the descriptions of diseases" to be found in books "are for the most part taken not from observation and matter of fact, but from the Authors' Brains".[157] As Baglivi defined the *Medicina Prima*, in a passage which also introduced the accompanying *Medicina Secunda*, the "curative part":[158]

> The *Medicina Prima* is a particular science of a peculiar form, which does not owe its principles or improvements to other sciences, but ... depends upon a diligent and patient description of all such things as the learned observator has marked down concerning the invasion, progress and exit of diseases, and committed to writing, with the same simplicity and sincerity that he used in observing them, without adding any thing of his own, or of the doctrines of books or other sciences.... In effect, all that part called the *Medicina Prima*, which is the basis of the *Medicina Secunda* or curative part, ought to be treated of so as that it be derived from the true nature of things and not from the nature of our thoughts, as many have done....

Thus the *Medicina Prima* was to be developed by setting aside all theoretical conjectures and by constructing instead "a pure and exact History of Diseases, I mean such as shows from the very Nature of things and is described" — Baglivi reiterated — "by the patients themselves".[159] In short, the basis of the *Medicina*

Prima was empirical observations, of a kind which specifically and explicitly privileged *the experiences of the patient*; and the "aphoristic way" was the appropriate way of recording such observations.

Having extolled the virtues of the aphoristic method, Baglivi proceeded to illustrate it from his own experience. "Now the way of setting down the solid and reported observations of diseases in a short and aphoristical style", he remarked, "will sufficiently appear from the succeeding diseases, which were examined by patient and repeated observations made in the Italian Hospitals".[160] There followed brief accounts of some twelve or so diseases, of which "a pleurisy" was the first. From what has been said so far, we should surely expect that Baglivi defined pleurisy symptomatically (since "a pure history of diseases" is "related by the patients themselves"), and that he did so strictly on the basis of his own experiences (that is, his "patient and repeated observations made in the Italian Hospitals"). Yet in fact Baglivi's conception of pleurisy was straightforwardly anatomical — and his opening remarks followed Galen! Here is the first paragraph of Baglivi's account:[161]

Of a Pleurisy

If you would discover a pleurisy, place your chief care in observing the nature of the pulse. The hardness of the pulse is almost an infallible sign of all pleurisies; and while the pleurisies are sudden, or complicated with other diseases of the breast, if you observe a hardness in the pulse, i.e. too great a distension or vibration of the artery, tho' the other signs are absent, you may assure yourself that the patient is under a pleurisy; for a hard pulse is an inseparable companion of all inflammations upon the nerves or membranous parts.

Obviously enough, both the hard pulse and its rationale echoed Galen (albeit with a slight modulation, from "a nervous part" to "the nerves or membranous parts"[162]), and I shall attend to this seeming paradox in a moment. But what is just as important is the massive depth of taken-for-granted assumptions built into Baglivi's remarks. To begin with, Baglivi simply assumed that pleurisy is an inflammation, and that his readers would share that premise; indeed, so tacit was this knowledge that he did not even trouble to spell out what he doubtless had in mind, that pleurisy consisted specifically in an inflammation of the pleural membrane. (We may surely infer that this was Baglivi's meaning, for he classed pleurisy as one of the "diseases of the breast" — and significantly, this appeared merely in an aside, which is another indication of how much he was taking for granted.) Similarly, he made no attempt to describe pleurisy's characteristic suite of symptoms — "the other signs", as he put it — for these too were common knowledge. Instead Baglivi concentrated upon just one sign, namely the hardness of the pulse, which he was privileging on account of its diagnostic power; and so too it emerged in the next sentence that "the difficulty of breathing" was a typical symptom of pleurisy, but this was mentioned specifically because of its special prognostic significance. It seems, then, that Baglivi had no need to enumerate the full list of pleurisy's symptoms, for those symptoms were taken as implied by the very word "pleurisy". Sure enough, Baglivi's subsequent discussion,[163] which was devoted to prognostics[164] and to therapeutics,[165] mentioned several of those symptoms — fever, spitting, and (obliquely) pain-in-the-side — but always in passing, as things which were already well-known.[166] In short, just as Baglivi could take it as read that pleurisy consisted in inflammation of the pleural membrane, so also he could assume that his readers were familiar with its characteristic signs and symptoms.

Thus Baglivi's discussion of pleurisy exemplified several times over the utter impossibility of his own project of pure observation, of what he called "diligent and patient description", uncontaminated by "the nature of our thoughts".[167] In the first place Baglivi, like any observer, was of course necessarily observing through inherited *categories*, categories which were so ingrained that he did not realize that they *were* categories: in this instance, the category "pleurisy". Secondly, that particular category as Baglivi deployed it embodied the conviction that pleurisy consists in an inflammation of what had now come to be called the pleural membrane — a conviction which by its very nature derived not from "sole observation at the sick man's bedside", but on the contrary from "our thoughts". It was of course this very conception of pleurisy, inherited from the later ancients, which Vesalius had contested in his *Venesection letter*. Evidently Vesalius's attempt to restore the symptomatic conception of pleuritis had failed, at least in Baglivi's particular setting; for the anatomical conception had somehow — we do not know how — attained the status of a convention. Indeed, so conventional had it become that Baglivi deployed it *malgré lui*: in the very attempt to illustrate his argument that medicine should be based on "a pure history of diseases, obtained by sole observation at the sick man's bedside, and related by the patients themselves", he actually defined pleurisy in anatomical terms.

Thirdly, precisely the same was true of the *diagnostic* claim which Baglivi was putting forward — that "the hardness of the pulse is almost an infallible sign of all pleurisies". For Baglivi justified this aphorism not by practical experience (either his own or that of others), but instead by appealing to underlying mechanisms: "a hard pulse is an inseparable companion of all inflammations upon the nerves or membranous parts."

Last but not least, this rationale was itself derived from Galen, yet Baglivi was seemingly unaware of the fact. He could have acknowledged Galen as his source, and indeed this would have been grist to his mill: for *De praxi medica* bracketed Galen with Hippocrates as laudable ancients, accurate observers, and Baglivi was also at pains to detach the virtues of Galen himself from the vices of the "Galen*ists*".[168] Yet as a matter of fact he did not mention Galen here; and the simplest explanation for this apparent oversight is that Baglivi had so internalized this particular Galenic message — perhaps derived from his teachers, rather than directly from Galen himself — that he really believed that it was his own observation. On this reading, it would seem that when Baglivi *felt* a hard pulse, he also and in the same moment *felt* an "inflammation upon the nerves or membranous parts", and specifically an inflammation of the pleural membrane. In other words, Baglivi had this particular doctrine of Galen's literally in his fingertips.

To sum up so far: In respect of pleurisy the medical men of the Renaissance inherited from the ancients two distinct conceptions, the one symptomatic (in the Hippocratic texts), the other anatomical (conveyed to them especially in Galen's works). These two approaches were surely in tension with one another, and this is indeed what we have found; yet that tension expressed itself in very surprising ways. In the case of Vesalius, we would expect to find the anatomical conception at work; yet in fact Vesalius defined pleuritis in symptomatic terms, that is, as pain-in-the-side, and explicitly argued against the anatomical interpretation of the disease. And in the case of Baglivi, we would expect to encounter a deliberate application of the symptomatic definition; yet Baglivi actually defined pleurisy anatomically, and moreover he did so quite unwittingly. In short, the relation between symptomatic and anatomical conceptions was remarkably subtle and complex — and this for just a "single" disease.

Nevertheless there seems to be a certain logic to the story of "pleuritis": for to judge by all that Baglivi was taking for granted, it would appear that Vesalius had been defeated over the definition of pleuritis just as he was over the naming of the membrane. That is to say, it seems that the anatomical conception of pleuritis — in its "Erasistratean" form, with the Galenic addition of the hard pulse — had prevailed in the course of the Renaissance just as it had in later Antiquity. Once again, however, we are in for a surprise, as we shall see by turning from Baglivi to Morgagni.

2.2.3. *Morgagni*

Giambattista Morgagni's *De sedibus* of 1761 was perhaps the most important work, and certainly one of the most original and profound works, in the whole Western medical tradition.[169] What characterized that great book was not only the painstaking correlation of symptoms with post-mortem findings, for, in addition, *De sedibus* was a vast meditation upon the entire corpus of Western medical writings, from Hippocrates to Morgagni's own day. Further, Morgagni's historical sense was far more subtle and sophisticated than that of, say, Baglivi (with his naïve assertion that "Hippocrates speaks in the words of Nature, rather than those of man")[170] or Boerhaave (with his Galen-like claim that Hippocrates was an anatomist).[171] Indeed, Morgagni dissected texts just as skilfully as he anatomized dead bodies and interpreted symptoms; that is, he was a master of analytical exegesis in three distinct domains: symptomatic, anatomical and textual. And the signal achievement of *De sedibus* was that it *united* these three layers or dimensions: that is, Morgagni systematically correlated (i) symptomatology with (ii) anatomy, meanwhile interweaving (iii) previous discussions of the disease in question. Consequently, *De sedibus* was a treasury not just of new observations but also of commentary upon old ones, stretching throughout Western medicine's history. Yet the vast riches of the book remain largely untapped by medical historians, at least those writing

300

in English.[172] In part this neglect reflects the inherent difficulty of the text, for Morgagni's prose is at first sight rebarbative and forbidding. At the same time, that neglect can be taken as a "symptom" (to use the obvious metaphor) of the very point which I am trying to argue: that medical history has strangely overlooked the history of medicine proper. Certainly there is a vast and troubling disparity between the recognized importance of *De sedibus* and the amount of attention that the book has received in English.[173]

But let us turn to Morgagni's discussion of pleurisy, which appeared — along with peripneumony — in Letters 20 and 21 of *De sedibus*.[174] (Letter 20 was concerned with the cases, dissections and observations of Morgagni's erstwhile teacher Antonio Maria Valsalva; Letter 21 with those of Morgagni himself.) It will be helpful to begin by comparing Morgagni's working definition of pleurisy with that of Baglivi, which we have just been examining. On the one hand, Morgagni differed radically from Baglivi in that he conceived pleurisy in rigorously *symptomatic* terms. On the other hand, Morgagni curiously echoed Baglivi in that he too *took for granted* the defining symptoms of pleurisy: that is to say, he never listed those symptoms in a formal way, but instead let them emerge piecemeal in the course of his case-histories and discussions. Thus the implied premise of his account was that there existed a consensus as to pleurisy's characteristic symptoms. We shall see in a moment what those allegedly-consensual symptoms were; first it is important to notice why Morgagni defined pleurisy symptomatically.

The point of Morgagni's symptomatic definition of pleurisy was this: that the very theme which Baglivi had *assumed* (at least, in the particular case of pleurisy), namely the anatomical seat of the disease, was what Morgagni wanted to *investigate*. In this respect Morgagni's approach to pleurisy was identical to his approach to diseases in general: he always defined diseases symptomatically and then tied them to anatomical seats as indicated by dissection — accomplishing this link by means of an intricate logical operation which rested on the comparison of different individual case-histories.[175] Hence the fact that Letters 20 and 21 of *De sedibus* were described as "the discourse of pain in the breast, sides, and back", that is, as being concerned with *experiences of the patient*. And this gives us a good indication of the nature of Morgagni's enterprise in general, and of his approach to pleurisy in particular. We have seen that pleurisy had been tied in Antiquity to the "*membrana hypezocota*", that is, to the membrane which later came to be called the "*pleura*", and that Baglivi had uncritically echoed this conception. But Morgagni, while being highly favourably disposed to anatomical localization, wanted to *reopen* the whole question as to the site of that localization. And for this purpose it was essential to begin with a strictly symptomatic definition, for only in that way could anatomical localization be investigated *de novo* as Morgagni was seeking to do.

The central symptoms-of-pleurisy which Morgagni was assuming, as best I can reconstruct them, were as follows (in purely arbitrary order): (1) a "pungent" pain in the side, (2) a fever, (3) a hard pulse, and (4) difficulty in lying on the unaffected side. In fact the last symptom on this list was attended with certain complexities; for some patients, paradoxically, experienced difficulty in lying not on the unaffected side but, on the contrary, "on the pained side". This anomaly occasioned a typically subtle and fruitful Morgagnian digression;[176] but for present purposes we can ignore it, since Morgagni acknowledged that the difficulty was indeed usually in lying on the unaffected side, just as the ancient dogmatics had claimed.[177] Now this occasional qualification aside, Morgagni's cluster of pleuritic symptoms was entirely conventional. Or to be more precise, Morgagni was here echoing those before him — from the later ancients to Baglivi — who had seated the disease in the "*membrana hypezocota*" / the "*pleura*"; for these were the very symptoms which had been identified by that anatomical tradition. Thus Morgagni's implicit definition of pleurisy overlapped with both Vesalius's conception and Baglivi's conception, while differing from them both. Like Vesalius, Morgagni defined pleurisy symptomatically — but Vesalius's symptomatic conception had been Hippocratic (pleuritis is pain-in-the-side), whereas Morgagni's conception followed that of the dogmatic tradition (pleuritis is a constellation of symptoms, of which pain-in-the-side is only one, and that pain is specifically "pungent" in character). And like Baglivi, Morgagni drew his suite of pleuritic symptoms from the dogmatic tradition, including the "hard pulse" which Galen had added — but Baglivi had defined pleuritis anatomically, whereas Morgagni defined it by its symptoms.

In short, Morgagni *accepted* that definition of pleurisy's symptoms which had been constructed by the ancient "dogmatic" tradition stemming from Erasistratus and culminating in Galen; but he *put in suspense* the anatomical localization which had been decreed by that same tradition, precisely because his purpose was to *reconsider* the site of pleurisy's localization. And in effect — to oversimplify brutally what was an immensely complex and subtle discussion — Morgagni took up again the very argument which had raged between Erasistratus *et al.* and Herophilus *et al.*, that is, the question as to whether pleurisy is seated in the membrane lining the ribs (which had now, of course, become a double membrane named the *pleura*[178]) or in the lungs. To this end he carefully compared the symptoms and post-mortem findings of pleurisy (traditionally seated in the membrane) with those associated with peripneumony (traditionally seated in the lungs). And he came up with the answer that pleurisy and peripneumony were not distinct diseases at all; rather, they were two aspects of a single disease, which Morgagni called *pleuripneumony*. Yet he did not present this conception as his own invention; rather, he ascribed it to his Paduan predecessor of the early seventeenth century, Vincent Baronius.[179] In short, the effect of Morgagni's argument is that the very category of pleurisy is a mistake, and that this has been known — albeit forgotten — for over a century! Notice Morgagni's rhetorical tactics: he could, of course, have begun with Baronius, but instead he chose to end with him. What he actually began with was the symptomatic content of the standard definition of pleurisy; and the point of this vast opening concession was that it rendered all the more forceful his eventual demolition of that definition.

302

In Morgagni's hands, then, pleurisy has literally disappeared: it is no longer a distinct disease at all. Rather, it is a mistaken interpretation of certain symptoms, symptoms which commonly (but not always) go together, and which are sometimes (but by no means always) associated with inflammation of the pleural membrane. So too peripneumony as conventionally conceived has to be re-thought, for the distinction between pleurisy and peripneumony is invalid. The real disease, pleuripneumony, is an inflammation of the lungs which is associated with various and irregular complications, such as the exudation of fluid, adhesion of the pleural membranes, and — as just one such complication amongst many others — inflammation of those membranes. Depending on the precise course of the disease in the particular patient, different patterns of symptoms are observed; but those patterns called "pleurisy" and "peripneumony" are merely arbitrary, for the supposed differences between them are often contradicted in particular cases. And danger to the patient arises not from the involvement of the pleura but solely from the inflammation of the lungs. Furthermore, these seemingly heretical doctrines are in fact consistent with all that has been learnt about pleuritis and peripneumony, both in Antiquity and since — as Morgagni shows through a careful contemplation of the medical writings of the ancients and moderns alike.[180]

Incidentally we should notice that by introducing us to Baronius, Morgagni has also muddied the waters of the previous stage of our story. We saw earlier that between the lifetimes of Vesalius and Baglivi, the meaning of "pleuritis" apparently stabilized much as it had done in later Antiquity: that is, it became an inflammation of the "pleura", the two-layered descendant of the *membrana hypezocota*. But now that we have come across Baronius, it is clear that the history of "pleuritis" between about 1550 and 1700 involved further complexities. Was Baronius responding to a previous debate? By what methods did he arrive at his concept of "pleuripneumony"? Was his work simply forgotten, was it debated and explicitly rejected, or was it in fact received more positively than Baglivi and Morgagni have led us to assume?[181] Such questions give concrete form to what we already know on grounds of principle: that an adequate history of "pleurisy" would require us to investigate a host of intermediate figures between Vesalius and Baglivi (not least Baronius), and for that matter, between Baglivi and Morgagni (for instance, Boerhaave).[182]

So too we could, of course, pursue the history of pleurisy after Morgagni. And if we were to take up the later history of pleurisy, we would find that Morgagni's discussion was by no means decisive; for in fact both pleurisy and peripneumony survived his putative dissolution of the distinction between them. Subsequently, in the hands of Laennec, pleurisy changed yet again, seemingly remaining within the pleural membrane yet with several novel twists. As the inventor of the stethoscope, Laennec found for pleurisy a distinctive auscultative sign, namely "egophony", a bleating sound as of a goat;[183] he therefore accorded special importance to the physical state which he took that sound to reflect, namely an effusion of fluid in the thoracic cavity;[184] further, pleurisy's other signs and symptoms were rather different from those which Morgagni had deployed;[185] and last but not least, Laennec distinguished between "pleuritis" and "pleurisy", for *pleuritis* was inflammation of the pleural membrane, whereas *pleurisy* was the larger disease-condition which such inflammation produced.[186] Nor did pleurisy in this new form achieve stability; for as we learn from Russell Maulitz's study of pleurisy in the Paris *clinique* of the 1830s,[187] Laennec's immediate successors such as Auguste François Chomel redefined pleurisy/pleuritis yet again.[188] Although they still regarded inflammation of the pleural membrane as definitive, it seems that they placed particular diagnostic emphasis upon the pleuritic pain;[189] they certainly loosened the tie between that pain and the pleural effusion,[190] thereby diminishing the pathognomonic significance of Laennec's egophony;[191] and they linked pleurisy with phthisis (tuberculous consumption),[192] whereas Laennec had made a point of separating pleurisy from phthisis.[193] (Notice too that this link between diseases of the pleural membrane and of the lungs was quite different from that which Morgagni had sought to establish — for Morgagni had connected pleurisy with peripneumony, not with phthisis,[194] and there is no indication that Chomel and his colleagues were seeking to dissolve pleurisy as Morgagni had done.) And meanwhile the clinicians of the 1830s were applying to pleurisy, as to other diseases, the new statistical methods introduced by Pierre Louis,[195] thereby adding a novel analytic dimension which Laennec had barely envisaged,[196] and which was of course quite alien to Morgagni's focus upon individual case-histories.[197]

Thus throughout the three centuries from the Renaissance to the Paris "clinic", the history of pleurisy reveals a repeated *refusal of closure*. Vesalius sought to restore a symptomatic definition of the disease, but he apparently failed in this just as he did in his attempt to preserve the Hippocratic meaning of "pleura"/"pleuron"; Baglivi took it for granted that pleurisy was an inflammation of the pleural membrane (now membranes, plural), but Morgagni demolished this conception and dissolved the very being of pleurisy; Morgagni's account, for all its rigour, did not persuade his successors; Laennec tied pleurisy to the "egophony" revealed by his stethoscope, but this bond was immediately weakened. Indeed, it is doubtful whether pleurisy ever stabilized; but that is a question for another study, as is the associated and equally intriguing issue as to the meaning, or meanings, of pleurisy today. What is clear is that in the first two thousand years and more of pleurisy's history, any such stability of its meaning was always temporary and contingent.

3. CONCLUSION

What larger implications might follow from this all-too-incomplete survey of pleurisy's history? I suggest that eight points stand out.

First, my findings underline once more what was demonstrated long ago by Temkin (for all the limitations of his conception), by Canguilhem and above all by Fleck, and has been confirmed by various investigations in the last twenty years or so: namely that concepts-of-disease comprise an eligible domain for historical investigation in their own right. That domain is distinct from — though by no means

304

independent of — such more familiar history-of-medicine themes as the history of anatomy and of theories of normal bodily function. More particularly, it is quite different from the exercise of retrospective diagnosis; for retrospective diagnosis suppresses precisely what the history of disease-concepts brings to the fore, namely the *content* of *past* descriptive and diagnostic categories.

Second, this particular historiographic theme is not only possible but is also uniquely appropriate: it is in the literal sense *proper* to the history of medicine, since the business of medicine was-and-is to do with human illnesses. Indeed, the history of concepts-of-disease takes us to the very heart of medicine's history: for of course it was those very concepts that determined what medical practitioners saw, and which thus defined what medicine actually *was*. In short, the history of disease-concepts is just that segment of the history of ideas which is medical history's distinctive and special concern.

Third, to judge by the example of pleurisy, the history of disease-concepts is rich with possibilities and has many unexpected twists and turns. When I embarked on this investigation, in blissful ignorance of Wesley Smith's pioneering study published over ten years earlier, I had expected to find a simple transformation of pleurisy from symptomatic to anatomical, and I was vaguely locating that putative transformation in the eighteenth century, or perhaps in the early nineteenth century, with the work of Bichat. In only one respect did those expectations prove correct: for while there was indeed a shift from a symptomatic conception to an anatomical one, it had taken place (as I learnt from Professor Smith's essay) over two thousand years earlier than I had thought, it was by no means simple, and it did not produce the closure that I was assuming. And my subsequent explorations have yielded further surprises at every point — for instance ramifying from pathology into anatomical discovery-and-nomenclature, and repeatedly raising the problem as to how medical consensus was established, if indeed such consensus was established at all.

Fourth, as has just emerged, this subject is by no means bounded by the history-of-ideas conception to which I have restricted myself here. On the contrary, both shifts and stability in the concept of pleurisy, or of any other disease, raise explanatory questions which could be addressed only by a widening of focus, a shift of attention outwards from the concepts themselves to the many other matters which might have influenced them — for instance, practices of healing and of pedagogy, corporate relationships, patronage networks, religious and philosophical allegiances. Indeed, one of the attractions of a history of disease-concepts is that it can provoke us to connect the cognitive and the social dimensions of medicine's history[198] — precisely in line with Fleck's conception of knowledge.

Fifth, and relatedly, the history of disease-concepts brings into play the perspectives of both patients and doctors, and what is more, it necessarily *combines* those perspectives. It is now, of course, well-recognized that medical history embraces the viewpoint of the patient as well as that of the practitioner.[199] And concepts-of-disease as an historiographic theme hold out the promise of enriching this insight, for one might well say that those concepts were and are the very ground upon which those two viewpoints come to meet and merge.[200] This is well attested by what we have seen of pleurisy's history, for while the various definitions of the disease all emanated from medical practitioners, those definitions always bore some imprint of the patient's experience, even if (as with Baglivi's conception) only in attenuated form. To recapitulate, "pleuritis" began as neither more nor less than an experience of the patient; its symptomatic content was actually *enlarged* — remarkably enough — by the adoption of an anatomical definition; and even in the Paris clinic of the 1830s, the supreme site of the anatomical conception of illness, the patient's experience in the form of pain-in-the-side retained a crucial diagnostic significance. In short, just as the sufferings of patients are the very occasion for medicine, so the history of disease-concepts entails attention to those sufferings and to the dialectic between the patient's experience and the practitioner's categories.

Sixth, the case of pleurisy has put in a very different light the picture developed in Foucault's *Birth of the clinic*. We saw at the outset that Foucault's programme was putatively constructed along strictly syntactic lines, and that this approach, were it actually possible to implement it, would foreclose the very possibility of writing a history of disease concepts; and now that we have glimpsed how complex was the development of the concept of "pleurisy", it has become only too apparent what a wealth of possibilities Foucault thereby excluded. But this is by no means all, for pleurisy's history radically qualifies the substantive story of *Birth of the clinic*. For one thing, pleurisy shows that the kind of anatomical localization pursued by Bichat — the siting of diseases not in the organs but in the "membranes" or "tissues" — had a model which began in Antiquity. For another, the shift in Antiquity from a symptomatic definition of pleurisy to an anatomical conception was associated with a transformation of medical categories just as radical as the "mutation in discourse" associated with *la clinique* itself. And finally, the relation between a medicine of symptoms and a medicine based on anatomy was far more complex than Foucault supposed: for rather than the one giving way to the other, whether in the years around 1800 or at any earlier point, the two were *in productive tension* for almost the entire history of Western medicine, that is to say, from the time of Herophilus and Erasistratus onwards. Nor was that tension abolished by *la clinique* — for as Jacalyn Duffin has recently shown, Laennec himself was deeply aware of the limitations of the very anatomico-clinical conception which he did so much to consummate,[201] and we have seen that the relation between symptoms, signs and anatomy continued to trouble his successors of the 1830s.

Seventh, the history of concepts-of-disease is a field of vast scope. To begin with, we have at our disposal literally hundreds of diseases whose history could be traced; but this, which we might call "special pathology history" (the history of concepts of particular diseases), is only part of the subject. For there also beckons the possibility of "general pathology history", that is, the history of pathological theory at large; and the latter theme, which was the very concern of Canguilhem's

306

The normal and the pathological, is every bit as important as "special pathology history". As just one illustration of the many opportunities that present themselves in "general pathology history", we may take the case of eighteenth-century *nosology*. Although Foucault rightly drew attention to nosology in *Birth of the clinic*, and although it has attracted a handful of studies since that work appeared, we still remain almost wholly in the dark as to the origins of nosology (just *why* did Sauvages invent it?);[202] about its relations with traditional "pathology" (how exactly did nosology differ from pathology?);[203] about the sites of its success and failure (which medical schools used nosologies in their teaching, and which did not?);[204] about its mutations and inflections in the course of the eighteenth century (how and why did Pinel's "nosographic" categories differ from the "nosological" categories of Sauvages or of Cullen?); and last but not least, about its historical impact (was nosology, as Foucault argued, the essential preliminary to *la clinique*, or was it, as Porter has suggested, of little or no long-term significance?).[205]

Finally, the history of disease-concepts is a theme which should lend itself to *comparative* investigation. For instance, to stay for convenience with the example of pleurisy, we might ask: is there any analogue of pleurisy in Chinese medicine or in Ayurvedic medicine?[206] Have Ayurvedic practitioners and Chinese practitioners encountered "pain in the side" at all, and if so, how have they described it, interpreted it and treated it? It is of course beginning to be recognized that "history of medicine" can no longer be narrowly equated with the history of Western medicine alone; but historians of medicine have not found it easy to bring different medical traditions within a common focus, because the cognitive structures of those traditions are so very different. But concepts of disease, with their necessary focus upon patients' experiences, hold out the promise of establishing points of intersection between different diagnostic categories, which should shed light upon the larger conceptual styles which characterize each of the three great medical systems. And it may be ventured that such a comparative perspective will make still clearer the historically-constructed character of disease-concepts in the Western tradition itself.

ACKNOWLEDGEMENTS

I thank my colleagues in the HPS Division of the School of Philosophy at Leeds for the chance to present this paper at an informal seminar, and for their very helpful comments on that occasion. For advice, support and particular information I am grateful to Otávio Bueno, Seán Burke, Mark Jenner, Russ Maulitz, George Macdonald Ross, Margaret Pelling, Migaela Scorah, Steve Sturdy and Roger White. Special thanks go to Wesley D. Smith, for substantial help on issues relating to ancient conceptions of pleuritis; to Graeme Gooday and Jon Hodge, both of whom have greatly clarified the argument of the paper; to three anonymous referees for *History of science*, whose valuable criticisms have led to significant revisions; and above all to Jackie Duffin, for support, for detailed advice and for her penetrating comments on earlier drafts. All remaining errors are my own responsibility.

225

REFERENCES

1. L. Fleck, *Entstehung und Entwicklung einer wissenschaftlichen Tatsache: Einführung in die Lehre vom Denkstil und Denkkollektiv* (Basel, 1935); *Genesis and development of a scientific fact* (transl. by F. Bradley and T. J. Trenn, ed. by T. J. Trenn and R. K. Merton, Chicago, 1979).

2. O. Temkin, *The Falling Sickness: A history of epilepsy from the Greeks to the beginnings of modern neurology* (Baltimore, 1945). On the limits of Temkin's vision see below, at ref. 40.

3. G. Canguilhem, *Le normal et le pathologique* (Paris, 1966); *The normal and the pathological* (transl. by C. R. Fawcett and R. S. Cohen, Dordrecht, 1978; New York, 1991). On the enduring relevance of Canguilhem's work see M. Nicolson, "The social and the cognitive: Resources for the sociology of scientific knowledge", *Studies in history and philosophy of science*, xx (1991), 347–69.

4. K. Figlio, "Chlorosis and chronic disease in nineteenth-century Britain: The social construction of somatic illness in a capitalist society", *Social history*, iii (1978), 167–97 (*cf.* below, at ref. 53); P. Wright and A. Treacher (eds), *The problem of medical knowledge: Examining the social construction of medicine* (Edinburgh, 1982).

5. For instance M. Pelling, *Cholera, fever and English medicine 1825–1865* (Oxford, 1978); S. Jarcho, *The concept of heart failure: From Avicenna to Albertini* (Cambridge, Mass., 1980); W. F. Bynum and V. Nutton (eds), *Theories of fever from Antiquity to the Enlightenment* (*Medical history* Supplement no. 1, London, 1981); R. C. Maulitz, *Morbid appearances: The anatomy of pathology in the early nineteenth century* (Cambridge, 1987); W. D. Smith, "Pleuritis in the Hippocratic Corpus and after", *Proceedings of the Sixth International Hippocratic Colloquium, Quebec, September 1987* (Quebec City, 1989); M. Nicolson and C. McLaughlin, "Social constructionism and medical sociology: A study of the vascular theories of multiple sclerosis", *Sociology of health and illness*, x (1988), 234–61.

6. For a helpful conspectus and a guide to recent literature see W. F. Bynum and R. Porter (eds), *Companion encyclopedia of the history of medicine* (2 vols, London, 1993), Part III (vol. i), particularly the essays by M. Pelling, L. G. Wilson, R. C. Olby, T. M. Brown, M. Worboys, D. Cantor and R. Porter (chaps. 16, 19–21, 24–25, 27). (The *Companion encyclopedia*, it should be remarked, is exceptional amongst recent textbooks in the attention it devotes to this theme.) See also R. C. Maulitz, "In the clinic: Framing disease at the Paris hospital", *Annals of science*, xlvii (1990), 127–37; essays of C. Lawrence and S. Peitzman, cited in refs 15, 18 below; and J. Duffin, *To see with a better eye: A life of R. T. H. Laennec* (Princeton, N.J., 1998).

7. On what "chlorosis" meant in relation to twentieth-century categories see I. Loudon, "The diseases called chlorosis", *Psychological medicine*, xliv (1984), 27–36.

8. See for instance S. L. Gilman *et al.*, *Hysteria beyond Freud* (Berkeley, 1993).

9. Fleck, *Genesis and development of a scientific fact* (ref. 1), 1–19.

10. The corollary was that in Fleck's view, "*Spirochaeta pallida* should ... be defined by syphilis rather than the other way around" (*ibid.*, 18).

11. *Ibid.*, 14, my emphasis.

12. "*The relation between the Wassermann reaction and syphilis — an undoubted fact*" entailed "*several adaptations and transformations of concepts*": *ibid.*, 97–98, Fleck's emphases. See also the extended discussion in note 5 (pp. 178–9) to p. 102.

13. *Ibid.*, 39.

14. J. Gabbay, "Asthma attacked? Tactics for the reconstruction of a disease concept", in Wright and Treacher (eds), *The problem of medical knowledge* (ref. 4), 23–48.

15. C. Lawrence, "'Definite and material': Coronary thrombosis and cardiologists in the 1920s", in C. Rosenberg and J. Golden (eds), *Framing disease: Studies in cultural history* (New

308

Brunswick, N.J., 1992), 50–82.

16. See the remarks of Paul White in 1931, quoted by Lawrence, "'Definite and material'", 67.

17. At least, so far as this has been traced — for the loose end left by Lawrence's study is the question as to how "consensus" over the ECG was reached (*ibid.*, 72).

18. S. J. Peitzman, "From Bright's disease to end-state renal disease", in Rosenberg and Golden (eds), *Framing disease* (ref. 15), 3–19.

19. *Ibid.*, 9, 11, 16.

20. The most notable exception is A. Cunningham, "Transforming plague: The laboratory and the identity of infectious disease", in A. Cunningham and P. Williams (eds), *The laboratory revolution in medicine* (Cambridge, 1992), 209–44.

21. C. Quétel, *Le Mal de Naples* (Paris, 1986); *History of syphilis* (transl. by J. Braddock and B. Pike, Cambridge, 1990). "Syphilis as a cultural phenomenon" is the title of the introduction (pp. 1–8).

22. *Ibid.*, 53, 67, 75, 81, 108.

23. This from the *Oxford English dictionary* — for characteristically, *Le Mal de Naples* does not mention the meaning of the term.

24. "Thus syphilis came to be recognised as syphilis, gonorrhoea as gonorrhoea" (Quétel, *Le Mal de Naples* (ref. 21), 111). *Cf.* and contrast Fleck, *Genesis and development of a scientific fact* (ref. 1), 7–8.

25. The point is touched upon just once and in passing: Quétel, *Le Mal de Naples* (ref. 21), 97.

26. Fleck, *Genesis and development of a scientific fact* (ref. 1), 41. See also, for instance, pp. 15–16 ("The discovery of the causative agent, *Spirochaeta pallida*, was the result of steady, logical work by civil servants"), 22, 69–70. For a general formulation see p. 123: "the true creator of a new idea is not the individual but the collective."

27. *Ibid.*, 98.

28. *Ibid.*, 99.

29. These mechanisms involved a spectrum of communication-media, from what Fleck called "journal science", through "vademecum science" and "textbook science", to "popular science": see *ibid.*, 111–25. At one extreme, "journal science", which is precisely the "vanguard" of science (p. 123), is "provisional, uncertain, and personally colored" (p. 119); at the opposite extreme, "popular science" entails "valuation" (p. 113), "simplicity" and "vividness" (p. 115). The key intermediate category was "vademecum science" (pp. 119–24), which represents the "collective, generally valid" aspect of research science (p. 120), and "requires a *critical synopsis in an organized system*" (p. 118, Fleck's emphasis); on this see refs 31, 34 below.

30. *Ibid.*, 112.

31. *Ibid.*, 122–3. Here I am simplifying Fleck's picture, for at this point he was in fact discussing "vademecum science" rather than "popular science". However this simplification is not inappropriate, for three reasons. In the first place, Fleck argued that popular science has a "general epistemological significance", since its qualities of "certainty, simplicity, vividness" are precisely the goals of "the expert" as well (pp. 114–15) — whence the fact that "the conviction that there is no development of thought", which as we see below is characteristic of popular science, is "a conviction that also influences the expert" (p. 116). Secondly, vademecum science and popular science as Fleck depicted these have many features in common: for instance, vademecum science resembles popular science in seeking to constitute a "closed system" (p. 119); in involving "exoteric" as well as "esoteric" knowledge (p. 123); and in constructing a mythical, individualized history (pp. 122–3; *cf.* p. 116, as quoted immediately below). Third, Fleck described vademecum science as developing out of "journal science" through processes of communication, including the stabilizing of nomenclature (pp. 120–3); and

he had already insisted that "*Every communication and, indeed, all nomenclature tends to make any item of knowledge more collective and popular*" (p. 114, Fleck's emphasis). See also ref. 34 below.

32. *Ibid.*, 116 (here referring to "popular science" itself).

33. On the same page Fleck reproduced a potted history of syphilis (from Gottstein's book of 1929) and commented: "From descriptions such as this, the conviction emerges that there is no development of thought."

34. *Ibid.*, 120–1. Strictly speaking, this anecdote concerning retrospective diagnosis was presented not as an aspect of "popular science" but rather within Fleck's account of "vademecum science", and not as a characteristic of such science but rather for a specific technical reason (i.e., as an illustration of the collective, "impersonal", origin of collectively-accepted concepts). But my appropriation of Fleck's brief discussion of retrospective diagnosis is, I submit, consistent with the claims he had already made about the apprehension of "syphilis" in "popular science" (p. 116). See also ref. 31 above.

35. *Ibid.*, 82–83, 165.

36. *Ibid.*, 140; *cf.* p. 111 (ref. 24 above).

37. For a rare exception whose very brevity confirms the rule, see *ibid.*, 5–6.

38. Above, at ref. 20.

39. For example, the main reference work on the history of science cites Fleck's work three times, in each case as a major conceptual resource, whereas the comparable (and substantially longer) reference work on the history of medicine refers to Fleck only once, and even then as what amounts to an addendum on the history of Fleck's own field, immunology. See respectively R. C. Olby, G. N. Cantor, J. R. R. Christie and M. J. S. Hodge (eds), *Companion to the history of modern science* (London, 1990), 64, 91, 164, and Bynum and Porter (eds), *Companion encyclopedia of the history of medicine* (ref. 6), 203. Even Cunningham's fine essay "Transforming plague" (ref. 20 above), the central historiographic point of which is entirely consonant with Fleck's approach, does not cite Fleck. Fleck was first noticed in English by T. S. Kuhn, *The structure of scientific revolutions* (Chicago, 1962), pp. vi–vii; the 1979 English translation was produced at the behest of historians and sociologists of science, notably R. Merton.

40. See for instance G. Brieger, "The historiography of medicine", in Bynum and Porter (eds), *Companion encyclopedia of the history of medicine* (ref. 6), i, 24–44, p. 31.

41. Temkin, *The Falling Sickness* (ref. 2), Preface, p. vii, my emphasis.

42. R. Koch, *The aetiology of tuberculosis* (German original 1882; transl. by Dr and Mrs M. Pinner, New York, 1932), 44. Tuberculosis was originally "consumption" or "phthisis" (touched upon in refs 110 and 194 below); Koch's redefinition of the disease transformed its meaning in complex ways, precisely in line with what Fleck was to write about syphilis (above, at ref. 13).

43. M. Foucault, *Naissance de la clinique* (Paris, 1963); *Birth of the clinic: An archaeology of medical perception* (transl. by A. M. Sheridan Smith, London, 1973).

44. See for instance D. Armstrong, *Political anatomy of the body: Medical knowledge in Britain in the twentieth century* (Cambridge, 1983).

45. Foucault, *Birth of the clinic* (ref. 43), pp. x, xv, xi.

46. For "imaginary investments" see *ibid.*, p. x.

47. *Mutatis mutandis*, the same is true of N. Jewson's classic study, "Medical knowledge and the patronage system in eighteenth-century England", *Sociology*, viii (1974), 369–85.

48. Foucault, *Birth of the clinic* (ref. 43), p. xi.

49. *Ibid.*, p. xi; my emphasis.

50. *Ibid.*, pp. xvi–xvii.

310

51. *Ibid.*, 196, p. xii; my emphases.

52. Thus for all that Foucault consistently distanced himself from structuralism, his archaeological *oeuvre* is open to precisely the kind of critique that P. de Man levelled at structuralism in various of his works; see for instance *Blindness and insight: Essays in the rhetoric of contemporary criticism* (first edn, 1971; revised edn, London, 1983); *Allegories of reading: Figural language in Rousseau, Nietzsche, Rilke and Proust* (New Haven, 1979); and *The resistance to theory* (ed. by W. Godzich, Minneapolis, 1986). See further the penetrating discussion of Foucault in S. Burke, *The death and return of the author: Criticism and subjectivity in Barthes, Foucault and Derrida* (Edinburgh, 1992; 2nd edn, 1998).

53. Figlio, "Chlorosis and chronic disease in nineteenth-century Britain" (ref. 4).

54. *Ibid.*, 173–5.

55. *Ibid.*, 175.

56. *Ibid.*, 193.

57. See respectively pp. 178 nn. 32, 34; 181; 185; 174 n. 21; and many subsequent citations (*Black's medical dictionary*).

58. *Ibid.*, 174–5.

59. See for instance *ibid.*, 179: "Constructing the illness ... was the other face of discovering adolescence."

60. Notably at *ibid.*, 177–8, invoking Laslett's argument that the age of menarche declined in the nineteenth century.

61. See for instance F. Boissier de Sauvages, *Nosologia methodica sistens morborum classes juxta Sydenhami mentem and botanicorum ordinem* (2 vols, Amsterdam, 1768), ii, 440–3.

62. F. H. Garrison and L. T. Morton, *A medical bibliography: An annotated check-list of texts illustrating the history of medicine* (4th edn, Aldershot, 1983), 418–19.

63. Rosenberg and Golden (eds), *Framing disease* (ref. 15).

64. Charles E. Rosenberg, "Framing disease: Illness, society, and history", *ibid.*, pp. xiii–xxvi, at pp. xiv–xv.

65. *Cf.* above, at ref. 42. On the shifting meanings of "cholera" and on the problems attending retrospective diagnosis of "tuberculosis", see M. Grmek, *Diseases in the ancient Greek world* (transl. by M. Muellner and L. Muellner, Baltimore, 1989), 7, 183–4. The latter work, it should be observed in passing, has an ambiguous significance in relation to my theme. On the one hand, it rests entirely upon retrospective diagnosis and pays little attention to ancient disease-concepts — thereby participating in the naturalist-realist tradition. On the other hand, Grmek stresses throughout (for instance, in the passages just cited) that modern concepts of disease are incommensurate with ancient ones — this in harmony with the historicalist-conceptualist approach.

66. See further Rosenberg, "Framing disease" (ref. 64), p. xvi, where this anti-relativist position was reiterated. Here the argument became rather more complicated, for Rosenberg rightly argued that "the process of disease definition" merited attention, thereby seemingly abandoning the framing metaphor. See also ref. 68 below.

67. For instance an essay on silicosis, bearing the promising title "The illusion of medical certainty", nevertheless began by asserting — with no intended irony — that "Silicosis is a chronic lung disease caused by the inhalation of silica dust". G. Markowitz and D. Rosner, "The illusion of medical certainty: Silicosis and the politics of industrial disability, 1930–1960", in Rosenberg and Golden (eds), *Framing disease* (ref. 63), 185–205.

68. Similarly, when introducing Peitzman's essay Rosenberg summarized its argument by saying that "the evolving framework of pathological assumptions describing and explaining 'Bright's disease' has been gradually integrated and reintegrated into a series of differently focused

explanatory frameworks for *the same clinical pictures*" (my emphasis), and remarked that "It is precisely this process of definition and redefinition that demands scholarly attention". Here the initial assumption of clinical constancy, associated again with the metaphor of framing-and-pictures, was immediately (and commendably) undermined by the notion of "definition and redefinition". See Rosenberg and Golden (eds), *Framing disease* (ref. 63), 4, and *cf.* ref. 66 above.

69. Until recently an analogous situation obtained within the sociology of medicine, the scope of which was traditionally restricted by giving a particular twist to the supposed distinction between "illness" and "disease". "Illnesses", it was said, were the subjective experiences of patients; they fell within the realm of "culture", and were therefore seen as forming a proper theme for sociological inquiry. "Diseases", in contrast, were conceived as real pathological processes, taken to coincide with their (supposed) medical definitions; they were regarded as inhabiting the realm of "nature", and therefore as lying beyond the bounds of sociological investigation. For this point, and for a cogent argument against this framework of assumptions, see P. Atkinson, *Medical talk and medical work: The liturgy of the clinic* (London, 1995), chap. 2. The burden of Atkinson's argument is that just as diseases are the constructs of medicine, so the supposed objectivity of those diseases was the construct of traditional medical sociology itself. Like Rosenberg, Atkinson has deliberately avoided the term "construction"; but significantly, he replaces it not by "framing" but instead by "production" (*ibid.*, 45); and unlike Rosenberg, he refers to Fleck (pp. 143, 147). Similar points had already been made, from a rather different perspective (concerned with the sociology of illness rather than the sociology of knowledge), by R. Dingwall, *Aspects of illness* (London, 1976), chap. 2. As for the "illness"/"disease" distinction, both words are so elastic that it can be made in many different ways, or avoided altogether, according to one's rhetorical purposes: see A. L. Caplan, H. T. Engelhardt, Jr, and J. M. McCartney (eds), *Concepts of health and illness: Interdisciplinary perspectives* (Reading, Mass., 1981), and C. Currer and M. Stacey (eds), *Concepts of health and illness and disease: A comparative perspective* (Leamington Spa, 1986).

70. S. Shapin, "History of science and its sociological reconstructions", *History of science*, xx (1982), 157–211, p. 157.

71. Smith, "Pleuritis" (ref. 5). I thank Professor Smith for e-mailing me a copy of this paper and of his translations from the ancient texts, and for helpfully discussing my various queries.

72. Foucault, *Birth of the clinic* (ref. 43), 122.

73. Smith, "Pleuritis", quoted here from typescript.

74. Particularly the *Aphorisms* (below, at ref. 121).

75. *Regimen in acute diseases* (below, at ref. 123).

76. This was the thrust of the discussions of pleuritis in *Diseases I* (the work known to Galen as *Internal suppurations*): 26 and in *Places in man*: 14. See respectively the Loeb edn, *Hippocrates*, v (transl. by P. Potter, London, 1988), 98–183, pp. 166–71, and Smith, "Pleuritis" (ref. 5), Appendix. This aspect also appeared in *Affections*: 7, which however was one of the texts that did define pleuritis, as next discussed.

77. *Affections*: 7. See Loeb edn, *Hippocrates*, v, 6–91, pp. 15–16.

78. *Diseases II*: 44–46. See Loeb edn, *Hippocrates*, v, 191–333, pp. 262–7.

79. *Diseases III*: 16. See Loeb edn, *Hippocrates*, vi (transl. by P. Potter, London, 1988), 6–63, pp. 38–57.

80. *Ibid.*, 38–39; Smith's translation, in the appendix to his "Pleuritis" (ref. 5).

81. Loeb edition, *Hippocrates*, vi, "Index of symptoms and diseases", 336.

82. *Ibid.*, translator's note, 334.

83. *Diseases I* and *Places in man*, as cited in ref. 76 above; *Aphorisms*, quoted below, at ref. 121.

312

84. See below, at ref. 123; Smith, "Pleuritis" (ref. 5), 3–4; and D. Jacquart, "Theory, everyday practice, and three 15th-century physicians", *Osiris*, 2nd ser., vi (1990), 140–60, p. 154.

85. Below, at ref. 87.

86. Here my reading differs from that of Smith, "Pleuritis", who characterizes *Diseases III* as discussing "a single disease with various manifestations".

87. *Diseases II*: 44–46 (Loeb edn, *Hippocrates*, v, 264–7); *cf.* above, at ref. 85.

88. In one text only, namely *Places in man*: 14, pleuritis was given an internal anatomical location, specifically in the lung. This work was also unique in conceiving pleuritis as the one-sided version of peripneumony: "When both sides are painful and the affections of both sides are similar, that is peripneumony; the other is pleuritis" (Smith's translation, "Pleuritis" (ref. 5), Appendix). Although many of the Hippocratic texts discussed pleuritis and peripneumony in sequence and offered overlapping therapies for them, they usually defined them in quite different ways. In particular, pleuritis was always defined with reference to pain in the side, as we have seen; but the defining symptoms of peripneumony were fever, cough and expectoration, with pain being mentioned only erratically. In short, the entire thrust of the discussion of pleuritis and peripneumony in *Places in man* was well outside the Hippocratic mainstream. (Accounts of peripneumony appeared in *Affections*: 9, *Diseases I*: 27, and *Diseases II*: 47, all in Loeb edn, *Hippocrates*, v; see pp. 17, 171, 267–9.)

89. Traditionally, Praxagoras is regarded as the teacher of Herophilus. With respect to the localization of pleuritis, Diocles may well have preceded Erasistratus, though this is not to say that he was Erasistratus's teacher. The possible roles of Praxagoras and (especially) Diocles in the story of pleuritis are discussed by Smith, "Pleuritis" (ref. 5); here, however, as a convenient simplification, I shall depict the anatomical tradition as stemming from Herophilus and Erasistratus, setting aside Praxagoras and Diocles. (The views of Diocles and Praxagoras on peripneumony are quoted in ref. 92 below.)

90. Caelius Aurelianus, *Acute diseases*, II.xiii–xxiv, in I. E. Drabkin (ed. and transl.), *Caelius Aurelianus: On acute diseases and On chronic diseases* (Chicago, 1950), 181–227, chap. 16 (pp. 189–93). In fact, my claim that the dogmatics "defined" pleuritis in anatomical terms is a projection backwards from stage (iii) of ancient medicine (see below, particularly the discussion of Aretaeus at ref. 115); strictly speaking, it is possible that the dogmatics defined pleuritis in symptomatic terms and added an anatomical seat (or rather, seats). But for convenience I am eliding this particular subtlety.

91. On peripneumony *cf.* ref. 88 above.

92. "In the case of people suffering from peripneumonia, Diocles says the veins of the lung are affected, while Erasistratus says the arteries are affected, and Praxagoras the parts of the lung which are joined to the spine. But Herophilus says the whole lung is affected. If the patients [also] suffer from fever, he says, it causes pleurisy." Caelius Aurelianus, quoted in H. von Staden, *Herophilus: The art of medicine in early Alexandria* (Cambridge, 1989), 378 (T.215). *Cf.* Caelius Aurelianus, *Acute diseases*, ed. by Drabkin (ref. 90), II.xxviii (p. 231).

93. This emerges from a passage from Galen's *De locis affectis*, as discussed by Smith in "Pleuritis" (ref. 5).

94. Caelius Aurelianus, *Acute diseases*, ed. by Drabkin (ref. 90), II.xiv [91] and II.xvi [96–98] (pp. 185, 189–91).

95. With a interesting qualification: that those who placed pleuritis in the membrane, or some of them, apparently believed that "some patients find it impossible to lie on the side affected, while others, on the contrary, rest more easily on that side": *ibid.*, II.xvi [98] (p. 191). To complicate the matter, the justifying argument does not match the claim itself, as Drabkin observes in an editorial footnote. This very issue would be revived by Morgagni: see below, at ref. 176.

96. *Ibid.*, II.xvi [96] (p. 189).

97. *Ibid.*, II.xvi [98] (p. 191). Also of interest is the passage which records the views of Soranus /Caelius himself, for here there emerged an additional dimension of this symptom, one which I have not encountered in any other text: "when they turn on the opposite side they experience pain and actually *feel the inflamed organs hanging and being drawn down by their own weight*": *ibid.*, II.xiv [91] (p. 185), emphasis added.

98. Caelius Aurelianus, *Acute diseases*, ed. by Drabkin; at ref. 73 on p. 284.

99. Cited below, from ref. 120 onwards.

100. Aretaeus, *On the causes. and symptoms of acute diseases*, in F. Adams (ed. and transl.), *The extant works of Aretaeus, the Cappadocian* (London, 1856).

101. For the original Greek and Latin words see Drabkin's introduction (*ibid.*, pp. xi–xxvi, at p. xix).

102. In the case of cardiac disease Soranus/Caelius was anti-localist (*ibid.*, II.xxxiv, 257–61, p. 259); with respect to hydrophobia, he adopted an intermediate position (III.xiv, 371–5, pp. 374–5).

103. *Ibid.*, II.xvi [100] (p. 193).

104. It should be mentioned, however, that Soranus's (Caelius's) citations of Hippocrates were somewhat haphazard and erratic: see *ibid.*, Drabkin's note 1, p. 62 and note 10, p. 353.

105. *Ibid.*, II.xix [113–24] (203–15).

106. Smith, "Pleuritis" (ref. 5), 5.

107. *Ibid.*, 6–7.

108. "*Stimulosus ac pulsuosus et igneus*": Caelius Aurelianus, *Acute diseases*, ed. by Drabkin (ref. 90), II.xiv [91], 184.

109. 'Nygmatodes' (νυγματωδης) is so translated in R. J. Durling, *A dictionary of medical terms in Galen* (Leiden, 1993).

110. The tricky issue concerns the term 'nygmatodes', used by Galen to characterize the pains of pleuritis. Aretaeus also used this word in connection with pleuritis, but he did so not in his generic description of the disease but rather as a sign that it had progressed to empyema: see Aretaeus, *Acute diseases*, ed. by Adams (ref. 100), I.x, 17 (Greek), 257 (English). Thus for Aretaeus, pains of the "nygmatodes" type were in fact characteristic not of pleuritis, but of empyema. And it would appear that Soranus had done something similar; for in Caelius Aurelianus's Latin rendition, he wrote that the transition from pleuritis to empyema is associated with "pungent pains" (*dolore pungenti*), as distinct from the pain of pleuritis itself, which in this particular context he described not as "pungent" but merely as "acute" (*dolor acutus*): see Caelius Aurelianus, *Acute diseases*, ed. by Drabkin (ref. 90), II.xvii [101–2] (p. 194). If (as later usages indeed imply) the Latin *pungens* was equivalent to the Greek *nygmatodes*, then the account of Soranus/Caelius differs from that of Galen much as that of Aretaeus does.

111. See above, at ref. 86.

112. On Archigenes see further below, at ref. 128.

113. This is Wesley Smith's interpretation. The matter is complicated by the relation between the "pricking" quality of the pain and the progression of pleuritis to empyema: see ref. 110 above.

114. Immediately after announcing the conclusion that "it is the *hypezocos membrana* which is the seat of this disease", Soranus/Caelius added: "And this membrane is the source of severe pains (*dolorem vehementem*), for it is fibrous and attached to the side." This came *within* a passage framed as a summary of the views of those who place pleuritis in the "hypezocos membrana", which indicates that Soranus/Caelius was here paraphrasing Erasistratus *et al.* See Caelius Aurelianus, *Acute diseases*, ed. by Drabkin (ref. 90), II.xvi [98–100] (pp. 191–3).

314

115. Aretaeus, *Acute diseases*, I.x, ed. by Adams (ref. 100), 16, 255–6; word-order modified slightly.
116. This with the phrase "all these symptoms", in the third sentence.
117. Foucault, *Birth of the clinic* (ref. 43), 137; A. Cunningham, "Getting the game right: Some plain words on the identity and invention of science", *Studies in history and philosophy of science*, xix (1988), 365–89, pp. 373–5.
118. *Cf.* M. Heidegger, *Being and time* (German original 1928; transl. from the 7th German edition by J. Macquarrie and E. Robinson, Oxford, 1962), section 7, p. 52, and below, at ref. 122.
119. See W. D. Smith, *The Hippocratic tradition* (Ithaca, N.Y., 1979). For a different reading see J. Longrigg, *Greek rational medicine: Philosophy and medicine from Alcmaeon to the Alexandrians* (London, 1993).
120. *Aphorisms*, V.viii (*cf.* also xv), in Loeb edn, *Hippocrates*, iv (transl. by W. H. S. Jones, London, 1931), 98–221, p. 159; Galen, *Commentary on Hippocrates' Aphorisms* (17B 399 K.), as cited and translated by Smith, "Pleuritis" (ref. 5).
121. Contrast the translation in G. E. R. Lloyd (ed.), *Hippocratic writings* (Harmondsworth, 1978/1983), 222: "If sufferers from pleurisy do not cough up material within fourteen days, the inflammation produces empyema." The "inflammation" here appears to have been interpolated by the translators (J. Chadwick and W. N. Mann). On the transition of pleuritis to empyema, compare Aretaeus's discussion (ref. 110 above).
122. Although certain of the Hippocratic texts had speculated as to the internal events underlying pleuritis (see above, at ref. 76), they had not installed these posited internal events as definitive of the disease; rather, the disease was identified *as* its symptoms. Hence the fact that those symptoms were never turned into "signs"; nor indeed were they conceived as "symptoms" in our sense (*cf.* above, at ref. 118), for they lay on the same ontological level as the disease.
123. Hippocrates, *Regimen in acute diseases*: 16, in Loeb edn, *Hippocrates*, ii (transl. by W. H. S Jones, London, 1923), 75; Galen, *Commentary on Regimen in acute diseases* (15.488 K), as cited and translated by Smith, "Pleuritis" (ref. 5).
124. Smith, "Pleuritis" (ref. 5) discusses several of these passages.
125. Galen, *De causis pulsuum*, IV.viii, in F. Blondel and A. Le Moine (eds), *Hippocratis Coi, et Claudii Galeni Pergameni archiatron opera* (13 vols in 9, Paris, 1639–89), viii, 223–5; *De praesagitatione ex pulsibus*, IV, *ibid.*, 298–9; *De pulsibus ad tyrones*, cap. xii, *ibid.*, 8–9; *Galeni Synopsis librorum suorum de pulsibus, ibid.*, 326.
126. So we may infer from the fact that the Soranus/Caelius passage cited earlier (above, at ref. 90) made no mention of the pulse in connection with the dispute over the localization of pleuritis.
127. See von Staden, *Herophilus* (ref. 92), 262–88. All observers credited Herophilus with the basic pulse-nomenclature, but none of them mentioned the "hard" pulse (or its opposite, the "soft" pulse) amongst the various terms he had developed.
128. It seems that the terms "hard" and "soft" pulse were introduced by Archigenes (see Galen, *De pulsuum differentiis*, III.vii, in Blondel and Le Moine (eds), *Hippocratis et Galeni opera* (ref. 125), viii, 77–79); but it is unclear whether Archigenes had applied these terms to the particular cases of pleurisy and peripneumony. On Galen's debts to Archigenes in respect of pulse-lore, see von Staden, *Herophilus* (ref. 92), 284 n.156; on Archigenes and pleuritis see above, at ref. 112.
129. Galen, *De causis pulsuum*, IV.xii, in Blondel and Le Moine (eds), *Hippocratis et Galeni opera* (ref. 125), viii, 227; *De pulsibus ad Tyrones*, cap. xii, in *ibid.*, 10.
130. Galen, *De causis pulsuum*, IV.viii, in *ibid.*, viii, 224.
131. *Ibid.*, viii, 223.
132. J. B. Saunders and C. D. O'Malley, *Andreas Vesalius Bruxellensis, The Bloodletting Letter of 1539: An annotated translation and study of Vesalius's scientific development* (New

York, 1946), 15. See also A. Cunningham, *The anatomical renaissance: The resurrection of the anatomical projects of the ancients* (London, 1997), 101–2, 110–11. The issue had medieval precedents: see Jacquart, "Theory, everyday practice, and three 15th-century physicians" (ref. 84), 158.

133. Saunders and O'Malley, *The Bloodletting Letter* (ref. 132), 74.

134. *Ibid.*, 81–82; *cf.* ref. 136 below.

135. *Ibid.*, 70, reading "pleuritis" for "pleurisy" throughout.

136. The membrane did enter Vesalius's discussion at a later point (*ibid.*, 81–82), but not as the seat of the disease; rather, to demonstrate that *dolor lateralis* tends most often to occur where that membrane is "less firmly attached", that is, in the vicinity of the fifth to the eighth ribs. See further ref. 144 below.

137. Cunningham, *The anatomical renaissance* (ref. 132), 124.

138. *Cf. ibid.*, 102.

139. *Cf.* Saunders and O'Malley, *The Bloodletting Letter* (ref. 132), 8, and ref. 144 below.

140. This in a later text, from 1546; see ref. 144 below.

141. Immediately after the passage just quoted Vesalius remarked: "In addition the name pleurisy derived from the ribs — also called πλευραι, because they form the side — by no means indicates a primary position, since the ancient Latin writers called the disease *dolor lateralis*, not *dolor costalis*..." (Saunders and O'Malley, *The Bloodletting Letter* (ref. 132), 70; here I have modified the translation and punctuation for greater clarity).

142. A strong contender was Mondino dei Liuzzi: see Jacquart, "Theory, everyday practice, and three 15th-century physicians" (ref. 84), 156.

143. *Cf.* G. E. R. Lloyd, "The development of Greek anatomical terminology", in his *Science, folklore and ideology: Studies in the life sciences in ancient Greece* (Cambridge, 1983), 149–67.

144. Vesalius, *De humani corporis fabrica*, VI.ii. A few years later (1546), in the course of his *Epistola rationem modumque propinandi radicis Chynae decocti* (*Letter on the China root*), Vesalius returned in passing to the topic of pleurisy, mentioning two fatal cases, each of which he had examined *post mortem*. The first case (in which the patient was said to have died of "*dolor lateralis*") seems at first sight to embody a shift from Vesalius's views of 1539, for this showed inflammation of the *membrana costas succingens* on the left side. But the second case (described as "*morbus lateralis*") suggests that his conception was unchanged, for here the inflammation was not tied to that membrane, but rather "occupied the whole posterior part of the thorax" and followed the distribution of the unpaired vein. Combining the two cases, we may infer that Vesalius regarded the *succingens* membrane as just one possible seat of "*dolor lateralis*" or "*morbus lateralis*", a view which harmonized perfectly with what he had written in 1539. Nevertheless it is worth remarking that both these post-mortems showed *inflammation*, whereas in 1539 Vesalius had mentioned only an "affection"; it is not clear whether this represents a change in his views or whether it was merely a matter of verbal tactics. See Vesalius, *Opera omnia anatomica et chururgica*, ed. by H. Boerhaave and B. S. Albinus (2 vols, Leyden, 1725), ii, 664, and Morgagni, *The seats and causes of diseases* (ref. 169), 623.

145. See G. Whitteridge (ed.), *The anatomical lectures of William Harvey* (Edinburgh, 1964), 236, 246. When William Harvey lectured on anatomy in 1616, taking Bauhin as his starting-point, he accepted this use of "pleura". (Incidentally, Bauhin also used "pleura" in a quite different way: as a designation for fibrous bands connecting the lungs to the chest wall. Harvey contested Bauhin's assumption that such fibrous bands were normal, but he did not dispute this further use of the term "pleura": see *ibid.*, 275.)

146. *Ibid.*, 236; Cunningham, *The anatomical renaissance* (ref. 132), 103.

316

147. G. Baglivi, *The practice of physick, reduc'd to the ancient way of observations. Containing a just parallel between the wisdom and experience of the Ancients, and the hypothesis's of modern physicians. Intermix'd with many practical remarks upon most distempers* (transl. anon., London, 1723), chaps. 9 and 103.

148. Cunningham, *The anatomical renaissance* (ref. 132), chap. 4.

149. Baglivi, *The practice of physic* (ref. 147), 2, 120–1.

150. *Ibid.*, *passim*, esp. pp. 20–21, 115–16.

151. *Ibid.*, 60. *Cf.* also pp. 103, 104 ("scattered sentences", "snug sentences").

152. *Ibid.*, 59.

153. *Ibid.*, 103, 60.

154. *Ibid.*, 105.

155. See F. Bacon, *The advancement of learning*, I.v.5, in Bacon, *The advancement of learning and New Atlantis*, ed. by A. Johnston (Oxford, 1974), 34. On Baglivi's admiration for Bacon see J. Martin, "Sauvages' nosology" (cited in ref. 202 below), 115–18.

156. Baglivi, *The practice of physic* (ref. 147), 188. *Cf.* also p. 22, where Baglivi offered his formal definition of the *Medicina prima*.

157. *Ibid.*, 197.

158. *Ibid.*, 22.

159. *Ibid.*, 197.

160. *Ibid.*, 60.

161. *Ibid.*, 60–61.

162. See above, at ref. 130.

163. Baglivi, *The practice of physic* (ref. 147), 61–66.

164. For instance, "A good respiration is a good omen, but a bad one is always to be dreaded.... But prognostics taken from the pulse are not so certain..."; and "Such pleuritical patients as were seized with a pain in the inner part of the ear, followed by an imposthume and pus, were all cured, pursuant to my repeated observations in the Italian Hospitals" (*ibid.*, 61). Again, "After the cessation of the pain of inflamed parts (especially in the case of a pleurisy or the inflammation of membranous parts), if the fever still continues, or increases, being attended with a low, intermitting and frequent pulse, cold sweats, etc., 'tis a fatal omen..." (p. 63).

165. Baglivi recommended bleeding (without considering its site, and so without mentioning the controversy which had raged in Vesalius's day) and expectoration, and argued against purgatives and diaphoretics: *ibid.*, 62, 64–65.

166. *Ibid.*, 62, 63, 65.

167. *Ibid.*, 22, quoted above, at ref. 158.

168. *Ibid.*, 20–21, 114–16, 118, 126–7, 197.

169. G. Morgagni, *De sedibus et causis morborum per anatomen indagatis* (Venice, 1761); *On the seats and causes of diseases, investigated by anatomy* (transl. by B. Alexander, 3 vols, London, 1769).

170. Baglivi, *The practice of physic* (ref. 147), 2.

171. See G. A. Lindeboom, *Herman Boerhaave: The man and his work* (London, 1968), 274–5, and contrast Morgagni, *On the seats and causes of diseases* (ref. 169), 613.

172. True, we have two excellent, complementary recent discussions: M. Nicolson, "Giovanni Battista Morgagni and eighteenth-century physical examination", in C. Lawrence (ed.), *Medical theory, surgical practice* (London, 1992), 101–34, and A. Cunningham, "Pathology and the case-history in Morgagni's 'On the Seats and Causes of Diseases Investigated Through Anatomy' (1761)", *MedGG*, xi (1995), 37–61. But a great deal more remains to be learnt from the 2,242 pages

of *On the seats and causes of diseases.*

173. On Morgagni see also *The clinical consultations of Giambattista Morgagni: The edition of Enrico Benassi* (1935), translated and revised by S. Jarcho, with new preface and supplements (Boston, 1984).

174. Morgagni, *On the seats and causes of diseases* (ref. 169), ii, 546–80 (Letter 20), 581–643 (Letter 21).

175. On Morgagni's logic see S. Jarcho, "Morgagni, Vicarius, and the difficulty of clinical diagnosis", in L. G. Stevenson and R. P. Multhauf (eds), *Medicine, science and culture: Historical essays in honor of Owsei Temkin* (Baltimore, 1968), 87–95; on the anatomical and case-historical dimensions of Morgagni's enterprise see Cunningham, "Pathology and the case-history" (ref. 172).

176. By explaining the anomaly Morgagni was able to advance a hypothesis as to the source of the pain-in-lying-down (*On the seats and causes of diseases*, 555), a hypothesis which fed into his larger subsequent discussion (see for instance p. 558).

177. *Ibid.*, 569–70. Here Morgagni duly noticed that the anomaly he had observed was also of ancient record, in Caelius Aurelianus's *Acute diseases* (ref. 94).

178. See above, at ref. 145.

179. Morgagni, *On the seats and causes of diseases*, 627.

180. *Ibid.*, 621–30.

181. In all probability, Morgagni had grossly exaggerated Baronius's contribution, and had suppressed the writings of many other authors, for in fact this conception went back to the sixteenth century and was well known in the early eighteenth century: see the citations under the entry for "pleuro-pneumonia" in the *Oxford English dictionary*. Nevertheless this licence on Morgagni's part was justified, for pleurisy and peripneumony were regarded as distinct diseases by Boerhaave, by van Swieten, and by all the leading nosologists, among them Sauvages, Linnaeus, Vogel and Cullen. See G. van Swieten, *The commentaries upon the aphorisms of Dr. Herman Boerhaave concerning the knowledge and cure of the several diseases incident to human bodies* (transl. anon., 18 vols, London, 1744–73), viii and ix (separate and extended treatments of peripneumony and pleurisy respectively); W. Cullen, *Synopsis nosologicae methodicae* (Edinburgh, 1769), 30, 33, 103, 105, 171, 260–1.

182. Garrison remarked: "It is said of him [Boerhaave] that he was the first to establish the site of pleurisy exclusively in the pleura...": F. H. Garrison, *An introduction to the history of medicine* (first published 1913; 4th edn, Philadelphia, 1929), 317, giving no reference. I have not identified the origin of this particular claim.

183. Duffin, *To see with a better eye* (ref. 6), 145–7, 216–17.

184. *Ibid.*, 205.

185. (1) The pain-in-the-side was described as being intensified by inspiration (J. Duffin, personal communication); this had already been identified earlier (see van Swieten, *Commentaries* (ref. 181), ix, 1). (2) The hard pulse had apparently been dropped as a diagnostic sign; I have not established when this took place. (3) Survivors of chronic pleurisy had retraction of one side of the chest; this was discovered by Laennec himself (Duffin, *To see with a better eye* (ref. 6), 161).

186. *Ibid.*, 158.

187. Maulitz, "In the clinic" (ref. 6).

188. Most of what follows rests specifically on Chomel's observations, of which Maulitz gives examples drawn from students' lecture-notes (*ibid.*, 134–5), but the link between pleuritis and phthisis was apparently characteristic of the Paris school at this time (p. 133). The quotations in the next four references are from Chomel, in *ibid.*, 134–5.

318

189. "The stitch in one's side [that is] worsened by inspiration and by cough is characteristic of pleurisy."

190. "Phthisical patients from time to time are subject to pleuritic stitches without effusions." See also the quotation in the next reference.

191. "Certain cases of pleurisy are accompanied only by a pseudomembranous exudate, in which case there is neither dullness nor egophony." Conversely, Andral had already argued in the 1820s that (as Duffin puts it) "egophony could exist under false positive circumstances, when there was no effusion at all" (Duffin, *To see with a better eye* (ref. 6), 205).

192. See the quotation in ref. 190 above, and also: "In chronic pleurisy we have often found tubercles in the chest of those who have succumbed."

193. Duffin, *To see with a better eye* (ref. 6), 158–9.

194. In the next letter of *De sedibus* (Letter 22), Morgagni discussed phthisis along with empyema; here he linked "pleuripneumony" (the concept which had now replaced both pleurisy and peripneumony) with empyema, and not with phthisis (*On the seats and causes of diseases* (ref. 169), 650, 655; *cf.* refs 110, 121 above). True, he suggested that some of Valsalva's "peripneumony" cases (which he had discussed in Letter 20) actually "related rather to consumption" (p. 645); but this was as near as he came to linking pleurisy or "pleuripneumony" with consumption. It should also be observed that *De sedibus* included only a few cases of phthisis, because both Valsalva and (even more so) Morgagni were "cautious" about dissecting the bodies of consumptives, evidently through fear of contagion (pp. 645, 661).

195. Maulitz, "In the clinic" (ref. 6), 130–1.

196. Duffin, *To see with a better eye* (ref. 6), 247.

197. See above, at ref. 174.

198. *Cf.* L. Jordanova, "The social construction of medical knowledge", *Social history of medicine*, viii (1995), 361–81, particularly p. 374.

199. See for instance R. Porter (ed.), *Patients and practitioners: Lay perceptions of medicine in pre-industrial society* (Cambridge, 1985); L. McC. Beier, *Sufferers and healers: The experience of illness in the seventeenth century* (London, 1987); R. Porter and D. Porter, *In sickness and in health* (London, 1989); D. Porter and R. Porter, *Patient's progress: Doctors and doctoring in eighteenth-century England* (Oxford, 1989).

200. For a fine illustration of this point see M. Nicolson, "The metastatic theory of pathogenesis and the professional interests of the eighteenth-century physician", *Medical history*, xxxii (1988), 277–300.

201. *Cf.* Duffin, *To see with a better eye* (ref. 6), 302–3.

202. For two very different accounts see R. French, "Sickness and the soul: Stahl, Hoffman and Sauvages on pathology", in A. Cunningham and R. French (eds), *The medical enlightenment of the eighteenth century* (Cambridge, 1990), 88–110, and J. Martin, "Sauvages' nosology: Medical enlightenment in Montpellier", *ibid.*, 111–37. For the most recent word on Sauvages, see L. Brockliss and C. Jones, *The medical world of early-modern France* (Oxford, 1997), 427–9, p. 435 and *passim*.

203. This crucial issue has been raised by French, "Sickness and the soul" (ref. 202), who stresses the differences; but Martin, in "Sauvages' nosology" (ref. 202), can be read as emphasizing the continuities between the two.

204. For an overview see W. F. Bynum, "Nosology", in Bynum and Porter (eds), *Companion encyclopedia of the history of medicine* (ref. 6), i, 335–56.

205. Foucault, *Birth of the clinic* (ref. 43), chap. 1 and *passim*; R. Porter, "The eighteenth century" in L. I. Conrad *et al.*, *The Western medical tradition* (Cambridge, 1995), 371–475, pp. 409–10. See also Maulitz, "In the clinic" (ref. 6), *passim*, and Duffin, *To see with a better eye* (ref. 6), 68–69, 251,

who both find that nosology remained very much alive in the Paris clinic.

206. Dr Shyamsunder Rao Chepur assures me (personal communication, 1998) that there are in the Ayurvedic tradition at least two standard diagnostic categories which correspond to, or overlap with, pleurisy: (1) *Parshuka roga* ("disease of the sides"); and (2) *Utpullika* (a "respiratory disorder" associated with "painful swelling in the right hypochondrium and intercostal space"). But I have yet to discover just how those categories developed historically within that tradition.

VIII

Porter versus Foucault on the 'Birth of the Clinic'

Texts and contexts

It is well known that Roy Porter's *oeuvre* in the history of psychiatry was partly stimulated by, and in no small measure pitched against, Michel Foucault's *Madness and Civilization (Folie et déraison)*. But what was Porter's response to Foucault's *Birth of the Clinic (Naissance de la clinique)*?[1] By the 'birth of the clinic', let us recall, Foucault referred to the remarkable change in medicine that took place in the Paris École de Santé between 1800, when Xavier Bichat's *Traité des membranes* initiated his new doctrine of tissues, which rapidly invigorated pathological anatomy, and 1817, when René-Théophile-Hyacinthe Laennec (1781–1826), one of the most influential pupils of the new school and himself a master of pathological anatomy, invented the stethoscope. Foucault himself, as we shall see, regarded this as the most important transformation in Western medicine's entire history, and although not all commentators would go this far, none would deny that pathological anatomy made giant strides in the Paris school, or that the stethoscope gave an unprecedented impulse to physical examination, with permanent effects. Thus we are dealing here with a momentous set of events, which means that Porter's view of *Birth of the Clinic* is of considerable interest.

If we concentrate on the directly corresponding passage in *The Greatest Benefit to Mankind* we find considerable harmony, for with respect to physical examination, Porter seems to have been persuaded by Foucault's version of events.[2] But when it comes to the other dimension of *la clinique*, namely the development of pathological anatomy, Porter's account was radically different from Foucault's. The way in which this becomes apparent is in their respective treatments of Bichat's precursors, notably – though not only – Giovanni Battista Morgagni, author of the monumental *De Sedibus et Causis Morborum per Anatomen Indagatis* (1761). This could be brought out using the appropriate passage from *Greatest Benefit* itself;[3] but it is simpler to use for this purpose another Porter work of the 1990s, part of his contribution

Originally published in *Medicine, Madness and Social History: Essays in Honour of Roy Porter*, eds Roberta Bivens and John V. Pickstone. Basingstoke: Palgrave Macmillan, 2007. Reproduced with permission of Palgrave Macmillan.

26

to the collectively authored *The Western Medical Tradition*, in which Porter was responsible for the chapter on the eighteenth century.

In this chapter, therefore, I shall juxtapose two texts – Foucault's *Birth of the Clinic* (mainly, though not only, its Preface) and Porter's discussion of eighteenth-century 'Pathology' (by which he meant pathological anatomy) in *The Western Medical Tradition*.[4] We shall see that these display both a systematic divergence and a subtle and surprising agreement, and that in each respect the Foucault/Porter comparison is emblematic of wider historiographical trends.

Foucault's picture

As I have remarked elsewhere, Foucault depicted the 'birth of the clinic' as a step from non-knowledge to knowledge.[5] The corollary of this, or indeed its prerequisite, was that the transition from the old medicine to the new was portrayed as a *discontinuous* development. Yet this fundamental posited discontinuity was never argued; rather, it was installed rhetorically, by the devices of metaphor and selective exemplification.

Metaphor

The very title *Naissance de la clinique* was, of course, a metaphor of discontinuity; further metaphors of this kind proliferated throughout Foucault's Preface, which invoked in turn a 'sharp line', a 'moment', a 'mutation in discourse' and a 'turning-point';[6] and last but not least, the climax of the book – a passage that I shall have occasion to examine later – spoke of 'the great break in the history of Western medicine'.[7] These multiple metaphorical resources (birth, line, moment, mutation, turning-point, break) range across the living and the non-living, the spatial and the temporal, the physical and the mathematical, but they have this in common, that each of them is an image of discontinuity.

Exemplification

The governing structure of *Naissance de la clinique* was set up in the Preface by means of a contrast between two texts, from 1769 and 1825, both concerned with 'membranes' but in very different ways: the first by Pierre Pomme (1735–1812), recounting a treatment for hysteria which caused 'membranous tissues' to be expelled from various bodily orifices; the second by Antoine-Laurent-Jesse Bayle (1799–1858), describing the meninges of the brain. According to Foucault's gloss, Pomme 'speaks to us in the language of fantasy', whereas in the work of Bayle and his contemporaries 'language has turned into rational discourse', making it 'possible . . . for the patient's bed to become a field of scientific investigation'. A little later in the Preface Foucault introduces another contrast, whose purpose is slightly different but whose structure is the same: here J. F. Meckel (1724–74), weighing portions of the brain in 1764, is counterposed to Bichat and his contemporaries (roughly simultaneous with Bayle), who examined the brain in qualitative terms. The effect of this twofold comparison is to install as representatives of mid-eighteenth-century medicine the forgotten figures of Pomme and Meckel, and conversely to depict 'medicine as a clinical science' as beginning with Bichat, Bayle et al. – that is, in the early nineteenth century.[8] But the force of all this hinges on the choice of the examples, as can be indicated by a thought-experiment: imagine replacing Pomme and Meckel with their contemporaries Morgagni (1682–1771) and Leopold Auenbrugger (1722–1809) and the entire contrast collapses. For as Foucault half-acknowledges elsewhere in the book (I shall touch on this in due course), the grand themes which defined *la clinique* – pathological anatomy and physical examination – had already flourished in the 1760s, when Morgagni published his incomparable *De Sedibus* and Auenbrugger announced his discovery of thoracic percussion. No wonder, therefore, that the Preface (and, for that matter, most of the book) rigorously excludes Morgagni and Auenbrugger, and *a fortiori* Morgagni's teacher Antonio Maria Valsalva (1666–1723) and his seventeenth-century predecessors such as Johann Jacob Wepfer (1620–95, author of the classic work on cerebral haemorrhage) and Théophile Bonet (1620–89, compiler of the 1679 *Sepulchretum*, a massive digest of cases and autopsies): the achievements of these individuals contradict the very premises of Foucault's argument.

Porter's picture

Porter, in sharp contrast, depicts the development with which he is concerned – pathological anatomy – as a *continuous* process with a protracted history. Yet his radically different picture has this in common with Foucault's: that its literary form is perfectly attuned to its content. The simplest way to bring this out is to inspect the key points of the story as Porter tells it:

> Since Vesalius, the idea had grown that the good practitioner must be proficient in gross anatomy. An inevitable consequence was that increased attention began to be paid to the connexions between the sick body and the disease signs afforded by the corpse. Anatomy, in other words, paved the way for morbid anatomy...
> The trail was blazed by ... Morgagni .... Building on earlier necropsy studies by ... Wepfer ... and ... Bonet ... Morgagni ... published in 1761 his *De Sedibus et Causis Morborum (On the Sites and Causes of Disease)*...
> In *De Sedibus*, Morgagni demonstrated that ... disease symptoms tally with anatomical lesions .... It was Morgagni who thus finally clinched the direct relevance of anatomy to clinical medicine...

242

28

> Others continued his work. In 1793, Matthew Baillie... published his *Morbid Anatomy*....
>
> Pathology became more fully systematised with the publication in 1800 of the *Traité des Membranes* (*Treatise on Membranes*) by... Bichat... As developed by Morgagni, pathology had dealt with organs. Bichat changed the focus [to the tissues]....
>
> Around 1800... thanks to developments in pathology, attention was newly being paid to normal and abnormal structures and functions, a trend that would come to fruition in the nineteenth century.

Again there are two rhetorical elements in play, which it is convenient to treat in the opposite order from that which I used for Foucault.

Exemplification

Porter deploys a very different cast of characters from that used by Foucault. Not only does he begin with Andreas Vesalius (1514–64), thereby giving pathological anatomy a vastly extended lineage; he also makes Morgagni his key eighteenth-century character, with the effect that the medicine of the nineteenth century is linked with that of the eighteenth, rather than separated from it as in Foucault's picture. In addition there are several other individuals who, so to speak, fill up the historical spaces: Wepfer and Bonet stand for the seventeenth century, Matthew Baillie (1761–1823) for the late eighteenth. Finally, at the very end of the story, comes Bichat – the solitary point of overlap with Foucault's picture, an overlap which is no accident, for Bichat was the individual in whom Foucault located the origin of modern medicine, as we shall see.

A vocabulary of continuity

The very presence of Porter's temporally extended cast list – Vesalius, Wepfer, Bonet, Morgagni, Baillie, Bichat – conveys a message of continuity. But more than this, whereas Foucault separated the characters of his non-story, Porter systematically connects them; and the way that he does so is consistently through a rhetoric of continuity. In the opening and closing phases of the story that rhetoric is largely metaphorical – *idea had grown, paved the way, trail was blazed, building on, come to fruition*; in the heart of the passage, that is to say when dealing with the eighteenth century, Porter abandons metaphorical language and uses direct representation: *continued his work, became more fully systematized*. Yet both forms of writing achieve the same effect, namely, continuity – the precise opposite of what Foucault had constructed with his panoply of metaphors.

In short, where Foucault depicted discontinuity, Porter installed a continuous story. And this disagreement is by no means confined to these two authors, for much the same contrast is to be found between the writings of Russell Maulitz (who treats pathology as effectively beginning with the Paris school, apart from a nod to Morgagni) and Othmar Keel (who has argued vigorously against Foucault's claims for the novelty of the Paris school).[9]

A hidden consensus

Thus far it appears that the stories told by Foucault and Porter have nothing in common, apart from their unsurprising convergence on the figure of Bichat and of course their considerable rhetorical mastery. Yet I shall now suggest that between those stories there subsists a subtle and interesting agreement, one that resides not so much in what they say as in what they tend to exclude.

The theme that I have in mind is the project of *relating postmortem findings to the prior symptoms of the living patient.* Let us first notice that by the time of *la clinique* that project was well over two centuries old. It had already been attempted quite commonly, albeit occasionally, in the sixteenth century;[10] it was formulated explicitly by Francis Bacon in 1605[11] and was pursued by many seventeenth-century medical men, among them Wepfer and Bonet; in the eighteenth century it was carried forward with particular rigour by Morgagni, whose efforts show, incidentally, how complex and difficult this undertaking was.[12] And in the epoch of *la clinique* this same project was attested, appropriately enough, by both Bichat and Laennec – the one the effective founder of the morbid anatomy which flourished in the Paris school, the other the begetter of that school's crowning invention, the stethoscope. Here is how Bichat, writing in 1801, depicted the future of pathological anatomy (with my emphases):[13]

It seems to me that we have reached an epoch in which morbid anatomy is bound to experience a new and rapid development. This science is not only that of the organic derangements which arrive slowly, as principals or as sequelae, in chronic illnesses; [rather] it consists of the examination of all the alterations which the parts can experience, at whatever stage their illnesses are examined. Thus apart from certain fevers and nervous affections, almost everything in pathology is within the competence of this science. How slight are the reasonings of famous physicians when we examine them not in their books, but in the dead body! Medicine was long excluded from the circle of the exact sciences; it will have the right to be associated with them, at least in respect of diagnostics, when *rigorous observation* [sc.: of symptoms] *is everywhere united with* the examination of the alterations suffered by the organs. This direction is beginning to be taken by all reasonable minds; it will without doubt soon become general. What is observation, if we are ignorant of the place where the evil is seated? For twenty years from morning to evening you have taken notes at the bedside of patients, on the affections of the heart, the lung, the gastric

244

30

viscera, etc., and all is confusion for you in the symptoms, which, having no common connection, exhibit only a series of incoherent phenomena. Open some cadavers, and you will soon see disappearing the obscurity which observation alone could not have dispelled.

For Bichat, then, morbid anatomy alone was not a sufficient basis for bringing medicine into 'the circle of the exact sciences'; rather, it had to 'be united with' the observation of disease in the living patient. And some ten years later, by which time Bichat's vision had already been realized in Paris by Jean-Nicolas Corvisart (1755–1821, the reviver of Auenbrugger's percussion) and many others, Laennec made much the same point (emphases mine):[14]

Pathological anatomy is a science whose aim is the knowledge of the visible alterations produced on the organs of the human body by the state of disease. The opening up of corpses is the means of acquiring this knowledge; but in order for it to become of direct use . . . it must be *joined to observation of the symptoms or alterations of functions that coincide with each alteration in the organs.*

In short, both Bichat and Laennec proclaimed that *morbid anatomy was not enough on its own*, but had to be 'united' or 'joined' with the study of symptoms in the living patient. This is all the more striking when it is remembered that these two men were, at least in the judgement of posterity, the most eminent practitioners of morbid anatomy produced by the Paris school. Yet at the same time their formulations betray a curious omission or elision: neither of them made explicit what was in fact the precondition for linking symptomatology with pathological anatomy, namely that *the same individual* be studied first when alive (as a patient) and then when dead (as a corpse).[15] This oversight, I suggest, was no accident, but rather reflected the inherent difficulty of the subject: just as the enterprise of linking postmortem findings with prior symptoms presented an immense challenge both practically and conceptually (as the work of Morgagni vividly attests), so also the theorization of that enterprise – the articulation of what it involved – was a troublesome task in its own right. For instance, this activity had no identifiable locus within the medical disciplinary matrix: it was connected with all three of pathology (the theory of disease), pathological anatomy and the observation of symptoms, but could not be subsumed within any of these.

How has this theme – the integration of postmortem findings with prior symptoms – been figured by Foucault and by Porter? We anticipate, of course, that Foucault will depict it (falsely) as the sudden product of the Paris school, whereas Porter will (correctly) give it an extended lineage, and this expectation is indeed borne out; yet as will emerge, their formulations also display an unexpected harmony.

245

Naissance de la clinique engages with the matter in chapter 8, which deals with what Foucault calls 'the age of Bichat'[16] and is entitled – significantly, as we shall see – 'Open up a few corpses' (*Ouvrez quelques cadavres*). A measure of the importance of this chapter is that it is precisely here that Foucault announces, in a phrase that I noted earlier, 'the great break in the history of Western medicine'.[17] It is appropriate to consider the chapter as a whole in order to see how my theme (which appears almost halfway through) is introduced.

The opening section of the chapter elaborates two theses in turn, the first historiographic, the second substantive. The *historiographic* argument is pitched against a longstanding medical myth: that before the Paris clinic, pathological anatomy had been held back by 'the opposition of religion, morality, and stubborn prejudice to the opening up of corpses'.[18] In rebutting that myth Foucault has to invoke the very figures that his Preface had so carefully suppressed: Bonet, Valsalva, Morgagni and Auenbrugger.[19] But the discontinuity constructed by the Preface is reinstated through Foucault's next, *substantive* claim: that the pathological anatomy initiated by Bichat was different in kind from Morgagni's. In place of 'the densities of the organs' investigated by Morgagni, Bichat substituted what Foucault calls 'the thinness of the tissue': that is, 'volumes' were replaced by 'surfaces'.[20] And this leads Foucault to the pivotal thesis of his book: that this new focus on 'tissual surfaces' made it possible to transfer the nosographic project of the late eighteenth century, based on Condillac's 'method of analysis', from the universe of symptoms – another 'surface', but a surface of a very different type – into the physical body.[21] This claim is rich in implications, both benign and baleful. On the one hand, it has the great virtue of making intelligible the fact (overlooked by some other commentators, including Porter) that the new, tissue-based pathological anatomy initiated by Bichat was entirely consistent with the continuation of the nosographical project.[22] On the other hand, it permits Foucault to advance a new myth of his own making, one which stands as the precise substitute for the one he had refuted a few pages earlier: that only now, in the 'age of Bichat', was pathological anatomy related to prior symptoms.[23] Accordingly, the remainder of the chapter is devoted to the ways that Bichat and his immediate successors – Corvisart, Gaspard-Laurent Bayle (uncle of Antoine-Laurent-Jesse Bayle, whom Foucault had used in his Preface), Laennec, Petit, Bouillaud – handled this (supposedly novel) task of relating postmortem findings to antecedent symptoms in the living patient.

Foucault depicts that task as presenting two aspects:[24] the integration of the spatial (anatomy) with the temporal (symptoms); and the need to overcome the distorting effect of postmortem changes, which confuse the significance of what is found at autopsy. Notice that this analysis drastically reduces the scope of the problem – for neither of these formulations begins to capture the awful and ineffable gulf that separates the dead

32

body, which knows no pain and neither feels nor speaks, from the living, breathing, suffering patient. Nevertheless, that problem is initially in focus, as is signalled by the fact that Foucault here includes Laennec's injunction (which I reproduced above) that pathological anatomy has to be 'joined to observation of the symptoms or alterations of functions that coincide with each alteration in the organs'. Yet as Foucault's discussion proceeds (by way of an elegant meditation on death in the writings of Bichat, supplemented by those of Bayle and Laennec), the problem gradually slips out of view,[25] until it is finally erased in the punchline of the chapter – the very passage which announces 'the great break in the history of Western medicine'. For here Foucault quotes from Bichat's view of morbid anatomy, just as he had earlier quoted that of Laennec, but in doing so he *omits* Bichat's requirement that 'the examination of the alterations that our organs suffer' should be 'everywhere united with' the 'rigorous observation' of patients' symptoms:[26]

> the great break in the history of Western medicine dates precisely from the moment clinical experience became the anatomico-clinical gaze. Pinel's *Médicine clinique* dates from 1802 . . . the rules of analysis seem to triumph in the pure decipherment of symptomatic totalities. But a year before, Bichat had relegated them to history:
> for twenty years, from morning to night, you have taken notes at patients' bedsides on affections of the heart, the lungs, the gastric viscera, and all is confusion for you in the symptoms which, refusing to yield up their meaning, offer you a succession of incoherent phenomena. Open up a few corpses: you will dissipate at once the darkness that observation alone could not dissipate.
> The living night is dissipated in the brightness of death.

The elegance of Foucault's concluding paraphrase should not blind us to the fact that we have been robbed: for the effect of this selective quotation is to obliterate Bichat's recognition of the need to *unite* postmortem findings with the observation of symptoms. And it can now be seen that the chapter's title is faithful to its trajectory: the injunction 'open up a few corpses' conveys precisely half, but only half, of what Bichat had in fact enjoined. Thus the effect of the chapter, ironically enough, is to eliminate from view the very activity which Foucault himself has claimed distinguished *la clinique* from all that went before it, namely the integrating of symptoms with anatomy.[27]

Turning to our Porter text we find the same suppression but in a different form, corresponding to the fact that Porter – quite rightly, and in radical opposition to Foucault – depicts anatomico-symptomatic correlation as a longstanding activity. What happens here is that this theme repeatedly enters and then disappears, submerged within the figure of pathological anatomy. This movement takes place at the very outset:

Since Vesalius, the idea had grown that the good practitioner must be proficient in gross anatomy. An inevitable consequence was that increased attention began to be paid to *the connexions between the sick body and* the disease signs afforded by the corpse. Anatomy, in other words, paved the way for *morbid anatomy*.

Here the living patient has been introduced in the form of 'the sick body', and Porter rightly points to the 'connexions' between this and 'the disease signs afforded by the corpse'; yet in the very next sentence all of this is lost, for the focus shifts to the mere corpse ('morbid anatomy'). And precisely the same transmutation takes place at the key moment of the passage, that is to say, in the discussion of Morgagni and his impact. Porter's account of Morgagni's *De Sedibus* is admirably explicit as to the importance within that work of anatomico-symptomatic correlation:

In *De Sedibus*, Morgagni demonstrated that . . . *disease symptoms tally with anatomical lesions* . . . . It was Morgagni who thus finally clinched the direct relevance of anatomy to clinical medicine.

Yet this insight is instantly cancelled in what follows. For as an example of those who 'continued' Morgagni's work, Porter offers Matthew Baillie – whose *Morbid Anatomy* in fact contained no case histories, and in its original edition (1793) did not even mention symptoms.[28] Thus the price of assimilating Morgagni to Baillie is neither more nor less than the elimination of anatomico-symptomatic correlation as a significant dimension of Morgagni's enterprise. And this is the same contradiction (*mutatis mutandis*) which we have seen at the climax of Foucault's *Birth of the Clinic*.

Whence this shared elision? I suggest that it reflects the inherently recalcitrant nature of the matter in question. We saw earlier that anatomico-symptomatic correlation was extremely difficult to carry out; that it cut across medicine's internal boundaries, involving at least three different areas and therefore falling into none of them; and moreover that this activity resisted theorization, for even Bichat and Laennec fell short of articulating fully what it entailed. The fact that Foucault and Porter, from their very different perspectives, have both written out this theme can be regarded as the historiographic echo of this same difficulty: that is, the activity of relating symptoms to post-mortem findings has been as difficult for historians to grasp as it was for early modern medical men to practise and to theorise. Similarly, neither Maulitz nor Keele has brought anatomico-symptomatic correlation into focus; instead, for all their disagreement, they are united in taking 'pathology' as their theme.[29]

34

Conclusion

The convergence that we have just been noting makes all the more remarkable the contrast with which we began – between Foucault's discontinuity picture and Porter's story of continuity. By way of conclusion, I want to suggest that neither of these accounts is sufficient in itself, and yet each of them captures a very important aspect of the problem. That is to say, there was indeed a sudden shift, as Foucault would have it, yet that shift had profound roots in earlier medical practices, as Porter claims.

We can reconcile the two pictures in this way if we posit that the activity of anatomico-symptomatic correlation, though it had often been *attempted*, attained a new level of *success* in the context of the Paris Ecole de Santé. And there are indeed good grounds for believing that this is the case. The earlier attempts of course require an extended discussion, for which there is not space here; but what can be said in a brief compass is that connecting symptoms with postmortem findings was an extraordinarily *difficult* enterprise, far more demanding than normal anatomy. Even for just a single illness it required at an absolute minimum: (a) observation and recording of the living patient's symptoms; (b) the death of the patient (this is by no means trivial, for even in early modern medicine most patients survived most of their illnesses); (c) the opportunity to dissect the body; (d) not just one such patient-and-corpse but many of them, because both symptoms and post-mortem findings were complex and variable; and finally (e) a rigorous method for collating the results. And it turns out that this combination of conditions was seldom satisfied: for instance, in eighteenth-century England most hospital patients survived (because the hospitals selected patients as curable), while conversely many and perhaps most anatomized bodies came with no record of symptoms (because corpses for teaching were probably secured by grave-robbing). The effect of such constraints was exactly *as if* there had existed either the supposed taboo on dissection (the myth demolished by Foucault) or the failure to attempt anatomico-symptomatic correlation (the alternative myth which Foucault installed). But in the Paris Ecole de Santé, these constraints were broken – not because this had been intended, but simply as a result of the fortuitous triple combination of practices and circumstances that emerged there. In the first place, hospital patients were used as clinical teaching material on an unprecedented scale. Second, it so happened that these hospitals were places of very high mortality. And third, from 1798 the bodies of those same patients were made available to anatomy teachers – initially purely for normal anatomy, which is all that the formal curriculum envisaged. The effect of this conjunction was that the preconditions for anatomico-symptomatic correlation were satisfied in the Paris Ecole to an unprecedented degree: hence the activities and achievements of Bichat, Corvisart, Laennec and their contemporaries.

If in this respect Foucault's picture of discontinuity is accurate, we should also recall that Porter's continuity story has a powerful element of truth; and it is appropriate, in a volume of this kind, to give Porter the last word. Let us therefore go back once more to the beginning of our little Porter passage:

> Since Vesalius, the idea had grown that the good practitioner must be proficient in gross anatomy. An inevitable consequence was that increased attention began to be paid to the connexions between the sick body and the disease signs afforded by the corpse. Anatomy, in other words, paved the way for morbid anatomy . . .

In thus launching his continuist picture, Porter captured a crucial element of seventeenth-century anatomy, and one which has strangely been marginalized by the specialist historians of anatomy. For the nub of his argument was that pathological anatomy was neither a new development in the eighteenth century nor a separate enterprise from normal anatomy, but rather an integral part of anatomy as such; and there is every reason to believe that this picture is correct. The historians of seventeenth-century anatomy have tended to overlook this by implicitly (and without discussion) defining 'anatomy' as 'normal anatomy';[30] but the anatomists of the seventeenth century (and to some degree at least those of the sixteenth as well) deployed a broader definition of anatomy, one which *included* what would later become the specialism of pathological anatomy. For bringing this out, as for so much else, Roy Porter – a historian of the eighteenth century, telling us something of profound importance about an earlier period – deserves our permanent gratitude.

250

Notes

A preliminary version of this chapter was given to the Glasgow Wellcome Centre for the History of Medicine; I thank the Centre for their invitation and the participants, particularly Malcolm Nicolson, for their comments. I am also grateful to Jackie Duffin and Roger White for help with the chapter. Errors are my own responsibility.

1. Michel Foucault, *Naissance de la clinique* (Paris, 1963); *Birth of the Clinic: An Archaeology of Medical Perception*, transl. A. M. Sheridan Smith (London: Tavistock, 1973), hereafter *BC*
2. Roy Porter, *The Greatest Benefit to Mankind: A Medical History of Humanity from Antiquity to the Present* (London: HarperCollins, 1997), pp. 306–14.
3. Porter, *The Greatest Benefit to Mankind*, pp. 263–5.
4. Lawrence I. Conrad, Michael Neve, Vivian Nutton, Roy Porter and Andrew Wear, *The Western Medical Tradition* (Cambridge: Cambridge University Press, 1995), pp. 410–12.
5. Adrian Wilson, 'On the History of Disease Concepts: The Case of Pleurisy', *History of Science* 38 (2000), 271–319.
6. *BC*, pp. xi, xv, xviii.
7. *BC*, p. 146.
8. *BC*, pp. xii, xv.
9. Russell C. Maulitz, *Morbid Appearances: The Anatomy of Pathology in the Early Nineteenth Century* (Cambridge: Cambridge University Press, 1987); Othmar Keel, 'Was Anatomical and Tissue Pathology a Product of the Paris Clinical School or Not?' in Caroline Hannaway and Ann La Berge, eds, *Constructing Paris Medicine* (Amsterdam: Rodopi, 1987/Clio Medica 50), pp. 117–83, and other works there cited.

10. Nancy G. Siraisi, *Medicine and the Italian Universities 1250–1600* (Leiden: Brill, 2001), chs. 11 and 15 *passim*, esp. pp. 237–8, 360.

11. 'In the inquiry which is made by anatomists I find much deficience . . . And as for the footsteps of diseases, and their devastations of the inward parts . . . they ought to have been exactly observed by multitude of anatomies, and the contribution of men's several experiences, and carefully set down both historically according to the appearances, *and artificially with a reference to the diseases and symptoms which resulted from them, in case where the anatomy is of a defunct patient;* whereas now upon opening of bodies they are passed over slightly and in silence.' Francis Bacon, *The Advancement of Learning* (1605), taken from Oxford University Press edition (ed. Arthur Johnston, 1974/1980), p. 110, emphasis added. In this respect Bacon's castigation of previous anatomists was almost certainly unfair, but we so far lack a clear picture of this aspect of sixteenth-century anatomical research.

12. See especially Saul Jarcho, 'Morgagni, Vicarius, and the Difficulty of Clinical Diagnosis', in Lloyd G. Stevenson and Robert P. Multhauf, eds, *Medicine, Science and Culture: Historical Essays in Honour of Owsei Temkin* (Baltimore, MD: Johns Hopkins Press, 1968), pp. 87–95; also Malcolm Nicolson, 'Giovanni Battista Morgagni and Eighteenth-century Physical Examination', in C. Lawrence, ed., *Medical Theory, Surgical Practice* (London: Routledge, 1992), pp. 101–34; Andrew Cunningham, 'Pathology and the Case-history in Morgagni's "On the Seats and Causes of Diseases Investigated Through Anatomy" (1761)', *Med Ges Gesch* XI (1995), 37–61; Wilson, 'On the History of Disease Concepts'.

13. *Anatomie Génerale, appliquée à la physiologie et à la médecine*, (Paris, 1812 edition), vol. i, pp. xcviii-xcix, my translation.

14. Laennec, 'Anatomie pathologique', in *Dictionnaire des sciences médicales* (1812), Vol. II, p. 47, quoted by Foucault, *BC*, p. 135 (Foucault's ellipsis; I have not seen the original text).

15. Thus Laennec's earlier manuscript 'Traité d'anatomie pathologique' (*c.* 1804–8) had illustrated each of its anatomical categories (the various 'accidental productions') with one or more cases of named patients: see Jacalyn Duffin, *To See with a Better Eye: A Life of R. T. H. Laennec* (Princeton, NJ: Princeton University Press, 1998), Table 3.3 (p. 71).

16. *BC*, p. 122.

17. *BC*, p. 146.

18. The opening passage is *BC*, pp. 124–33; quotations here are from pp. 122 (end of the previous chapter), 124.

19. *BC*, p. 126.

20. Quotations here are from *BC*, pp. 127–8.

21. *BC*, pp. 129–32.

22. Oddly, Bichat himself seems to have wavered over this issue, for he advocated a tissue-based classification of diseases in *Anatomie pathologique* and implicitly endorsed this idea in *Anatomie générale*, yet in the *Anatomie Descriptive* he expressed indifference towards classification. See respectively Foucault, *BC*, p. 129; Bichat, *Anatomie générale*, vol. iv, p. 415; Foucault, *BC*, p. 177. But both Bayle and Laennec were enthusiastic about the idea, and Corvisart used it to organize his classic treatise on heart disease: see Duffin, *To See with a Better Eye*, pp. 38, 97–8; Foucault, *BC*, p. 177; J. N. Corvisart des Marets, *Treatise on the Diseases and Organic Lesions of the Heart and Great Vessels*, trans. C. H. Hebb (London, 1813), *passim*.

23. This assertion becomes explicit at *BC*, p. 135. Here Foucault suggests that the application of the 'diacritical principle' to the 'dimension . . . in which the recognizable forms of pathological history [i.e. symptoms] and the visible elements that it reveals on completion [i.e. postmortem anatomical findings] are articulated' required the 'medical gaze' to '*travel along a path that had not so far been opened to it*' (my emphasis). The 'diacritical principle', he has just argued (pp. 134–5), was not in itself new, but as applied in pathological anatomy it had hitherto been confined to comparisons (a) with normal bodies; (b) with postmortems of other patients who had died from the same disease; and (c) 'between what one sees of an altered organ and what one knows of its normal functioning'. Notice, incidentally, that (b) actually implies comparison with symptoms, which undermines the discontinuity claim; but this contradiction, being at one remove, is barely visible. Cf. note 25 below.

24. *BC*, pp. 133–4.

25. Specifically, what happens is that symptoms are replaced in Foucault's discourse by pathological processes, with the implication – though this is nowhere explicitly asserted – that this mirrors what happened historically. As Foucault himself puts it (*BC*, p. 139), 'the density of pathological history' was introduced 'into the specified volume of the body'; this formulation is no doubt accurate in itself, but the implication that the study of symptoms was thereby replaced (or displaced) is fallacious. For an eloquent counter to this picture, see Duffin, *To See with a Better Eye*, p. 303.

26. *BC*, p. 146, replacing 'anatomo-clinical' with 'anatomico-clinical'.

27. To put this another way, Foucault's account of what he calls the 'anatomo-clinical method' has depicted this as wholly anatomical, emptying it of its clinical dimension.

28. Matthew Baillie, *The Morbid Anatomy of Some of the Most Important Parts of the Human Body* (1793).

29. See the works cited in note 9 above.

30. This can be illustrated by selective results of a recent Internet search. In the Catholic Encyclopedia, for instance, it is under the heading of 'ANATOMY IN THE EIGHTEENTH CENTURY' that both Wepfer and Bonet appear; and the reason for this is that pathological anatomy is there presented as an eighteenth-century activity. Another encyclopaedia (Wikipedia), under 'history of anatomy in the seventeenth and eighteenth centuries', does have a few scattered references to 'morbid anatomy', but treats this as a separate activity, quite distinct from anatomy proper. See, respectively, http://www. newadvent.org/cathen/10122a.htm (accessed 1 March 2004); http://en2.wikipedia. org/wiki/History_of_anatomy_in_the_17th_and_eighteenth_centuries (accessed 8 April 2004).

Postscript to 'Porter versus Foucault on the "birth of the clinic"'

This paper, I now feel, wasn't entirely fair to Foucault. It was deficient in not directing at the primary sources – specifically, at Bichat – the rhetorical analysis that it applied to the secondary sources (Porter and Foucault). And it overlooked a key point that actually supported an aspect of its own argument.

These are three ways of saying the same thing, as I shall now explain.

The paper argued that anatomico-symptomatic correlation was and has been a *difficult* activity in three ways:

(a) it was difficult in practice to carry out in the eighteenth century (and earlier);

(b) it was hard to conceptualize at the time; and

(c) it has proved elusive historiographically, for the tendency has been to transmute it into mere 'pathological anatomy' – as we see in the discourses of both Porter and Foucault.

To illustrate (c) in the case of Foucault's *Naissance de la Clinique* (*Birth of the Clinic*), I drew attention to Foucault's abbreviated quotation from Bichat. Foucault's version, I pointed out, wholly suppressed Bichat's point that what was required, in order for medicine to take its place amongst the sciences, was that 'rigorous observation' [of symptoms] should be *united* [my emphasis] with the examination of the alterations suffered by the organs'. But what I overlooked was that *the same suppression had already been made by Bichat himself*. For immediately after what I've just quoted, Bichat wrote:

For twenty years, from morning to night, you have taken notes at patients' bedsides on affections of the heart, the lungs, the gastric viscera, and all is confusion for you in the symptoms which, refusing to yield up their meaning, offer you a succession of incoherent phenomena. Open up a few corpses: you will dissipate at once the darkness that observation alone could not dissipate.

The second of these two closing sentences contains two mutually-contradictory meanings:

[1] If "open[ing] up a few corpses" will "dissipate... the darkness" *at once*, then no correlation of its findings with symptoms is required: thus Bichat himself has here obliterated his own earlier point.

254

POSTSCRIPT TO VIII

> [2] However, such anatomico-symptomatic correlation then makes a covert, implicit and – it has to be said – feeble re-entry by way of the word 'alone'. For the remark that 'observation *alone*' could not 'dissipate' the 'darkness' implies that observation *together with* 'open[ing] up a few corpses' can do so.

Even in [2], the actual 'uniting' (Bichat's earlier formulation) of post-mortem findings with prior symptoms has not been mentioned, and to that degree the two sentences are consistent. Nevertheless there is a very real tension between 'at once' and 'alone', a tension which corresponds to the absence and presence respectively of anatomico-symptomatic correlation. The very phenomenon which we observed in both Porter and Foucault – the tendency for anatomico-symptomatic correlation to slip out of focus and to be replaced by the mere performance of the post-mortem – here appears within the discourse of Bichat himself.

Let us notice in passing that all the more credit accrues to Laennec, who was perhaps the first to articulate fully, clearly and unambiguously what was required.[1] (It is a nice irony that it is Foucault who brings this remark of Laennec's to attention, just as it is typical of Foucault's highly obscure way of writing that he presents the Laennec quotation from 1812 *before* the Bichat quotation from 1801: pp. 135, 146.) I suspect that this is no accident; we already know that Laennec carried all aspects of anatomico-symptomatic correlation to a new level (not only did he invent the stethoscope, he also produced more detailed morbid anatomical descriptions than Bichat or Baillie had), and it would be of a piece if, as seems to be the case, he did the same for *the understanding of* that enterprise.

To return to where we were with Bichat: Bichat's slippage surely to some extent excuses Foucault, who merely echoed and amplified it. But the fact that I overlooked that slippage is not so easy to excuse, for it can only mean that I wasn't reading the primary texts with the same attention – and in particular the same *kind* of attention – that I was devoting to the secondary sources. And the cost was that I missed a major trick, for Bichat's elision was a perfect illustration – indeed a better one than I came up with in the paper - of my point (b).

This failure on my part can be taken as an ironic and unintended illustration of my point (c): anatomico-symptomatic correlation not only *was* difficult – both to practise and to theorize – but also *is* difficult, specifically difficult to grasp historically.

---

[1] It may be, however, that Morgagni – who was certainly at least as much of an intellectual giant as Laennec – had already articulated a similar understanding in his *De Sedibus* of 1761: this possibility is something that I hope to investigate in the future.

INDEX

256

INDEX

Birth (cont.)
See also specific headings immediately
below, *and*: lying-in; male paths
to childbirth; man-midwifery;
midwifery; midwives; revival of
newborn child
Birth, historiography of, *see* Historiography
Birth, major complications of 2, 15, 75–7
Convulsions 3, 27, 75
Haemorrhage 3, 10, 73, 75, 78
Birth, methods of delivery in 81–2
Difficult births, *see* cephalic version;
craniotomy; midwifery forceps;
placenta, extraction of; podalic
version; twins, delivery of
Normal births, *see* midwife's stool;
postures for delivery; placenta,
extraction of; revival of newborn
child; twins, delivery of
Birth, minor complications of 2–3
Birth, obstructed 2–3, 10, 15, 19, 26, 34,
72–3, 75–9, 86–8, 102 n.30, 103 n.35
Birth, varieties of presentation
Arm / shoulder (including 'compound
presentation') 2, 3, 16, 16 n.8, 73,
75–9, 85
Breech (including footling) 2, 15, 73,
75–80, 84–92, 94
Head 2–3, 26–7, 70–78, 82, 83, 85, 88,
90, 92, 101 n.15
Blackmore, Sir Richard 134–5
Bladder stone 142
Blenkinsop, Henry 5, 81
Blundell, Nicholas 37, 38, 61
Bolingbroke, Henry St John, First Viscount,
127
Bonet, Théophile 241–3, 245
Book of Common Prayer 39, 65 n.108
Booking of calls, *see* Male paths to childbirth
Borough franchises 154–5, 164
Borsay, Peter 167
Bouillaud, Jean-Baptiste 245
Boulton and Fothergill (manufacturers) 173,
175
Boulton, Jeremy 57
Boulton, Matthew 170, 173–5, 177, 186 n.60,
187 nn.86, 90
'Bourgeois public sphere' (Habermas) *see
Bürgerliche Öffentlichkeit*
Brady, Samuel 135–6
Bright's disease 190, 191, 194, 199
Brissot, Pierre 211
Bristol 149
Borough of 148, 150 n.5, 151 n.1
Bristol Infirmary 147, 148, 150

Brock, Helen 18, 22
Bromley, William 175
Broughton, Bridget (Lady Broughton), 24
Bueno, Otávio 224
Burdett, Sir Francis 131
Burke, Seán 68–9, 224
Bürgerliche Öffentlichkeit ('bourgeois public
sphere', Habermas) 167–9, 181–2
Burton, John 18
Bury St Edmunds 149
Byrom, Dr John 135–7
Byron, Lady (possibly Elizabeth, second wife
of Richard Byron, second Baron
Byron) 24, 106 n.102, 107 n.113

Caelius Aurelianus, *see* Soranus
Cambridge, Borough of 145, 148, 155
Cambridgeshire 32, 37, 148
Canguilhem, Georges 190, 221, 223
Canterbury, Borough of, *see* Kent and
Canterbury Hospital
Carles, Joseph 175
Cathedral chapters 165
Caudle 33–4, 36, 42, 54
Cellier, Mrs Elizabeth 95, 106 n.94
Cephalic version (turning the birth to the
head) 3, 81–4
Chamberlen family 4, 106 n.94, 140
Chamberlen, Hugh 6, 12, 18
Chambers, Ephraim 135
Charity Schools 112, 124–5
Chartism 112, 198
Cheshire 84, 148, 154
Chester
Borough of 136, 148, 151
Chester Infirmary 130, 139, 148, 154
Cheswardine, Shropshire, 39
Childbirth, *see* Birth
Chlorosis 197–9
Cholera 199–200
Chomel, Auguste François 221, 235 n.188
Chrisom cloth 40
Christian Churches 38, 52
Catholic 38, 129, 252
Church of England 38, 39, 52, 126, 127,
171, 188 n.99; *see also Book of
Common Prayer*
Orthodox 38
Churching 38–45, 48–53; *see also* purification
Cinchona bark 132
Clark, Alice 60, 110
Clarke, Alured 146, 150, 163
Clarke, Samuel 135
Close Vestries Bill (1716) 128
Cobbett, William 43, 131

INDEX

INDEX

INDEX

INDEX

INDEX

Sigerist, Henry 197–8
'Sir Tennebs Evanks lady', *see* Gervase
    Bennet and Mrs. Bennet
Sketchley, James 172
Skipwith, Thomas 172–3, 179
Sloane, Hans Sir 132–5, 139, 142
Smellie, William 1, 4–8, 10–15, 17–21, 23,
    25–6, 100, 140–41
Smith, Wesley D. 201–2, 205–6, 222, 224
Smollett, Tobias 141
    Aristocracy 40, 163, 171, 173, 177–8
    Gentry 8, 40, 163, 172, 174, 176–80
    Semi-gentry 8, 40
    Social classes and estates 8, 14, 40, 56–7
    Working class 48, 197
Soft pulse 210, 215; *see also* Hard pulse
Somerset 148–9
    County Infirmary 148
Soranus 202–6
South Sea Bubble 137
SPCK (Society for the Promotion of Christian
    Knowledge) 124–6, 150 n.4
Spirochaeta pallida 190, 192
Sponsors (in baptism), *see* godparents
Stafford 69, 71, 84–90, 92, 94–6, 100
    Borough of 148, 155 n.3
    Stafford County Hospital 148, 155 n.3,
        174
Staffordshire 24, 86, 94, 96, 102 n.22, 148,
    154, 161 n.2, 174–5, 177
    Collieries 178
Statutes
    Black Act (1722) 137
    Gin Acts (1736, 1751) 111–12
    Quarantine Act (1721) 134, 137
    Septennial Act (1716) 138
    Toleration Act (1689) 126
Steigerthal, Dr John George 133, 135
Stethoscope 220–21, 239, 243, 254
Stewart, Larry 139
Stow-cum-Quy, Cambs. 37
Sturdy, Steve 167, 182, 224
Surgeons 4, 5–6, 10, 16, 20, 22–3, 78, 80, 95,
    117, 119, 168
Surgeon-apothecaries 4, 117, 140, 168
Sutton family (inoculators) 130
Swaddling 35, 42, 43, 53
Syphilis 189–90, 192–4

Tate, W.E. 40, 62, 66–7
Taunton, Borough of 148, 155 n.3
Taylor and Lloyd (bankers) 170, 175–6, 185
    n.47, 186 n.63, 187 nn.84, 90, 91;
    see also John Taylor *and* Sampson
    Lloyd

Taylor, John 170, 175–6, 185 n.47, 186 n.63,
    187 nn.82, 84, 86, 90 and 91, 187
    n.96
Temkin, Owsei 189–90, 195, 221
Tenon, Jacques 115
'Textbook science' (Fleck) 226 nn.29, 31
Theatres 167; *see also* Birmingham: Play
    House
Therapeutics 201–2, 204, 216
Thomas, Keith 44–5
Thornton, Alice 101 n.4, 105 n.75
Thornton, John 127
'Thought styles' (Fleck) 194
Toft, Mary 41
Tom Jones (Fielding) 29
Tories 109, 113, 126–9, 134–6, 138, 141–3,
    149–50, 170–73, 177–80
Town corporations 165
Trebeck, Rev. Andrew 126 n.18, 127
Trevelyan, G.M. 112
Tristram Shandy (Sterne) 30
Tuberculosis 195, 199–200
Turning to the feet, *see* Podalic version
Turning to the head, *see* Cephalic version
Twins, delivery of 5, 11, 12, 15–17, 19, 20,
    34, 73, 75–7, 81–4, 87, 103 n.36

Undergirding membrane, *see* Membrana
    hypezocota; Membrana costas
    succingens
Unpaired vein, *see* Azygos vein
Upsitting 35, 36, 42, 54
'Urban renaissance' (Borsay) 167–9
Urban, Sylvanus, *see* Gentleman's Magazine
Utility, concept of 138

Vaccination 131–2
'Vademecum science' (Fleck) 226 nn.29, 31,
    227 n.34
Valsalva, Antonio Maria 218, 236 n.194, 241,
    245
Vesalius, Andreas 201, 211–14, 216–17,
    219–21, 241–2, 247, 249
Voluntary hospitals 115–29, 138–9, 142,
    145–65, 167–9
Voluntary hospitals, London:
    Foundling Hospital 63 n.75, 111, 184
        n.20
    General Lying-in Hospital 119 n.9
    Lock Hospital 116
    London Hospital 119, 150
    Lying-in Hospital, Brownlow Street
        116–18, 141
    Middlesex Hospital 18, 91, 141, 150, 154
    St George's Hospital 119–22

INDEX